LAW–MEDICINE NOTES

LAW–MEDICINE NOTES

Progress in Medicolegal Relations

William J. Curran

NEJM Books
Waltham, Massachusetts
1989

Library of Congress Cataloging-in-Publication Data

Curran, William J.
Law–Medicine Notes.

Reprints of articles by Curran, originally published in the New England journal of medicine, 1964–1987, with new commentary and updated references.
Includes bibliographies and index.
1. Medical laws and legislation—United States.
I. New England journal of medicine. II. Title.
III. Title: Progress in medicolegal relations.
[DNLM: 1. Ethics, Medical—collected works. 2. Forensic Medicine—United States—collected works. 3. Jurisprudence—United States—collected works. 4. Legislation, Medical—United States—collected works. 5. Malpractice—collected works. W 32.5 AA1 C9L]
KF3821.A75C87 1989 344.73′041 88-27204
347.30441

ISBN NUMBER: 0-910133-26-3

Printed in the United States of America
10 9 8 7 6 5 4 3 2 1

This book was set in Imprint by the Electronic Production/Composition Department of the Massachusetts Medical Society.

Printed and bound by Edwards Brothers, Ann Arbor, Michigan.

Design by Emily Cohen.

Contents

CHAPTER 2 ♦ HOSPITALS: THE NEW LEGAL DOCTRINES

CHAPTER 3 ♦ FORENSIC MEDICINE AND THE LAW

Chapter 6 ♦ Legal and Moral Problems in Human Reproduction

Chapter 7 ♦ Life and Death

APPENDIX

Preface

Twenty-four years ago, when Professor William J. Curran wrote his first "Law–Medicine Notes" column for the *New England Journal of Medicine,* the field of medical law was in its infancy. Only a few lawyers, and even fewer physicians, thought much about the relation between law and medicine. That was understandable, because malpractice litigation was far less common than now, government entitlement programs had not yet expanded very much, federal and state regulation of hospitals and medical practice was minimal, and the commercialization of health care was still largely in the future. Furthermore, the technology of medicine was relatively unsophisticated and had not yet gained its present power to determine conception and birth and the manner and moment of death.

All this has now changed. The increasing complexity and cost of the medical care system, the growing power of medical interventions to affect all aspects of life profoundly, and the expanding involvement of government and private corporations in the funding and delivery of health care have created problems requiring much new legislation and a large new body of case law. An increasingly litigious social climate and a diminution in the public's trust in health care providers have produced an epidemic of legal action against doctors and hospitals. As a result, medical law is now a large and growing field, engaging the attention of many lawyers and prompting many young physicians to seek legal training.

Medical law is not just for specialists, however. It deals with issues so pervasive and diverse that few physicians or health care administrators can afford to ignore them. The range of topics covered by Professor Curran's writings in the *Journal* illustrates the point. Over the years, in some 150 articles, he has commented on legal developments that have affected practically every aspect of health care. Regular readers of his columns have been afforded a broad overview of the subject, illuminated by his trenchant analysis and his forthright opinions.

Now, in this book, Professor Curran has collected 86 of the most interesting of his columns and arranged them under appropriate subject headings. He has provided new introductory material to put his notes in perspective and additional commentary to bring his exposition of certain topics up to date. The editors hope that readers already familiar with Professor Curran's contributions to the *Journal* will welcome the opportunity to study his collected works, organized in this manner and set in context. We also hope that this book will introduce its author to many new readers, who may be interested in receiving an introduction to the range of issues covered by medical law.

This is not a systematic textbook. Rather, it is an organized collection of columns by a noted authority on some of the most important actions taken in medical law in recent decades. The editors of the *Journal* believe that it will appeal to physicians, lawyers, health administrators, and all those interested in understanding the evolution of health law in this country.

Arnold S. Relman, M.D.
Editor-in-Chief
New England Journal of Medicine

INTRODUCTION

This book contains a selection of the medicolegal writing I have contributed to the *New England Journal of Medicine* over a span of more than 20 years. Responsibility for the selection is mine. In addition to the articles themselves, I have in each instance added a commentary containing current references in order to update the issues examined in the columns.

These contributions on medicolegal topics began quietly in March 1964. They were called "Law–Medicine Notes," an intentionally unpretentious description, indicating an informal and quite personal effort at interdisciplinary communication. The title and purpose of the writing have remained the same over these two decades.

My first column was called "The Armor of the Law," a reflection on the assassination of President John F. Kennedy by Lee Harvey Oswald and the trial of Jack Ruby for later killing Oswald. The title of the essay was drawn from a remark by Thomas Erskine, a famous English barrister, at the 1800 trial of James Hadfield for his attempted assassination of King George III. Hadfield was seized at the scene of his crime, acting in what was described as a disturbed and insane manner. Erskine pointed out in his opening statement to the jury that although the defendant was charged with a grievous crime against the head of state, not a hair on his head had been touched since his apprehension and arrest. He was, said Erskine, "covered all over with the armor of the law." I was very much impressed with this observation – it meant that, as a person obviously mentally ill, the defendant was afforded a high degree of legal protection, numerous procedural safeguards to ensure a fair trial, and the provision of competent, experienced legal counsel to represent his best interests in defense. This column was my first attempt to convey to a medical readership an understanding of the importance of legal rights and protections – and the long tradition behind such protections – in litigation concerning an allegedly mentally ill person accused of a sensational crime involving national security.

When these columns began in the 1960s, I was a young law professor just beginning a career as a specialist in the medicolegal field. The field was then quite small and lonely. Few practitioners were concentrating on this area, and legal scholars took even less interest. Like most law professors, I felt my legal skills in communication were being developed primarily to influence the body of the law itself, especially as pronounced in the higher appellate courts. I would speak and write on the law; the justices of the high courts would listen, read, and be impressed. They would adopt my views – with proper attribution, of course – in their judicial opinions. Thus, in the traditional manner, I would advance academically and influence the law in my still new and growing field. This was the accepted route to legal scholarly reputation. God forbid that we should, as law professors, address ourselves to nonlawyers.

Nevertheless, at the invitation of the *Journal*'s editor, Dr. Joseph Garland, I agreed to try my hand at medicolegal writing for a professional audience of physicians. I was assured that it would not be onerous or time-consuming. The trick would be, I was told, to select interesting legal problems and to analyze them clearly – without legalistic jargon, of course – with the very strict brevity demanded by the *Journal.*

The writing of these essays did not turn out to be the simple task I had bargained for, for a variety of reasons. In that earlier era, physicians tended to take a rather narrow view of the medicolegal area. Forensic medicine was largely felt to be limited to the public investigation of suspicious or violent deaths. There was also, perhaps, some slight recognition of the need for psychiatric evidence in appropriate legal cases, but much of this evidence was considered scientifically suspect. Otherwise, little notice was taken of medical law, least of all its civil aspects. Since I was determined to seek broader interest among medical readers, I knew I would have to expound on basic law and demonstrate the importance of less familiar legal subjects to physicians and to medical practice. I was determined not to imitate the few legal reports I had found in medical publications, in which law practitioners, often "house counsel" to the particular medical organization or specialty society, and only rarely professors of law or scholars, would produce extremely dull, often biased, highly technical accounts that could have been written by a law firm's most recent and least imaginative law clerk.

I also discovered that medical journals did not serve the same function for medical readers as law reviews did for lawyers. My natural reference point was, after all, the quarterly publications turned out by nearly every recognized law school in the country. They were generally of high quality and reflected laborious attention to detail and depth of citation to proper legal authority.

These law reviews were not, however, in a newsletter style suited for regular reading by practitioners as primary and immediate sources of current law, since lawyers were made aware of current developments in their field through subscriptions to the latest judicial opinions and advance copies of federal and state statutes and administrative rules and regulations affecting their practices. I found that practicing physicians and medical researchers read the leading weekly medical periodicals, such as the *New England Journal of Medicine,* to discover and assimilate important advances in their practices and research work, much as lawyers read current court decisions and statutes. Medical journals were clearly quite different from law reviews, which afforded a more leisurely pace, much greater space allowances, and far wider opportunity to comment on the work and theory of other legal scholars and authorities in one's field of specialization.

I therefore modified my writing approach even more. I determined to write only about the most current new decisions and laws, usually long before they were noticed or dealt with in the law reviews of the country. I could not wait to see what others thought; I could not comment on the comments of others. Like other departments of the *Journal,* the "Law–Medicine Notes" column had to lead the way and offer contemporary analysis; at the same time, the columns would need to contain clear expositions of legal matters for a medical audience without legal training. These are the main considerations that have shaped my medicolegal writing during my years at the *Journal.*

There is one more aspect of the *Journal* environment that deserves mention, since it is reflected in these essays. Through letters to the editor, the readership keeps the contributors within reasonable bounds. Those who disagree with my views or find errors of any kind in my brief presentations frequently write to the editor, and their letters are often printed in the weekly correspondence section, a regular forum for criticism without parallel in American law reviews. I am invited to respond to the letters to explain more fully my views on a point of law, to limit my own previous overstatements, or to admit and accept a correction with all the grace I can muster. These letters have always affected my later writing, since I resolve, in the face of these public reminders, to do better the next time. When one writes and comments as regularly and as briefly as I must on so many different medicolegal issues, there are bound to be disagreements, faults, and errors. To my regular readers I can only offer my apologies for errors and my resolutions to improve.

In this Introduction I would like also to provide an overview of the subject areas covered in this book. The columns reprinted here include both older and newer writings, with emphasis on the newer and most relevant to the modern medicolegal world. The older columns were selected largely to provide background and historical understanding to current problems. As indicated earlier, they have been updated with comments especially prepared for this book; in addition, some have been slightly revised to clarify chronologic references. In order not to overwhelm the columns themselves as the primary focus of the collection, these additions have been kept to brief commentary, with emphasis on useful current references. In some instances, the original titles of columns have been abbreviated or changed slightly to distinguish them from similar articles published in other years.

The subjects examined in the various chapters are those that have the broadest application to medical practice. As might be expected in today's legal climate, the largest number of commentaries concerns medical and hospital malpractice. Over the years, the columns on the subject of malpractice have attracted the most attention, provoked the largest number of letters to the editor — and to me personally — and had the most impact, as reflected in judicial and legislative response. I am sure that it was mainly because of these columns that I was appointed in the 1970s to the first national investigating commission on medical malpractice, as the only member who was a full-time academic lawyer. I later wrote two columns for the *Journal* about this assignment, both of which are included in this book.

Much of what is new in clinically related legal issues will be found in the first two chapters. The emphasis is on malpractice, but matters of hospital administration and research-related liability will be found here also. It must be admitted that power to make decisions regarding many aspects of patients' welfare is shifting away from attending physicians and toward hospitals, third-party payers, and government regulatory agencies. The columns in these two chapters describe many of the legal milestones in this transition.

Chapter 3 is made up of essays relating to the more traditional areas of forensic medicine and the applications of medical evidence in court. It contains several of my frequent public pleas for improvement in medicolegal death-investigation programs in the United States.

When I first began writing for the *Journal,* support for forensic pathology programs in metropolitan areas of the country, let alone rural communities, was abysmal, and I said so. The two columns from the early 1970s reprinted in this collection received the most widespread attention. I am pleased to say that the situation of medicolegal death investigation has greatly improved in the past 10 years. Today, most metropolitan areas — including even Chicago, the last bastion of politically appointed coroners — are served by qualified, competently trained medicolegal specialists. In New England, my own region of the country, every one of the six states has a statewide system of investigation under a chief medical examiner. In Massachusetts, I had the pleasure of drafting the legislation and serving as the first chairman of the new state Commission on Medicolegal Investigation.

Several other columns in this chapter touch on my continuing quarrel with the American courts about the admission into evidence of the results of medical and other scientific tests. It is my view that American judges are overly cautious about allowing juries (and themselves) to hear and evaluate evidence based on scientific test procedures. This practice can be contrasted with the far too ready acceptance by the same courts of the opinions of so-called experts of dubious qualifications who are called into court by both sides in the adversary process, and whose evidence is in many instances unsupported by any semblance of scientific verification.

In these quarrels with the law of scientific evidence over the years, however, I must admit to almost total defeat. The courts of the current period are even less receptive to change in the traditional rules than was true when I began these columns more than 20 years ago. In fact, *Harper* v. *State,* included in this chapter—from my perspective, the worst reasoned of these high court opinions in recent years—is more restrictive in its application than any earlier state supreme court decision passed down in this century.

The last group of columns in Chapter 3 is concerned with a disturbing phenomenon of our age: the mass-population disaster, as exemplified in a number of contemporary tragedies, in many, if not most, of which technological change played a part. The first of these columns deals with the huge number of deaths and other injuries resulting from the emission of poisonous gas at Bhopal in India in 1985. Among other medicolegal issues, this essay touches on the overzealous involvement of American personal-injury lawyers, who rushed to Bhopal to sign up the village victims as clients for compensation suits in the United States. Two other columns deal with the difficult and complex problems of the medicolegal investigation of airliner crashes that resulted in hundreds of deaths and led to investigations with a multinational political flavor.

The last column in this chapter presents what is probably the most bizarre story, the most aggravated and most tragic of all the public events discussed in these columns over the past 20 years. This was the mass suicide at Jonestown, Guyana, where more than 900 persons, members of an obscure religious cult, died rather than have their practices revealed to the world by a visiting U.S. congressman. The congressman was murdered by the cult leaders, who thereupon encouraged the mass suicide of the church community. The column explores the methods of medicolegal investigation employed at the site of the tragedy and warns of future problems in the investigation and handling of mass disasters involving 1000 or more persons.

Chapter 4 deals with forensic psychiatry, one of the most troubled of the fields of medicolegal relations. Many developments have come about in this field over the 20 years since I began writing for the *Journal*. The period opened with President Kennedy's assassination and the trial of Jack Ruby. The law of insanity has, however, been most seriously affected by a more recent presidential assassination attempt, made by John Hinckley on President Ronald W. Reagan.

Hinckley's trial and acquittal resulted in a wave of reform legislation that placed much tighter restrictions on eligibility for insanity defenses in criminal cases. I observed in my first column, in 1964, that the changes that had come about in insanity law in England and the United States over the past century had been particularly strongly affected by trials for assassination or assassination attempts against major political leaders and heads of state. I indicated that this legal opportunity had been lost because of the killing of Oswald by Ruby. This analysis proved correct; nearly two decades passed before the Hinckley affair, which resulted in a radical reexamination of the law of criminal responsibility of the mentally ill, both within the framework of the trial and in subsequent developments.

The insanity defense is not the only medicolegal issue examined in Chapter 4. Attention is also given to the problems involved in predicting dangerousness in mentally ill persons and disturbed criminal offenders, the rights of the mentally ill and the retarded in legal proceedings, and the importance from a legal standpoint of the movement away from long-term commitment in large, remote, high-security mental institutions. Each of these developments has touched on conflicting social values and beliefs, and in many cases the nation's highest tribunal, the Supreme Court of the United States, has been obliged to decide the issues on constitutional grounds. As may be imagined, commenting briefly on Supreme Court decisions, many of which involve multiple opinions, has been one of the more challenging tasks that I have undertaken in the "Law–Medicine Notes" columns over the years.

Chapters 5 and 6 contain essays on ethical responsibilities in medical practice and on more general issues of morality and law as they relate to human reproduction. These columns, like the previous chapter, touch on opinions of the U.S. Supreme Court, some of the most controversial in the Court's long history. The discussions form a rather closely knit pattern; one point naturally leads into another because the philosophical issues at stake keep turning out to be the same. What readers may find surprising is that this area of morality and ethics has been dealt with extremely comprehensively in court decisions and legislation, even though most of the issues are entirely new to the law in the sense that it is only within the past 20 years that they have come to be frequently raised in a legal framework.

This is not to say that the ethical principles or the lines of moral reasoning examined in these columns are in themselves new. The novelty lies in the much more frequent resort to the law for resolution of the conflicts brought on by new medical technologies and capabilities unknown to the ancient philosophers who, with a certitude made possible by their comparatively narrow experience, laid down the principles being reexamined today.

Chapter 7 contains writings on issues of life and death. As medical students come to realize early in the course of their professional education, the practice of medicine and patient care unremittingly involves the physician in matters of life and death. Accordingly, it must be expected that medicolegal problems will also arise in these areas. However, the legal system does not invariably use the same labels as the medical profession to classify these problems when they are the subject of court controversies. The litigation may involve new concepts of life and death, but the technical legal issues on which the decisions depend may be highly varied and complex. It is essentially this complexity that is reflected in the makeup of this seventh and last chapter, which may be too involved for some readers' liking, especially since very little of it deals with traditional areas of forensic medicine, such as forensic pathology.

The different subjects treated in this last chapter can be linked to separate stages in the 20-year historical period covered by these columns. In the early 1960s, the key conceptual controversy in the law related to the policy to be adopted in personal-injury and medical-malpractice litigation when damage occurred to a fetus during gestation or at delivery, or when a woman became pregnant unexpectedly after a sterilization operation or while using what she thought were effective birth-control pills. Should such cases result in large compensation awards when the infant is stillborn or lives for only a few minutes? Should any recovery at all be allowed when the mother delivers a healthy but unwanted child? These fascinating issues of compensation policy came to be known as questions of "wrongful birth" and "wrongful life."

The next major problem of legal policy in this field arose in the early 1970s as a result of the medical redefinition of death and, in particular, the introduction of the concept of brain death. The movement received its primary impetus in 1968 with the publication of the report of the Harvard Ad Hoc Committee on Brain Death (on which I was the lawyer member), headed by the late Henry K. Beecher, M.D. The first legislative action came in 1970 – a surprisingly short time later, considering the magnitude of the consequences – when the State of Kansas responded with a well-drafted statutory definition of brain death. The statute endorsed the concept and defined it in scientific terms but wisely did not spell out all the medical criteria, leaving these for determination by the medical profession over time. The new law also dealt directly with the need to keep the body prepared and on a respirator after the official declaration of brain death so as to allow time for permission to be given for the removal of vital organs for transplantation. I wrote a column strongly commending the adoption of the statute, and, over time, the position I took has received broad support in legislation enacted all over the world.

The final chapter also covers another, more recent, development of such importance that its continuing impact cannot be measured fully at this time. It concerns the law's involvement in critical medical decisions regarding efforts to sustain the lives of elderly patients, as well as severely damaged and disabled newborns. Issues related to this point have, with the possible exception of medical malpractice, probably aroused the greatest degree of controversy among physicians and lawyers of all questions raised in the pages of the *Journal* over the past 20 years. The responsibilities and powers of attending physicians, patients, guardians, and families have by no means been clearly and definitively sorted out. Over the next decade there will be more cases and more legislative action involving the legal obligations of the living to the dying and to persons deserving and demanding the protection of the law at various stages of life.

The two decades covered in this collection were rich in medicolegal developments; indeed, they may have witnessed the most important changes of this century. In the past 20 years, the courts have ceased to be reluctant reviewers of medical decisions previously considered private matters between doctors and their patients and have become regular intruders in many areas of medical concern. Moreover, the courts have not been alone in adopting this increasingly intrusive style; in recent years, economists and ethicists have taken what are probably still more critical stances and have been at least equally influential in forcing reforms in traditional areas of medical practice.

It is, therefore, not surprising that interest in the interfaces between medicine and the law has markedly increased among physicians over these same two decades. This should be regarded as a healthy trend, since it is clear that developments in this area in the 1980s and 1990s will not affect narrow circles only; their impact will undoubtedly be felt throughout medical practice. Accordingly, it is essential that the professional community participate in the legal process — in the courts, regulatory agencies, and legislatures — and that practitioners, researchers, and educators from all branches of medicine be represented, so that the views of the physicians most affected by the law can be heard.

As the writer of "Law–Medicine Notes," I should like to express the hope that the current healthy trend will continue and that medicolegal affairs will never again come to be the exclusive province of a parochial elite. It is my further hope that this collection of essays — which, while not making up a full history of medicolegal relations in recent times, does cover the main developments — will generate still greater interest in this area among physicians of all backgrounds and encourage a broad approach to the issues involved. I am grateful to the editors of the *Journal* for making this collection possible.

William J. Curran, J.D., LL.M., S.M.Hyg.
Boston, November 1, 1988

LAW–MEDICINE NOTES

1 ♦ Medical Malpractice

The Not-So-Good Samaritan Laws

One result of the increased rate of medical malpractice suits in this country has been the reported reluctance of physicians to stop and to render emergency medical treatment to victims at the scenes of accidents. It is alleged that the doctors fear malpractice suits may be brought against them by the ungrateful victim or his family.

The reaction of the state legislatures to these reports has been rapid. In 24 states laws have been passed granting some form of immunity to physicians who render aid in an emergency situation. Fourteen states have passed such laws in 1963, and the majority of the others were passed in 1962 and 1961.

The Massachusetts statute is exemplary. Chapter 112, Section 12B, of the *General Laws* provides that no licensed physician "who, in good faith, renders emergency care or treatment" at the scene to automobile-accident victims shall be liable in a suit for damages for any "acts or omissions" in giving such aid. Many of the laws are broader than that of Massachusetts, granting immunity in any emergency situation.

The first problem with these laws is in assessing the public need for them. Are doctors being sued who render emergency aid? There is *not a single case* of such a suit to have reached the appellate level of any jurisdiction in this country. Also, there is no information of any trial-court cases in the United States. (One action involving a Massachusetts physician has been reported in the Virgin Islands.) There are no published statistics on insurance claims to indicate this as an area of significant risk. Governor Kerner of Illinois vetoed such a bill in August 1963 and said, "So far as I can ascertain, the attendant danger [of malpractice suits] is largely, if not wholly imagined.

From the *New England Journal of Medicine*
1964; 270:1003-1004.

A systematic inquiry into all the reported malpractice decisions has failed to disclose a single roadside instance."

Governor Rockefeller of New York also vetoed a so-called Good Samaritan law in 1962 on similar grounds.

As can be seen, however, these two executive vetoes, both upheld, in important states did not stem the tide of this legislative movement. Some might argue, in fact, that the lack of reality in the basis of the physicians' fears is not important. The important thing is that the fear, which is real enough, has caused physicians to drive past the scenes of accidents. The legislation is a quick method of reassuring the physicians that they will not be sued. Or is it?

There are problems with these statutes, many of them hastily drawn and just as hastily enacted. What immunity is actually given by these laws? What does "good faith," the term used in most of the statutes, mean? Will it grant immunity only from suits for "ordinary negligence," or will "gross negligence" and "recklessness" also be excused? If only ordinary negligence is covered, as many commentators hold, very little actual protection from suit is accorded to the doctor. The plaintiff's attorney merely has to add the adjective "gross" to his complaint, and he can sue, get into court, and force the physician and his insurance carrier to litigate. In fact, such "Good Samaritan" legislation actually could encourage lawyers to plead and prove gross negligence or recklessness. For doctors concerned with their reputations first and their insurance-claims records only second, this is hardly a good trend in the law.

Another serious question on these laws must be faced. They may well be unconstitutional. The Massachusetts Constitution provides: "Every subject of the Commonwealth ought to find a certain remedy, by having recourse to the laws, for all injuries or wrongs which he may receive in his person, property, or character. . . ." Most of the states have similar constitutional provisions.

This is not to say that the legislatures cannot abrogate legal remedies under any circumstances. Some states have abolished actions for breach of contract to marry or for alienation of affections, on the grounds that they are used almost totally for purposes of extortion or bribery. The U.S. Supreme Court has said that the U.S. Constitution "does not forbid the creation of new rights or the abolition of old ones recognized by the common law, to attain a permissible legislative object."

It remains to be seen whether or not the courts will consider the Good Samaritan immunity justified by the facts indicated above. Even if justification is found, there is another constitutional question in these laws. Both Governor Kerner and Governor Rockefeller alluded to it in their veto messages. Why are physicians alone, or physicians and nurses in some states, given immunity? Constitutional law requires that if laws make classifications, these must be reasonable and nondiscriminatory. A good argument could be made that physicians are more apt to be sued. However, one may not want to discourage the laymen who might save a life. After all, the Bible does not say that the first Good Samaritan was a physician. Also, this parable of Christ's seems to have been intended as a lesson in nondiscrimination.

♦

COMMENTS

This was one of the earliest columns I wrote for the *New England Journal of Medicine* and one of the first in which I expressed disagreement with the prevailing "medical viewpoint" on a medicolegal issue.

At that time the great majority of physicians believed firmly that many malpractice suits had been brought against physicians for negligence in rendering aid at the scene of an accident or in a crowded sports stadium or theater, and I pointed out that there were no empirical data to support this widespread belief.

Twenty-four years have passed since this column was written, but there is still no recorded instance of a suit arising out of medical care given by a volunteer at the scene of an accident. Nevertheless, all 50 states now have some form of Good Samaritan law. In each case, the reason for enactment of this legislation was the evidence that physicians were not volunteering aid at accident scenes because, despite efforts to convince them otherwise, they feared that they would be sued. In other words, the statutes were indeed necessary, but the reason was not that an alarming number of malpractice suits were being filed, but that physicians needed to be encouraged to give voluntary emergency care outside their usual areas of practice.

In all 50 states, it was the U.S. Department of Transportation, with its state highway-safety programs, that encouraged the passage of statutes protecting physicians, and the Good Samaritan laws enacted in the 1960s applied mainly to highway accidents, along with other nonhospital situations. In more recent years, several states have amended these laws to include emergency care given by physicians responding voluntarily to "code" calls to hospital patients with whom they have not had any other relationship. These amendments were urged when courts refused to expand existing traditional Good Samaritan laws to include such voluntary actions. See *Guerrero* v. *Copper Queen Hospital,* 112 Ariz. 104 (1946) and *Colby* v. *Schwartz,* 78 Cal. Rptr. 624 (1978).

Despite the universal enactment of the laws in every state, there have been no legal challenges in any state to the constitutionality of the basic thrust of the legislation. In fact, as a result of the wide-ranging reforms in the malpractice laws of several states in recent years, the concept of providing at least partial immunity from lawsuits has been extended to other activities. The most common type of immunity provision currently being enacted or considered applies to members of hospital peer-review committees, whose duty it is to make judgments pertaining to the quality of medical care, patient-risk management, and containment of the costs of medical care. See later columns in this chapter for further examination of such legislation.

The Case of the Monumental Malpractice

An incident reported by the Medical Defence Union in Great Britain in its 1969 Annual Report might be considered the unkindest cut of all in the history of the deteriorating relations of physician and patient in situations involving alleged medical malpractice. The distraught and grieving father of an 18-year-old boy who had died in a hospital erected a tombstone over his son's grave and had the following inscription carved on its primeval granite face:

> Never given the chance to fight for his life due to the incompetence callous neglect and wrongful diagnosis by . . . [naming the general practitioner and hospital physician who had attended the youth in his last illness in the hospital].[1]

The physicians named on the stone complained to the medical-defense organization that represents British doctors in legal matters, and this group, along with the local church burials committee, was able to get the stone removed. The physicians contended that the boy had died of natural causes and that no negligence had occurred. No legal action was taken by the father against the physicians or any other medical personnel.

American law would probably react in similar fashion to such an incident, even though we accord more leeway to "free speech" than the British do. There are no American cases directly in point with this quaint English libel, but there are a few that are close. I particularly recall a Massachusetts case in which a customer who was greatly disappointed in the quality of an automobile he had purchased took to hanging lemons all over it, drove it around the town, and then left it parked in front of the dealer's showroom with suitable signs hanging on it. (In American automobile slang, a

From the *New England Journal of Medicine*
1970; 283:33.

"lemon" is a defectively built automobile.) The dealer brought an action in court and succeeded in forcing the purchaser to stop his demonstration of displeasure.

Very little is gained in publicly maligning persons against whom we have personal grievances. The legal system has been built as a means of peaceful, orderly redress of such wrongs, or alleged wrongs. Particularly in such delicate and intimate relations as that of physician and patient, there is a need for encouraging trust and confidence. Every effort is made by lawyers, courts, insurance carriers, and physicians to handle medical grievances, including malpractice actions, with fairness and with as little public display as possible. In many cities the newspapers also cooperate and do not publicize malpractice suits at the time of the claim or during trial. They will publish accounts only at the end of a trial and only if the plaintiff wins his suit.

It is sometimes said that physicians bury their mistakes whereas lawyers perpetuate and enshrine their errors in statutes and case precedent. This English case proves that physicians must also guard against longstanding monuments to their alleged misfeasance.

REFERENCE

1. *Annual Report.* London: Medical Defence Union, 1969:44.

♦

COMMENTS

I know of no later efforts to etch physicians' alleged errors of malpractice into tombstones.

This column, also an early one, was obviously written with tongue in cheek, but it brought an important message to American physicians about the British medical-defense organizations, the Medical Defence Union and the Medical Protection Society. As the anecdote makes clear, both of these nonprofit societies not only defend physicians and provide malpractice insurance, but bring countersuits and other affirmative legal action on behalf of physician and dentist members. They will, for example, bring actions of libel or slander on behalf of members whose professional reputations have allegedly been damaged as a result of defamation.

Until the mid-1980s, the British seemed to be escaping from the crisis of increasing malpractice insurance premiums. In those years, however, Britain was struck with a serious problem. See W.A. Harland and R.S. Jandoo, "The Medical Malpractice Crisis" (*Medicine, Science and the Law* 1984; 24:123-9). The standard premium rate for members of the Medical Defence Union practicing in the United Kingdom rose from £336 in 1986 to £576 in 1987. The premium is, of course, still much lower than in the United States and is charged at a flat rate applying to all types of practice.

The Medical Defence Union reported an increase of 65 percent in total damages paid out in 1985 over 1984, whereas the 1984 total damages had been 22 percent higher than those paid out in 1983. The highest award in 1980 had been £270,000. In 1986, the highest award was "in the region of £700,000." See *Annual Report, 1986* (London: Medical Defence Union, 1987:7). See also J.S. Lublin, "England Braces for a Jolt in Court Awards" (*Wall Street Journal.* June 6, 1988:16).

For a historical review of the development of the British defense organizations and of malpractice litigation in the United Kingdom, see Hawkins' *Mishap or Malpractice* (London: Blackwell Scientific Publications, 1985). The book was prepared to commemorate the 100th anniversary of the Medical Defence Union. See also the recent article by the American commentator F.H. Miller, "Medical Malpractice Litigation: Do the British Have a Better Remedy?" (*American Journal of Law and Medicine* 1986; 11:433-63).

Defense organizations for medical practitioners in Europe are not limited to the United Kingdom. A medical-defense group, called "Le Sou Médical" (because for many years the annual membership fee was one sou) has been in existence in France since 1897.

Peer-Review Programs of Physician Performance: The Question of Legal Immunity

In the midst of another medical-malpractice crisis, medical peer-review programs concerning the quality of physicians' performance are receiving renewed attention as at least partial solutions to the problem. State legislatures are mandating comprehensive programs of peer review in all licensed hospitals, health maintenance organizations, and other health care programs. Despite these enactments, however, the effectiveness of peer-review performance monitoring has been greatly undermined by a genuine fear of retaliatory lawsuits brought by physicians who are the subjects of disciplinary action. Some states have passed "shield laws" that are designed to provide a degree of legal immunity for hospital peer-review committees, hospital staffs, and witnesses.[1,2] President Reagan has recently signed new federal legislation that extends a limited degree of immunity to medical peer-review activities in regard to both federal and state lawsuits.[3]

In earlier years, most of the suits brought by physicians against peer-review committees and hospitals alleged inappropriate procedures or lack of due process in disciplinary proceedings. These suits were designed basically to obtain reinstatement, not to harass or punish fellow physicians involved in the monitoring process. As the system grew uglier, however, the physicians who were the targets of discipline or exclusion from the staffs of health care organizations brought defamation actions (libel or slander) and discrimination suits against the physicians who were on credentials and discipline commit-

From the *New England Journal of Medicine*
1987; 316:597-598.

tees or those who had appeared as witnesses against them. The physicians who were faced with these suits often found themselves without insurance coverage for either lawyers' services or paying awards.

As if this situation were not bad enough, in the past five years or so an even worse problem has emerged — the advent of suits for violation of the federal antitrust laws. As I discussed in some previous Law–Medicine Notes,[4,5] the courts have removed traditional barriers to such suits against the professions. Violation of the antitrust laws can be used not only to force admission or reinstatement to hospital staffs but also to obtain treble damage awards of hundreds of thousands of dollars.

The special difficulty of the antitrust laws is that they have a built-in policy against competitors (other physicians) having the power, by means of concerted action, to prevent entry into the relevant market (e.g., the hospital) by other new competitors or to discipline fellow competitors by exclusion or restriction of trade in the marketplace. Peer review by medical staffs in health care organizations fits this proscribed model. Thus, in recent years, when medical staffs or hospital governing boards have sought to refuse physicians' privileges or have restricted or revoked existing rights to practice in their institutions, they have regularly been threatened with antitrust lawsuits. Many suits have been brought and several have been successful. The litigation is usually complex and very hard fought, with allegations that the primary motive of the medical staff and hospital was to stifle competition, not to improve the quality of medical care or to rid the staff of incompetent or seriously impaired physicians.

For physicians and hospitals that follow developments in peer review, the most disturbing antitrust controversy in this field involves the *Patrick* case, which has been fought out for nearly 10 years in Astoria, Oregon. A full description of the accusations of unfair competitive practices and biased hospital peer-review actions, the investigations by state medical-licensing boards, and the court proceedings would fill far more pages than are available in the *Journal.* An account published in 1985 provides useful background on the controversy.[6] In addition, a physician from the Astoria clinic has commented in the *Journal*[7] on the verdict of the lower court.

A review of the activities of the principal figures in the case provides considerable evidence that anticompetitive motives were involved. A jury in the Federal District Court in Oregon certainly thought that such motives were present: in 1984 it returned a verdict (and granted a stunningly large financial award) for the surgeon plaintiff, Dr. Patrick, and against several physicians in practice in the Astoria area and against the Astoria Clinic. The defendants were found guilty of violations of the federal Sherman Antitrust Act, Sections 1 and 2, and of unreasonable interference with economically advantageous relations under state law. The jury granted treble damages under the Sherman Act that totaled $1,950,000. It awarded another $90,000 in punitive damages, $20,000 in compensatory damages, and $228,600 in attorneys' fees. The grand total of the award was $2,288,600.

In congressional testimony after the jury award, evidence was presented that one of the hospitals that had been involved in the suit had dropped out of the case (by making a settlement) before the verdict was rendered and had left the defendant physicians without insurance protection.[8] It was stated that at least one of the defendants had 100 percent of his professional income attached after the verdict.

The huge award in the *Patrick* case sent shock waves through the ranks of medical and hospital organizations concerned with monitoring physician performance. In the appeal to the Federal Court of Appeals for the Ninth Circuit, the Joint Commission on Accreditation of Hospitals, the American Medical Association, the Oregon Medical Association, and the Oregon Hospital Association all filed amicus curiae briefs.

The recently issued decision of the court of appeals was almost as surprising to many observers as the verdict in the trial court. After a comprehensive review of the case, the judges dismissed the finding against the defendants under the Sherman Act.[9] Their conclusion was that the defendant physicians were immune from suit because the members of the hospital medical staff had taken their disciplinary action against the plaintiff under a state law that required the type of peer review conducted. The court observed that "Oregon, by compelling physicians to review their competitors, affirmatively has expressed a policy to replace pure competition with some regulation."[10]

The court went on to declare a further immunity for one of the defendant physicians for his actions as a member of the state's medical-licensing agency. In each instance, the court held the immunity to be total and complete, even against allegations of bad faith and anticompetitive motives. The court also reversed the granting of attorneys' fees in the plaintiff's award.

The only aspect of the case left open for potential liability against the defendants was action outside the scope of the antitrust laws involving violations of state laws regarding anticompetitive conduct that were not covered by the immunities laid down in the opinion of the court of appeals. The case was remanded to the trial court to consider those aspects of the case.

Attempts were made in Congress after this decision to defeat the proposed federal "shield law" on the basis that the *Patrick* decision made such immunity unnecessary. Proponents of the bill denied the implications of the *Patrick* case and asserted that other circuit courts and the U.S. Supreme Court might not agree with the rulings of the Ninth Circuit Court of Appeals. Evidently, they were able to convince a majority of their colleagues and the President. The bill was passed.

Medical groups across the country seem pleased with the new law, but it comes with mixed blessings. Its primary thrust is not the provision of an admittedly moderate immunity. The fundamental objective was to install a detailed medical peer-review system for monitoring physicians' performance. It was no mistake that Sydney Wolfe, M.D., of Washington, D.C., was the first witness called before the committee that produced the bill. Dr. Wolfe complained vigorously about the total inadequacy of current monitoring and discipline systems in hospitals and medical-licensing boards in every state.

The law establishes a very extensive data-reporting procedure that requires all hospitals and state medical-licensing agencies to report directly to the federal government on all aspects of physician monitoring, discipline, and malpractice settlements and suits. Even proponents of the legislation admit that it has the potential to place substantial administrative burdens on hospitals and state agencies.

Worst of all, the legislation contains a quite confused and convoluted immunity provision – the result of many compromises in the original language of the bill. The intent may still be to provide a degree of protection from lawsuits, but the shield for physicians now contains a plethora of gaping holes through which many a guided legal missile can reach its human target. For example, the application of immunity cannot even be claimed unless four "tests" are passed; thus, the monitoring action must have been taken (1) in reasonable belief that it was done to promote the quality of health care, (2) after reasonable investigation of the facts, (3) with adequate due process and procedural safeguards afforded to the accused physician, and (4) in reasonable belief that the action taken to discipline the physician was warranted by the evidence. This is not all. The legislation exempts suits under state or federal civil rights laws and exempts other actions by state attorneys general, the U.S. Department of Justice, and several other federal agencies.

On the whole, the new federal legislation may prove to be worthwhile, but its merits will lie more in its encouragement of programs to improve the quality of medical care and of more effective monitoring of physicians' performance than in its immunity provisions. In this respect, the *Patrick* decision may turn out to be more constructive as a protective shield for physicians, especially if its full application is upheld by the U.S. Supreme Court.

REFERENCES

1. Florida Comprehensive Medical Malpractice Reform Act of 1985.
2. Oregon Rev. Statutes, Sections 441.030-441.055.
3. Health Care Quality Improvement Act of 1986.
4. Curran WJ. Exclusive hospital–medical service arrangements for anesthesiology: antitrust consequences. N Engl J Med 1984; 311:243-4.
5. *Idem.* Health planning, Blue Cross, and the federal antitrust laws. N Engl J Med 1981; 305:1194-5.
6. Holoweiko M. What competition can do to peer review. Med Econ 1985; 62:122-39.
7. Dolin LC. Antitrust law versus peer review. N Engl J Med 1985; 313:1156-7.
8. House of Representatives. Congressional Record, October 17, 1986:H11590.
9. Patrick v. Burget, 800 F.2d 1498 (9 Cir. 1986).
10. Patrick v. Burget, 800 F.2d 1498 (9 Cir. 1986:1505-6).

♦

COMMENTS

The *Patrick* case reviewed in this column was reversed in a unanimous decision by the U.S. Supreme Court. The Court held that the immunity granted to members of peer-review organizations does not apply to the anticompetitive actions alleged and proved in this litigation. The state law was held not to provide sweeping protection because the hospital's peer-review process was not "actively supervised" by a state agency, *Patrick* v. *Burget,* 108 S. Ct. 1658 (1988).

In the future, unless the malpractice suits and antitrust prosecutions quiet down, we can expect more legislation designed to carve out selective islands of immunity for physicians. It is likely that these immunities, at least those of them that have public support, will continue to be granted in areas where physicians are performing tasks of benefit to the larger community. These activities will include monitoring of the quality of care and cost-control surveillance. They may also be expanded to include medical services and clinical investigation in situations in which protection is needed in order to encourage physicians and other care givers to engage in these activities. It has also been suggested that immunity, or a "cap" on awards, be granted to clinical investigators and even to commercial enterprises (drug companies and biotechnology firms) in order to encourage the development of treatment for and vaccines against the acquired immunodeficiency syndrome (AIDS). See *Confronting AIDS: Directions for Public Health, Health Care, and Research* (Institute of Medicine, National Academy of Sciences. Washington, D.C.: National Academy Press, 1986:228-30). See also a progress report by the Institute of Medicine, *Confronting AIDS: Update 1988* (Washington, D.C.: National Academy Press, 1988).

INFORMED CONSENT AND *RES IPSA LOQUITUR*: SERIOUS PITFALLS FOR PHYSICIANS

Two recent medical malpractice cases passed down by important state courts illustrate the difficulties of physician defense against suits based on the two favorite plaintiff doctrines of courtroom attack: failure to obtain "informed consent" and *res ipsa loquitur*.

The first case, which has received a marked degree of attention among the personal-injury bar, is *Darrah* v. *Kite*.[1] This was a decision of the Appellate Division of the Supreme Court in New York reversing a jury verdict for the defendant and ordering a new trial on the issue of "informed consent." A neurosurgeon had recommended hospitalization for a diagnostic workup on a nine-year-old boy with a history of convulsive seizures. Included in the tests was a ventriculogram. The results of the tests were negative so far as any tumor or other pressure on the brain was concerned. The child was discharged but was later admitted again after further seizures, and a craniotomy was performed. A blood clot was removed. His condition deteriorated, and he is now institutionalized as mentally deficient.

The parents of the child claimed that the full nature of the procedures were never explained to them. They claimed to have been told only that "routine brain tests" would be performed.

At trial, the judge charged the jury that it could find damages for failure to inform fully about the procedures only if damages resulted to the child as a direct result of this failure to disclose risks inherent in the procedure.

The appellate division reversed the decision on the grounds that the above charge was erroneous. It was held that a failure to obtain

From the *New England Journal of Medicine*
1970; 282:36-37.

informed consent is "tantamount to no consent at all." The court concluded,

> As the trespass to the body arises from the unlawful touching itself there need be no showing of negligence or malice and the plaintiff is entitled to any damages which flow from the unauthorized procedure regardless of the fact that the operation was performed with the utmost care.

As can be seen, this is strong language. It goes against the most recent trend in "informed-consent" cases, in which the courts have treated the cause of action as having the effect of negligence rather than of battery. Such an interpretation of the law makes such an action extremely difficult to defend.

The second case, *Hand* v. *Park Community Hospital,*[2] was decided by the Court of Appeals of Michigan. Again, the appellate court reversed a trial-court finding for the defendant. In this case, the plaintiff was hospitalized with a stroke on the right side. Some three days later, he suffered burns on the right buttock, right thigh, right arm, and back. At trial, no proof of how the accident occurred was offered. The plaintiff himself testified but said he could not recall the cause of the injury. The trial court dismissed the action stating, "There has been no showing of negligence on the part of these people; there wasn't any showing at all. The mere fact he was in the hospital is not evidence of negligence."

The court of appeals thought otherwise. Without actually using the Latin phrase that strikes terror into the heart of every defense lawyer, *res ipsa loquitur,* the court held that on the above facts, the jury could reasonably infer negligence on the part of the hospital, its employees, and its agents. The court concluded, "We think the plaintiff proved all he could be expected to prove in this case."

The Michigan court seems to be saying that when the plaintiff goes as far as he can go, the defendant hospital must *disprove* the case. The burden of proof traditionally carried by the plaintiff is shifted over to the defendant. The courts cite other cases[3] supposedly holding a similar doctrine. However, these cases involved unconscious patients suffering unexplained injuries in the hospital. This case extends the doctrine to include conscious patients under other handicaps. The gates of the courts continue to be opened wider and wider to malpractice actions.

REFERENCES

1. 301 N.Y.S.2d 286 (1969).
2. 165 N.W.2d 673 (1969).
3. Ybarra v. Spangard, 25 Cal.2d 486, 154 P.2d 687 (1945); Danville Comm. Hosp. v. Thompson, 186 Va.746, 43 S.E.2d 882 (1947); Beaudoin v. Watertown Mem. Hosp., 32 Wis.2d 132, 145 N.W.2d 166 (1966).

♦

COMMENTS

The later decisions in American courts have not followed the direction of the *Darrah* case reviewed in this column. Nearly all state courts now classify the failure to obtain adequate informed consent as negligence, not as the intentional tort of trespass to the body. See the recent and quite complete study of the subject in F.A. Rozovsky, *Consent to Treatment: A Practical Guide* (Boston: Little, Brown, 1984). See also R.R. Faden and T.L. Beauchamp, *A History and Theory of Informed Consent* (New York: Oxford University Press, 1986). For a psychological review, see J. Katz, *The Silent World of Doctor and Patient* (New York: Free Press, 1984). Several other columns reprinted in this chapter review developments in the law related to informed consent to medical procedures.

Hand v. *Park Community Hospital,* the second case examined in this column, presented one of the most egregious instances of decisions against physicians in this era. The court virtually held the hospital and its staff liable without proof of fault for the plaintiff's injuries. In later years, several courts have refused to apply a *res ipsa loquitur* approach to liability without fault in most medical care situations. For a general review of the subject, see G.R. Podell, "Application of Res Ipsa Loquitur in Medical Malpractice Litigation" (*Insurance Counsel Journal* 1977; 44:634-49); and H.L. Hirsch, D. Shapiro, and J. Lustig, "Res Ipsa Loquitur and Medical Malpractice – Does It Really Speak for the Patient?" (*Medical Trial Technique Quarterly* 1984; 30:452-72).

The First Mechanical Heart Transplant: Informed Consent and Clinical Experimentation

In April 1969, Dr. Denton A. Cooley implanted the first totally mechanical heart into the chest of Haskell Karp. The mechanical device sustained the patient for approximately 64 hours, when a heart transplant from a donor was performed. Mr. Karp died 36 hours later.

Mrs. Karp brought an action for money damages against Dr. Cooley and Dr. Liotta, who had built the mechanical heart, alleging negligence (and gross negligence) resulting in the death of the patient, a lack of informed consent, and improper experimentation.

A nine-day trial took place in the Federal District Court in Texas at the end of which the judge directed a verdict for the defendants. Mrs. Karp appealed to the federal court of appeals, and, in a very important decision, a three-judge bench unanimously upheld the dismissal of the case against Drs. Cooley and Liotta.[1]

The basic medical facts of the case are well known to most physicians. Mr. Karp was 46 and had a 10-year history of cardiac problems, including 13 cardiac hospitalizations and the insertion of a pacemaker in May 1968. He came to Dr. Cooley's unit in Houston on March 5, 1969. Dr. Cooley recommended a heart transplant. Mr. Karp at first rejected this suggestion in favor of some other operation. Dr. Cooley agreed to perform an extensive operation called a wedge resection with extensive plastic restructuring of the ventricle, but thought he needed to be ready to do a heart transplantation as a backup if it was needed at the time of the operation. Some three weeks passed, and the patient's condition worsened considerably while a heart donor

From the *New England Journal of Medicine*
1974; 291:1015-1016.

was sought. About a week before the operation, Dr. Cooley began to discuss with Mr. Karp the possibility of a mechanical-device implant since a donor could not be found and the patient's condition was deteriorating very rapidly. Dr. Cooley testified that he told Mr. Karp about the heart pump in detail and said that it could be used to sustain him for a time until a donor could be obtained and a heart transplant performed. Dr. Cooley explained that the pump was experimental and had never been used in human beings. He told Mr. Karp that it had been successful in keeping a 135-kg calf alive for more than 40 hours. Dr. Cooley said that he told Mr. Karp that he was reasonably confident that the pump could keep him alive until a heart transplantation could be done. He firmly asserted that no guarantees were made.

On the day before the operation, a detailed consent form was brought to Mr. Karp, who signed it. Dr. Cooley was not present at the signing. The witnesses to the document were Mrs. Karp and the assistant administrator of the hospital, Mr. Reinhard.

Mrs. Karp based her action on her own allegations that she did not understand that her husband's heart was going to be removed and a new type of mechanical device implanted. She testified that Dr. Cooley told her that the device was like a heart–lung machine commonly used in open-heart surgery, and also that she was told that the success rate on the wedge operation was 70 percent and that Dr. Cooley had a failure rate of less than 5 percent.

Mrs. Karp's case was greatly undermined legally when the circuit court refused to go into the issue of Mrs. Karp's understanding of the procedure. The court examined the patient's own involvement and his consent. The court ruled that the wife's understanding and consent were not legally necessary. Even if the patient himself were not legally capable of giving consent, his wife would not automatically become the person whose consent was required. She would have to be legally authorized by a court as a guardian to exercise such powers. The court examined the evidence of the information given the patient on a number of occasions. An important witness on these aspects was a rabbi who had seen Mr. Karp on a number of occasions before the operation. The testimony of the rabbi, the medical staff, and Dr. Cooley were all consistent with the description of the procedures and risks in the consent form. The court found that the document was "the best evidence" of what the patient had been told. The court found that no evidence was introduced by Mrs. Karp to prove lack of informed consent by the patient or to show any breach of Dr. Cooley's duty to apprise Mr. Karp of the nature and risks of the operation under Texas law. (The Texas law required expert medical evidence of what risks a reasonable medical practitioner would explain, taking into consideration the patient's condition.)

On the issue of experimentation, the court found that the rules of medical-malpractice cases should apply, again requiring expert medical testimony to support allegations that the defendants had deviated from accepted norms of practice so as to be negligent or grossly negligent. No such testimony was produced by the plaintiff. The court observed, "The record contains no evidence that Mr. Karp's treatment was other than therapeutic and we agree that in this context an action for experimentation must be measured by the traditional malpractice evidentiary standards."

Other issues were raised by the appeal, but the above are the most important for medical readers, especially those engaged in any type of clinical investigation. On the whole, the case is much more favorable to investigation and therapeutic innovation than most of the other recent cases that I have reviewed in this column in recent years. In particular, the court continued to apply the majority rule, and Texas law, on "informed consent," which makes disclosure a matter of medical judgment under the circumstances and not an unpredictable and virtually uncontrollable question for the lay jury to decide years after the event, as is now the law in California and the District of Columbia. Also, the case gives heavy weight to what is contained in a well-drafted consent form that was specifically designed for the case at hand. Certainly, this point is reassuring for all medical and scientific investigators and institutional review committees who are now struggling with "informed consent" and trying to prepare and use documents that do provide fully informed consent. There has been much talk, some of it in judicial opinions, that consent forms are "worthless."[2] This court certainly did not think so, at least when the consent document is prepared especially for the situation at hand and specifically details the nature of the procedure, its purposes, and all risks and inconveniences reasonably to be expected.

It might be noted that a petition for certiorari has been filed to appeal this decision to the Supreme Court on the issues discussed above, but also some other matters involved in the case. The petition challenges the upholding of the lower court's refusal to call Dr. DeBakey as a witness in open court. (He was interrogated in chambers, where he asserted he was not willing to testify as the plaintiff's expert witness.) It also challenges the application of a Texas statute making the records of a Baylor University investigating committee in the Karp case confidential and not subject to subpoena.

REFERENCES

1. Karp v. Cooley and Liotta, 493 F.2d 408 (1974).
2. Curran WJ. Informed consent and blanket consent forms. Am J Public Health 1971; 61:1245-6.

♦

COMMENTS

Petition for certiorari in the *Karp* case was denied in the U.S. Supreme Court. The *Karp* decision remains the most important case in the American courts upholding informed consent as protection for clinical investigators in innovative surgery and medicine. Although a great number of clinical investigative procedures are performed each year, very little litigation has resulted. At the present time, federal regulations applicable to "experimentation on human subjects" are considerably more important in controlling activities in the field than are medical malpractice suits.

At the time of this case, the Congress had not yet enacted legislation authorizing much stricter requirements for premarket testing of experimental medical devices. The mechanical heart device used by Dr. Cooley would now come under the regulatory program set up under that law. For a review of patient-related issues, see R.A. Knox, "Heart Transplants: To Pay or Not to Pay" (*Science* 1980; 209:570).

The patient in this case, Mr. Karp, was desperately ill and seeking any chance he could find to prolong his life and to improve his quality of life. What is the ethical significance of using "first-time" experimental procedures on desperately ill patients? For an analysis of this issue, see F.A. Moore, "Therapeutic Innovation: Ethical Boundaries in the Initial Trials of New Drugs and Surgical Procedures" (*Daedalus* 1969; 98:502). Quite recently, the federal Food and Drug Administration issued new regulations expanding the opportunity for desperately ill patients to receive experimental drugs in situations in which no other treatment is known to be effective. See "Treatment IND: Making Investigational New Drugs Available to the Desperately Ill" (*Federal Register* 1987; 52(99):19466-77).

Informed Consent, Texas Style

The medical-malpractice insurance crisis of the mid-1970s produced some effective reforms in the litigation of claims as well as in the availability of adequate insurance coverage for beleaguered physicians and hospitals.[1] It also resulted in some oddities in medicolegal relations. One of the strangest has been the attempt of the Texas Legislature to bring certainty and predictability to one of the foggiest and deepest quagmires of all malpractice law, the requirements of informed consent.

The complaint of physicians has been that the scope of adequate or, even worse, of fully informed consent can never be satisfactorily defined or predicted. The judges in the most famous cases in the field have been little help. They have held that the consent must contain all material facts or all information a reasonable person would want or need to make a rational choice. But in any given situation, what is "material"? How is the doctor to disclose adequately all the material risks, and yet not so alarm the patient as to remove his chance to act rationally? The Hippocratic Oath demands that above all no harm be done to the patient. Informed consent in the hands of an insensitive physician seeking only to protect himself from lawsuit is a dangerous weapon aimed at the emotions—the fear and insecurity—of the patient as well as at his supposedly reasonable mind.

The Texas Legislature, at the urging of medical groups, enacted in 1977 a package of medicolegal reforms in the malpractice law. Among them was a statute requiring that all suits alleging failure to inform, or to inform adequately, be based on negligence rather than the intentional tort of battery.[2] This is not a radical reform in itself. It removed some vexatious suits, resulted in the application of a somewhat shorter statute of limitations, and made insurance coverage

From the *New England Journal of Medicine*
1979; 300:482-483.

more certain, since some policies did not afford protection against suits for intentional wrongs like battery. But the Texas statute went farther and broke new ground. It set up the Texas Medical Disclosure Panel, composed of six physicians and three lawyers, to make regulations about what must be disclosed and what need not be disclosed in all medical situations of treatment or surgery. In December 1978, the panel issued its first set of proposed regulations.[3]

The regulations contain two lists of medical procedures, one that the panel asserts requires full disclosure, List A, and another that requires no disclosure, List B. For List A, the panel mandates the use of a specific consent form contained in the regulations. Also, the panel specifies particular risks concerning these procedures that must be disclosed. The two lists are by no means complete. They are a first attempt at meeting the legislative directive. For procedures not listed in either group up to the time of a lawsuit, the prevailing Common Law will apply.

Physicians should be interested and, at times, may be puzzled and astonished at what procedures are placed in the two groups, especially the "no disclosure" list.

List A contains 11 major categories of "procedures and treatments," each with various subdivisions. The 11 areas are enumerated alphabetically, beginning with anesthesia and followed by 10 systems: digestive, ear, endocrine, eye, female genital, integumentary, male genital, musculoskeletal (one of the longest subcategories), nervous (also quite long), and respiratory (with no specific risks actually listed as requiring disclosure). All the subcategories under each system are surgical procedures; none are "treatments" as far as I can judge. No special risks except those contained in the standard consent form are listed for anesthesia. An example of a listing of risks is that for mastectomy: "(a) limitation of movement of the shoulder and arm; (b) swelling of the arm; (c) loss of the skin of the chest requiring skin graft; (d) possible recurrence of malignancy; (e) decreased sensation or numbness of the inner aspect of the arm and chest wall."

List B contains several major categories, including local and regional anesthesia, excision and ligation of varicose veins of the leg, lumbar puncture, needle biopsy or aspiration of bone marrow, cranioplasty, appendectomy, hemorrhoidectomy with or without fistulectomy or fissurectomy, resection of the colon, cleft-palate operations, cosmetic surgery of the face and neck, free skin grafts other than to the hand, cystoscopy, corneal transplant, ligation of the fallopian tubes, thoracotomy, intravenous pyelography, and urethrotomy.

It should be recalled that the regulations provide that procedures contained in List B require no disclosure of any risks or hazards. No mention is made of the condition of the patient as an additional consideration; nothing is said to indicate that the physician need ever tell the patient anything about the known risks or benefits of the procedures to any particular patient or in any particular circumstances. The required consent form applies only to procedures under List A.

The Texas statutes under which these regulations were adopted are not so clear or definite on the effect in court of the physician's compliance with these two lists. Some of the sections seem to make disclosure (not nondisclosure) in accordance with List A an effective defense to a charge that the disclosure was inadequate. Nevertheless, Section 6.07(a)(1) of the same law creates only a rebuttable presumption that disclosure under List A or nondisclosure under List B will be an effective defense. The effect of nondisclosure is the issue left most in doubt. Frankly, I would be worried about total nondisclosure of risks concerning many, if not all, of the procedures in List B.

The ambiguity of the Texas law seems to have been produced because the draftsmen wished to protect the physician with a rebuttable presumption in yet another type of situation: when the physician does not disclose as required under List A because of "an emergency or if for some reason it was not medically feasible to make a disclosure." By providing for this exception, the draftsmen allowed a rebuttable presumption to be applicable to both List A and List B. The physician is thus left with uncertainty when he or she dares to disclose nothing to the patient in compliance with List B.

The problem here, as I see it, is that this medicolegal panel was attempting to divide all common surgical and diagnostic procedures into either risk or no-risk categories. The listing just does not ring true; most of these procedures do involve some discernible risk. Fundamentally, only a total lack of risk or hazard can ethically justify complete nondisclosure when the physician need not consider or weigh the potential benefit of the procedure to the patient as offsetting the risk. This panel may have been acting in good faith under the mandate of the Texas Legislature, but it is not clear that it was following the realities of medical science in this proposal.

REFERENCES

1. Curran WJ. Malpractice crisis: the flood of legislation. N Engl J Med 1975; 293:1182-3.
2. Texas Revised Civil Statutes, Title 71, Art. 4590i, Section 6.02.
3. Texas Register, Vol. 3, No. 92. December 12, 1978:4293-6.

♦

COMMENTS

As might be expected, changes in the court-imposed doctrine of informed consent were a favorite target of the legislative reformers in the later 1970s. This column, published at the end of the decade, examined the most radical — some say the most bizarre — of the legislative remedies applied in this period. The statutes in question read something like a menu in a Chinese restaurant: a little something from List A; a little something from List B.

Despite the law's strangeness, the regulatory agency in Texas took the statutory plan seriously and issued regulations to implement its requirements. The program has remained on the code books in Texas and is making more sense than most commentators, including myself, thought that it would. The Texas courts have upheld the law's validity. See E.P. Richards and K.C. Rathbun, "Informed Consent and the Texas Disclosure Panel" (*Texas Bar Association Journal* 1983; 46:349-53). Most important, the Texas courts have ruled on the effect of the law when the particular procedure, and the injury incurred, were not included on either List A or List B at the time of the alleged injury. In such situations, the courts have imposed a very high standard of compliance, requiring full disclosure of "all risks" that could have influenced a reasonable person in making a decision to give or withhold consent. See the leading cases: *Peterson* v. *Shields,* 652 S.W. 2d 929, Texas (1983); *Sherrill* v. *McBride,* 603 S.W. 3d 929 Texas Civ. Appeals (1983). See also D.M. Wallach and S.J. Berry, "Informed Consent in Texas: A Proposal for Reasonableness and Predictability" (*St. Mary's Law Journal* 1987; 18:835-82).

The only state that has followed Texas in enacting a "listing system" for medical procedures and informed consent is Hawaii.

There, the State Board of Medical Examiners has been designated to set standards of disclosure for accepted medical procedures and treatments.

I have selected the Texas-style reform measure for examination, but I do not mean to ignore other efforts at legislative reform of the doctrine of informed consent. In both the 1970s and the 1980s, many states attempted to change judicial standards by enacting new definitions of informed consent that did not require the disclosure of very remote potentials for harm resulting from medical interventions. Several examples of these statutory approaches are collected in a chapter on reform legislation in the third edition of my law school textbook. See W.J. Curran and E.D. Shapiro, *Law, Medicine, and Forensic Science* (3rd ed. Boston: Little, Brown, 1982).

One of the legislative devices developed to provide more protection for physicians in malpractice suits based on a failure to obtain adequate informed consent has been to establish by law a presumption of the validity and adequacy of an informed consent that was obtained in writing and signed by a mentally competent patient not under duress at the time of signing. The presumption can, however, be rebutted by the plaintiff. These statutes are quite complex and, when fully understood and applied by experienced plaintiff's lawyers, may not change the law as practiced in the courts as much as the reformers expected. See, for example, the law passed in Ohio (Ohio Revised Code, Section 2317.54), which is typical of the enactments in question. This statute provides that a written, signed consent is to be presumed valid unless the plaintiff produces sufficient evidence that the physician was acting in "bad faith," that the consent was obtained by "fraudulent misrepresentation of material facts," or that the patient was unable to communicate in the language in which the written consent was expressed. Moreover, the written consent document must meet certain standards. It must describe in general terms the nature, purpose, and expected outcome of the proposed procedure and the "reasonably known risks" of the procedure; except in emergencies, the document must identify the treating physician and must indicate that the patient acknowledges that "the information" to satisfy the conditions of adequate consent has been provided and establish that all questions asked by the patient have been answered to the patient's satisfaction.

Informed Consent in Malpractice Cases: A Return to Reality in the 1980s

For at least two decades, American law in the malpractice field has often imposed unrealistic burdens on physicians in regard to informed consent.[1] The courts have, in my opinion, turned the proper ethical obligation of a physician into an expansive intellectual exercise that is of dubious benefit to sick and worried patients. In an angry essay some years ago, Franz Ingelfinger referred to the legal rules as creating informed, but uneducated, consent.[2]

Perhaps worse is the fact that the doctrine of informed consent in its most severe form—which requires a physician to inform the patient of all potential risks of a treatment or operation, no matter how remote—too often makes the physician a guarantor of good results when, unfortunately, events that are only remotely foreseeable do sometimes occur. Thus, when the courts, after the fact of severe injury and nondisclosure, impose the doctrine, they encourage application of the concept of strict liability of the physician, without proof of negligence, and require the payment of inflated tort-law damages, often in six- or seven-figure amounts. On the other hand, every proposal for the enactment of a no-fault system of medical liability at least replaces the tort-law rule with a much lower scale of recovery for actual damages suffered.[3]

Until the latest decision of the Massachusetts Supreme Judicial Court in *Precourt* v. *Frederick,*[4] the trend of unrealistic and oppressive damages decisions seemed unbroken across the country. In fact, it was not expected that the Massachusetts court would issue an

From the *New England Journal of Medicine*
1986; 314:429-431.

important opinion in this direction, because it had only recently adopted the modern rules of informed consent, including what seemed to be highly detailed standards of full disclosure.[5]

In the trial of the *Precourt* case, the evidence indicated that the patient, a 33-year-old electrical-construction worker, had been hit in the left eye at work. A piece of metal was removed from the eye at a local hospital, but a smaller piece remained deeply embedded. After removal of the larger piece, the patient was referred to the defendant, Dr. Frederick, at Massachusetts Eye and Ear Infirmary. The physician advised surgery for the removal of the smaller fragment and explained to the patient the risks and possible benefits of the procedure. The patient consented to the operation, which was successful in removing the metal. After the surgery, Dr. Frederick recommended a course of treatment with prednisone, a corticosteroid, to control inflammation. The patient took the prednisone for 90 days after the surgery. The court record and testimony did not indicate the dosage. The patient's vision improved at first but later deteriorated until he was blind in the injured eye. Despite this, the patient returned to work.

Several months later, the defendant and plaintiff discussed an operation to remove scar tissue from the eye. Dr. Frederick indicated that this second procedure had only a 10 percent chance of restoring vision. Nevertheless, the patient elected to undergo the surgery. The procedure was performed and much of the scar tissue was removed, but sight was not restored. After the surgery, Dr. Frederick again prescribed corticosteroid treatment, and the patient took the drug for 55 days. Again, the record of the case and the court opinion did not indicate the dosage.

About three years later, the plaintiff was found to have aseptic necrosis in both hips. By the time of the trial, he had had bilateral hip-replacement operations.

It was agreed at the trial that the defendant had not told the plaintiff of a risk of aseptic necrosis associated with prednisone treatment. The doctor indicated that he considered it a very remote risk. Dr. Frederick testified that, since 1963, he had treated 50 to 75 percent of the eye patients in his practice with corticosteroids after surgery and that aseptic necrosis had never developed as a result of administration of those drugs. He admitted, however, that aseptic necrosis was listed in the *Physicians' Desk Reference* as 1 of the 41 potential complications known to be associated with use of the drug. An expert witness for the plaintiff testified that the "high dose" and "long course of treatment" had, in his opinion, caused the aseptic necrosis in the patient's hips. The witness also said that physicians should warn patients about the "possibilities" that such conditions may result from sustained corticosteroid use by persons who, like the patient in this case, have a history of alcohol use and slightly elevated blood pressure.

On the basis of this evidence, the trial court refused to direct a verdict favorable to the defendant and sent the case to a jury. The jury returned a verdict of $1 million against the defendant ($800,000 to the plaintiff for his injuries and $200,000 to his wife for loss of companionship and marital relation—a so-called loss of consortium). The judge denied a motion for a new trial, with the condition that the damages to the wife be reduced to $100,000—a sum that she accepted to avoid a new trial. Dr. Frederick appealed the decision to the Massachusetts Supreme Judicial Court.

The trial court's action shocked and distressed many physicians in Massachusetts. An amicus curiae brief was submitted to the high court by the Massachusetts Medical Society, the Massachusetts Society of Eye Physicians, and the Massachusetts Eye and Ear Infirmary. The brief took the position that the case was of great importance in establishing standards for disclosure of risks in the "ubiquitous area of prescribing drugs and medications" and that the effect of the trial court outcome, if not clarified, would be to make Massachusetts physicians

> virtual insurers of all risks of every drug they prescribe and every medical procedure they undertake, however infinitesimally remote, unless they explain every potential side effect of every drug and procedure to every patient, at a cost of time and resources that will be detrimental to good patient care and medical practice in Massachusetts.[6]

The brief cited the testimony of an expert for the defense in the trial, who testified that the risks of "most of the side effects" of prednisone, presumably including those that led to the patient's condition, were extremely remote—i.e., they occurred in only about one of tens of thousands of cases. This witness also indicated that he had conducted a computer search of 29,000 articles on the subject and had not found a single report of aseptic necrosis resulting from treatment with prednisone after eye surgery. Other ophthalmologists also testified that they were unaware of any reports of such side effects of the use of corticosteroids after eye surgery. It was also asserted that the plaintiff's expert witness had not contradicted this observation.

The Massachusetts high court, in an opinion written by Justice O'Connor, held that the verdict in the case should be reversed in favor of the defendant. All the justices agreed with this opinion, although Justice Liacos did write a separate concurring statement on the case. He did, however, agree with the results.

Justice O'Connor concluded, "In this case, there was no evidence [submitted by the plaintiff] that a person would develop aseptic necrosis after taking prednisone or that [Dr.] Frederick knew or should have known that the likelihood was other than negligible." The court found that the opinion of the plaintiff's expert witness, who said that the risk of this side effect was "high," did not constitute adequate evidence to support a verdict for the plaintiff. Justice O'Connor also observed that "high" was a relative term and could mean "one in ten, but it could just as well mean one in a million." Presumably, the court found the evidence too speculative in this case, in which the plaintiff had the burden of proof.

Most important, Justice O'Connor stressed that the earlier *Harnish* case[5] had established the standard that there must be a balancing, an accommodation, among the patient's right to know, fairness to physicians, and society's interest that medicine be practiced "without unrealistic and unnecessary burdens on practitioners."

There seems little doubt that this decision will be helpful in moving American law away from serious collision with the realities of what physicians can and cannot do to inform their patients of the risks and benefits of proposed treatments.

I do not argue against reasonable disclosure of important risks of treatment, nor do I argue against the need to offer alternatives to patients when alternatives are available. Every physician has an ethical obligation to involve patients in decision making about their care.[7-9] However, prudent medical practice must incorporate limits to disclosure in regard to different types of procedures, as well as divergent emotional and intellectual assessments of a patient's capacity to deal with medical information at a particular time in an illness.

The *Harnish* case in Massachusetts, the forerunner to the present decision, involved elective surgery that was important primarily in relation to a young woman's physical appearance. Such a situation seems to call for full disclosure because the procedure is neither urgent nor highly effective in combating disease or disability. Under such circumstances, the patient should consider the remote but serious risks thoughtfully in deciding, for example, to undergo elective plastic surgery of the neck. In the *Precourt* case, on the other hand, the patient was seeking restoration of sight – a goal for which considerable risk might be justified and disclosure of negligible, remote risks might not be warranted in the view of either patient or physician.

I am, however, rather surprised at the brevity of the court's opinion in the *Precourt* case and at its failure to review the evidence in depth or to lay down a range of obligations for physicians in different types of clinical situations. My own suggestion in regard to the situational differences between the *Harnish* case and the *Precourt* case is not included in either opinion, nor are other examples given or evaluated. The decision of Justice O'Connor is more impressionistic than analytic. It clearly conveys the feeling that the justices thought that, in this case, the application of a full-disclosure standard would be unfair, and that the risk of necrotic hip disease was too remote to have required disclosure and culpability to the tune of nearly $1 million. Beyond this, however, the opinion offers little future guidance. We must await further decisions in the common-law traditions of the courts to flesh out the details of the true meaning of this step in the right direction.

REFERENCES

1. Rozovsky FA. Consent to treatment: a practical guide. Boston: Little, Brown, 1984.
2. Ingelfinger FJ. Informed (but uneducated) consent. N Engl J Med 1972; 287:465-6.
3. Curran WJ, Shapiro ED. Law, medicine, and forensic sciences. 3rd ed. Boston: Little, Brown, 1982:517-36.
4. Precourt v. Frederick, 395 Mass. 689 (1985).
5. Harnish v. Children's Hospital Medical Center, 387 Mass. 152 (1982).
6. Brief of Amicus Curiae, typescript copy to the court, October 23, 1985:3-4.
7. Rennie D. Informed consent by "well-nigh abject" adults. N Engl J Med 1980; 302:917-8.
8. Chapman CB. Physicians, law, and ethics. New York: New York University Press, 1984.
9. Katz J. The silent world of doctor and patient. New York: Free Press, 1984.

COMMENTS

In letters responding to this column, physicians uniformly supported my qualified praise for Justice O'Connor's decision, whereas lawyers, in the main, stoutly defended the earlier libertarian requirements of "full disclosure." Actually, this essay does not endorse the opinion in the *Precourt* case without reservation but points out several problems raised by the court's rather brief and cursory pronouncements.

This column also provided me with a welcome occasion to comment on an earlier dispute in Massachusetts, known as the *Harnish* case. In that instance, the court's decision received extensive notice in the medicolegal journals as an endorsement of full disclosure. None of the commentators seemed to attach due importance to the fact that elective surgery was involved and that in this situation there is more clinical justification for full disclosure than would be true under most other circumstances.

For some conflicting viewpoints on the merits of informed consent in medical practice, see F.J. Ingelfinger, "Informed (but Uneducated) Consent" (*New England Journal of Medicine* 1972; 287:465-6); G.J. Annas, "The Goals of Informed Consent" (*Medicolegal News* 1980; 3:13-5); D. Rennie, "Informed Consent by 'Well-Nigh Abject' Adults" (*New England Journal of Medicine* 1980; 302:917-8); and M.D. Kirby, "Informed Consent: What Does It Mean?" (*Journal of Medical Ethics* 1983; 9:69-75). For a review of both law and practice in Canada, see G. Robertson, "Informed Consent in Canada: An Empirical Study" (*Osgood Hall Law Journal* 1984; 22:139-61). For a comparison with the law in West Germany, see J. Shaw, "Informed Consent: A German Lesson" (*International and Comparative Law Quarterly* 1986; 35:864-90).

The studies listed above examine only the law of informed consent. What are the realities? Are patients protected from making rash decisions about their medical care by being given more complete information? Several empirical studies have been done in clinical situations. The studies indicate that most patients recall little of the technical information provided either orally or in writing in the context of ensuring informed consent, but that they do seem to understand the general procedures they have undergone. Data on risk were generally not well retained when the treatment had actually progressed well and the patients were satisfied with the care delivered. See, for example, B.R. Cassileth et al., "Informed Consent – Why Are Its Goals Imperfectly Realized?" (*New England Journal of Medicine* 1980; 302:896-900). Other studies evaluated understanding and retention in simulated situations not reflecting the clinical experience of actual patients. See W.E. Woodward, "Informed Consent of Volunteers: A Direct Measurement of Comprehension and Retentions of Information" (*Clinical Research* 1979; 27:248-52); A.H. Taub and M.T. Baker, "The Effect of Repeated Testing upon Comprehension of Informed Consent Materials by Elderly Volunteers" (*Experimental Aging Research* 1983; 9:135-8).

Package Inserts for Patients: Prescription-Drug Information in a New Form

Should patients be given direct information on the risks and benefits of prescription drugs in order to help them formulate an effective informed consent? An effort to move toward a system of patients' "package inserts" for all prescription drugs has been under consideration at the Food and Drug Administration (FDA) for some time. Earlier this year, the effort was further delayed when the Reagan administration called a moratorium on new regulations. The idea, however, is still strongly supported by many consumer and patient groups.

The legal battle over package inserts for patients came about when the inserts were proposed for oral contraceptives containing conjugated estrogens. Studies published in the mid-1970s had indicated an association between such estrogens and endometrial cancer. Changes were suggested in the standard package insert for physicians. In addition, the FDA suggested that a patient-information leaflet accompany the product.

The protest against this proposal was immediate and strong in the medical profession, especially among obstetricians, and throughout the pharmaceutical industry. The installation of such a program would break the barrier preventing direct communication (i.e., direct advertising) by the drug companies to patients concerning prescription products. The barrier had been laboriously constructed to protect the public from overselling, exploitive practices common among "patent-medicine hawkers" in earlier centuries. Avoidance of these practices had led to the term "ethical drug industry," which had become current in recent decades.

From the *New England Journal of Medicine*
1981; 305:1564-1566.

A suit was brought by the Pharmaceutical Manufacturers Association to stop the FDA from requiring a patient's package insert for oral contraceptives. Joining in the action were the American College of Obstetricians and Gynecologists, the Congress of County Medical Societies, the Oklahoma State Medical Society, the American Society of Internal Medicine, the American Pharmaceutical Association, the National Association of Chain Drug Stores, and others, as parties or amici curiae. The FDA was supported by the Consumers Union of the United States, by other consumer groups, and by women's health-advocacy organizations.

This formidable group of opponents of the requirement was not able to convince a federal district court in Delaware in early 1980 that the FDA had no legal authority to impose this new form of consumer protection.[1] The court dealt with the case as involving a requirement for such patient information only for a particular drug because of specific dangers in its customary use – not as involving the power of the FDA to install the system for all prescription drugs. It was determined that failure to warn patients directly of the danger of cancer could render the labeling false and misleading. This danger was found to be "sufficiently serious as to be material to the patient's decision on use of the drug."

The court also dismissed the medical groups' contention, supported by affidavits from noted physicians, that such a system would be deleterious to patient care and would conflict with the physician's constitutionally protected right to practice medicine without undue interference. The medical groups seemed particularly exercised by the fact that the FDA not only wished to prescribe the content of the information to be given patients but also would not allow physicians to override the requirement and deny the package insert to particular patients when it seemed undesirable to expose them to it. Also, it was alleged that since the FDA had conducted no field studies of the effects of this new approach to informed consent, the whole scheme was an arbitrary and capricious abuse of regulatory powers. The court dismissed these contentions as well. It was observed that these estrogens were prescribed mainly for menopausal symptoms, which, though sometimes severe, were not life-threatening. The objective of the warnings was to avoid prolonged use of the drugs and to alert women to watch for the side effects. Suggestion-induced side effects were believed to present little problem with this drug. On the whole, the patient information supplied in this case was found to have reasonable support and to be protective of patients.

The lower court's decision was appealed to the Court of Appeals for the Third Federal Circuit. In late 1980, the appellate court affirmed the lower court's decision in a unanimous per curiam opinion.[2] The court had no trouble with the determination and rendered a short opinion of affirmation. Stress was placed on the statutory powers of the FDA when it found that, without the patient package insert, the estrogen labeling would be "misleading." Since that time the parties in the case have decided not to appeal the case to the Supreme Court of the United States.

Even though both these courts dealt with the issues narrowly in regard to estrogen prescribing, the general impression in the medical community and in much of Congress has been that the FDA has been found to have the power to require that package inserts for patients be provided for all drugs.

The lower court specifically noted that it was not dealing with the "wisdom" of adopting the new system. Further consideration of the general policy of such package inserts should therefore not be precluded by this decision.

First of all, it would be an oversimplification to consider these package inserts as part of the primary process of obtaining the patient's informed consent for the treatment, even though the language of the court suggests it. The information conveyed in the leaflet is received by the patient much too late to influence the basic decision of whether to follow the physician's advice. The patient has already been seen and evaluated by the physician. A diagnosis has been determined and a course of treatment suggested. The patient has received a prescription and then receives this patient information, usually in quite technical language, as part of the drug package. If the patient is disturbed about what it contains, such as warnings that some patients may suffer serious side effects after short-term or long-term use, and these effects have not been fully explained by the physician, the patient may be in a quandary. The only protective course is then to decline the medication and call the doctor. The doctor may then interpret the matter more fully and reassure the patient or suggest an alternative medication or treatment. Some concerned patients may decide not to take the medication and also not to call the physician; they may wait for the next scheduled visit, or consult another physician. Failure to take the medication, or a substantial delay in following a course of treatment—either one without the physician's knowledge—could be severely detrimental to the patient's welfare.

The most innocuous of drugs, and those generally considered safe, effective, and best for a given problem may, nevertheless, produce serious side effects in some patients. A description of risks in a package insert drafted for the self-protection of the drug company and the FDA could disturb even the most sophisticated patient. Placing this type of information in the hands of patients after the course of treatment had been agreed on with the physician would add an uncontrollable and often unknown factor to the treatment process. The patient might make a new judgment not to take the medication as directed. Undoubtedly, some patients would be helped in this new process. Perhaps the prolonged use of oral contraceptives by women who are not sick or who know of the alternatives is one of the most effective and most self-protective areas for the application of such a program. In addition, such a system could improve the primary process of informed consent if the physician would more thoroughly review what the patient might read in a later-received package insert. Nevertheless, one wonders how widely such a program, with no allowable intervention or override by physicians, should be imposed on areas of practice in which the medications are used by sick patients who are not readily able to weigh either the possible risks or the estimated benefits of a prescribed treatment against those of the available alternatives. These issues remain unanswered in today's rapidly changing world of improving, but still sometimes dangerous, prescription-drug therapy.

REFERENCES

1. Pharmaceutical Manufacturers Assoc. v. Food and Drug Admin., 484 F.Supp. 1179.
2. Pharmaceutical Manufacturers Assoc. v. Food and Drug Admin., 634 F.2d 106.

♦

COMMENTS

For a comprehensive review of the law regarding obligations to provide information on medications directly to patients, see D.B. Brushwood and L.M. Simonsmeier, "Drug Information for Patients: Duties of the Manufacturer, Pharmacist, Physician, and Hospital" (*Journal of Legal Medicine* 1986; 7:279-340). For a more recent analysis of legal obligations to warn consumers about the dangers of oral contraceptives, see T.M. Schwartz, "Consumer Warnings for Oral Contraceptives: A New Exception to the Prescription Drug Rule" (*Food, Drug and Cosmetic Law Journal* 1986; 42:241-56).

The commissioner of food and drugs has recently published a paper describing the regulatory policy of the FDA in this decade. See F.E. Young, "FDA's Philosophy of Regulation in the 1980's" (*Food, Drug and Cosmetic Law Journal* 1987; 42:157-61).

Medical Malpractice in Diagnosis

It is commonly said that physicians cannot be held liable for "mere errors in professional judgment." This is taken to mean that there is no liability for an erroneous diagnosis. However, the courts have held that this doctrine applies only when the physician has examined the patient, taken an adequate history, and conducted the accepted diagnostic tests and procedures. In two important decisions, the federal courts have reaffirmed this qualification on the basic doctrine.

In *Clark* v. *United States*[1] the Court of Appeals for the Fourth Circuit was called on to interpret the leading case in the field, *Hicks* v. *United States,*[2] which had been decided in that circuit. The court, in a two-to-one split decision, upheld a district-court verdict for the plaintiff, who had been operated on to correct an ectopic tubal pregnancy. A chronic pelvic inflammation was ascertained. At surgery, certain organs were found to be severely distorted and out of position. To control the extensive bleeding, a number of ligations were required, and in the course of these procedures the right ureter was inadvertently sutured in two places. No negligence was found in this action. However, negligence was found in the failure to consult a urologist or to take an intravenous pyelogram to identify the problem until the sixth postoperative day. During all this time, the patient was complaining "of all types of pain." The symptoms seemed to point to a kidney infection or ureter blockage. When the diagnostic tests were performed and corrective surgery became necessary, it was found that there was considerable degeneration in the ureter. It later became necessary to remove the right kidney.

The other case, *Steeves* v. *United States,*[3] is particularly important because of its detailed examination of legal responsibilities in emer-

From the *New England Journal of Medicine*
1969; 281:312-313.

gency-department operation, medical staffing, supervision of interns, and consultation requirements. A full reading of the case is recommended for all physicians and medical care administrators interested in emergency medical programs.

The case involved an 11-year-old boy sent to a Naval Hospital by a physician who had examined him at an Air Force dispensary. The symptoms, strongly suggestive of acute appendicitis, were described on a consultation sheet sent to the hospital with the patient. The provisional diagnosis was "possible appendicitis — emergency." The patient was seen at the hospital by a physician, who sent him home. That night, at 2:30 a.m., the mother took him back to the hospital in great pain. He was examined briefly by an intern, who again sent him home without taking any laboratory tests or x-ray films and without seeking a surgical consultation. On the next afternoon, the mother took the patient back to the Air Force dispensary, where blood counts and urinalysis were conducted, further indicating appendicitis. At 11 p.m. that night, a physician at the dispensary sent him, now for the third time, to the Naval Hospital with the following notation: "Please do not let this child's appendix rupture."

The trial judge then asserts, "After interminable delays at the Emergency Room, the child was put to bed at 2:10 a.m." Surgery was performed the next morning beginning at 10:28 a.m., and the appendix was found to have ruptured.

The court found liability and negligence. It was held that the hospital owed a greater degree of care to a child than to an adult. It also found that more diligence is owed by a physician in conducting diagnostic procedures when the finding at the hospital is in "direct conflict" with the diagnosis suggested by a reputable physician who refers the patient to the hospital as an emergency surgical problem.

Many physicians have complained that recent court decisions in medical malpractice have caused too many unnecessary diagnostic tests to be ordered merely for the protection of the doctor, rather than for the patient's sake. Decisions such as those discussed above may reinforce this fear. These decisions do go farther than earlier cases in legally requiring specialist consultation and the use of a battery of at least the more commonly accepted diagnostic procedures. However, it may be difficult in any clinical situation brought before the courts to draw the line on what is "required" for the patient's welfare and what is unwarranted interference by the law in matters of medical judgment.

REFERENCES

1. 402 F.2d 950 (4 Cir. 1969).
2. 368 F.2d 626 (4 Cir. 1966).
3. 294 F.Supp. 446 (1968).

♦

COMMENTS

As we move into the 1980s, "error of judgment" continues to be one of the most commonly pleaded of all defenses in medical-malpractice cases, but the concept involved is extremely difficult to define. The courts appear to have recognized the "error of judgment" rule as applicable in regard to three stages of clinical management, at all of which the exercise of clinical judgment is clearly called for: (1) diagnosis of the patient's current illness; (2) decisions on initial treatment or surgery for the patient's illness or condition; and (3) further decisions on treatment or surgery when complications occur or when the patient does not respond to initial interventions. However, the majority of litigated cases have continued to involve allegations of error in the original diagnosis. When the diagnosis is corrected and proper treatment is begun before any damage or injury is done to the patient, no liability will be found. See *Dettman* v. *Flanary,* 86 Wisc.2d 728 (1979); *Lis* v. *Robert Packer Hospital,* 579 F.2d 819 (Federal Court of Appeals, Third Circuit, 1978).

Later decisions have closely followed the reasoning of the two decisions reviewed in this column. The "error of judgment" defense tends to be accepted in misdiagnosis cases when the patient has had a complete diagnostic workup and a reasonable basis exists for a differential diagnosis including the choice or choices selected by the defendant physician. See *Herskovits* v. *Group Health Coop.,* 664 P.2d 474 (Wash., 1984); *Speer* v. *United States,* 512 F.Supp. 670 (Fed. Dist. Ct., N. Texas, 1983); *Voegeli* v. *Lewis,* 568 F.2d 89 (Federal Court of Appeals, Eighth Circuit, 1977); *Borne* v. *Brumfield,* 363 So. 2d 79 (La. App., 1978); *Riddlesberger* v. *United States,* 406 F.Supp. 617 (Federal District Court of N. Dakota, 1976).

An important study analyzing a series of surgical procedures in a large teaching hospital over a period of one year suggests that the number of instances of adverse outcomes in general surgery due to error by the surgeon was very small (36 cases in 5612 surgical admissions). In their conclusion, the authors suggest that what they referred to as "the British distinction" between errors of judgment (errors related to flawed reasoning) and errors of negligence (errors due to inattention or lack of obligatory effort) be adopted by American courts. The authors argued that confining the concept of malpractice to instances of the latter type of error would result in a considerable improvement in American law and would "open discussion of such error (error of judgment) in all branches of medicine." See N.P. Couch, N.L. Tilney, A.A. Rayner, and F.D. Moore, "The High Cost of Low-Frequency Events: The Anatomy and Economics of Surgical Mishaps" (*New England Journal of Medicine* 1981; 304: 634-7).

Diagnostic Errors in Glaucoma and Streptococcal Pharyngitis

One of the "old saws" of the law of medical practice used to be that physicians were not liable for mere failure to diagnose an illness correctly. Defense lawyers were frequently heard to comfort their doctor clients by assuring them that they would not be required to pay damages in court for errors of judgment. Like most dogmatic statements in the law, this one was never fully true. Five years ago, several important cases were pointed out in which physicians were held liable for incorrect diagnoses.[1] Now, however, two very much more important new cases may well bury the old saw once and for all.

Both cases involved the failure to perform simple, harmless diagnostic tests: in one it was a pressure test for glaucoma; in the other it was a throat culture for streptococcal pharyngitis. In each case the patient had serious illness and incapacity.

In the first case, *Helling* v. *Carey and Laughlin,*[2] the Supreme Court of Washington State held as a matter of law that the defendants, two specialists in ophthalmology who were practicing as partners, were negligent in not doing a pressure test for glaucoma on the eyes of a patient during a period of treatment for eye complaints from 1963 to October 1968. During this time, the defendants allegedly believed that the patient's complaints were solely related to complications associated with her contact lenses, for which she had been fitted on her first visit to the specialists in 1959. On the last visit, the pressure test was done and was positive for glaucoma. The patient's sight was then severely impaired, central vision being reduced to 5 degrees vertical and 10 degrees horizontal. There seemed to be no

From the *New England Journal of Medicine*
1974; 291:508-509.

disagreement that the patient, then 32 years of age, had had the disease for 10 years or longer.

At the trial, the defendants produced uncontroverted expert testimony that the practice among ophthalmologists throughout the country was not to conduct a routine pressure test among eye patients under 40 unless they had symptoms indicating suspicion of glaucoma. One of the defendants, Dr. Carey, testified that the first complaint by the patient about visual-field problems was on August 30, 1968, just 30 days before the first pressure test was administered on her next and last visit on October 1. The jury returned a defense verdict, finding that no negligence occurred in the treatment.

On appeal, the Washington Supreme Court unanimously reversed the judgment, holding that the defendants should have tested for glaucoma in a "timely" fashion such as to have prevented the blindness. The court did not say when the test should have been given.

There was no expert evidence to support the reversal. The court did so of its own accord, virtually holding the entire specialty of ophthalmology to be negligent in not administering pressure tests routinely with all patients regardless of age. To my knowledge, this is the first time any state supreme court has applied this legal theory in a malpractice case. The court cited no precedent for doing so. The only two cases cited at all were a railroad case[3] decided in 1903 in the U.S. Supreme Court with the opinion by Justice Oliver Wendell Holmes, Jr., and a famous 1932 case involving tugboats in New York Harbor.[4]

Surprisingly enough, there were no dissenters from this audacious pronouncement from the Washington bench. Furthermore, three of the seven justices, though concurring in the result of reversal, would have gone further and imposed "strict liability without fault" in this situation rather than call it negligence. Quite baldly, these justices asserted that the reason for their opinion was that the defendants' liability insurance should pay for this damage to the plaintiff rather than have it fall on the plaintiff, unaided by compensation. Incidentally, the opinion does not even explore whether the defendants had adequate insurance. The verdict of a later retrial on the issue of how much money the defendants should pay was not limited to the defendants' available insurance coverage.

The casualty insurance companies and defense counsel all around the country have been stunned by this decision. The implications of both the majority opinion and the concurring opinion make rate setting in the malpractice field even more difficult than it has been in the past. The movement to establish some entirely new compensatory plan for medical situations may well be accelerated as a result of this case if it represents any trend of the courts in the future. As an example of sound legal reasoning or opinion writing, the decision leaves much to be desired. The majority opinion is only three pages long; the concurring opinion is less than two. The theories of liability in both are extracted wholly from other fields without any expressed justification for their application to medical practice. Space limitations make it impossible for me to provide further critique of the technical aspects of the opinion.

The second case was an approved settlement in the U.S. District Court for the District of Columbia in the amount of $250,000, a very high damage figure in malpractice litigation nationally. In this case, a three-physician partnership of pediatricians failed to do a throat culture on a 12-year-old girl. Her complaints were variously diagnosed, according to a report in the *Washington Post,* as a urinary-tract infection, old-fashioned grippe, and anemia.[5] Three months later, the child became severely ill and was diagnosed by other doctors as suffering then from rheumatic fever. The settlement seems to have been based on a theory close to that applied in the Washington case, though actual negligence may have been alleged and proof may have been available from experts on this issue. The case has no importance as precedent, of course, since it was settled before any trial or decision of a higher court.

The American Heart Association's Rheumatic Fever Committee called my attention to this latter case. The committee is concerned with encouraging physicians to administer a full course of antibiotic treatment in all cases of streptococcal infection as a preventive for rheumatic fever. In the instant case, the legal issue was related to failure to diagnose the illness properly. The matter of treatment of choice was not reached. Nevertheless, the settlement in the District of Columbia seems to be the first successful action for malpractice involving streptococcal infection and the complication of rheumatic fever — it was the complication that resulted in the huge monetary compensation.

REFERENCES

1. Curran WJ. Medical malpractice in diagnosis. N Engl J Med 1969; 281:312-3.
2. 519 P.2d 981 (1974).

3. Texas and Pac. Ry. v. Behymer, 189 U.S. 470 (1903).
4. The TJ Hooper, 60 F.2d 737 (2 Cir. 1932).
5. Washington Post. April 24, 1974:C5.

♦

COMMENTS

The decision discussed above, *Helling* v. *Carey and Laughlin,* proved — as predicted in the column — to be one of the most influential developments in malpractice litigation in that decade. It was undoubtedly a major factor in causing many insurance carriers to withdraw from the field of malpractice insurance, thus precipitating the insurance crisis of the mid-1970s, which is examined in later columns reprinted in this chapter. See a discussion of the influence of the decision in a Congressional study, U.S. Senate Subcommittee on Health, *Report on Continuing Medical Malpractice Insurance Crisis* (Washington, D.C.: Government Printing Office, December 1975). See also L.S. Charfoos, "Helling: The Law of Medical Malpractice Rewritten" (*Ohio Northern Law Review* 1975; 2:692-703); P.W. Keeton, "Medical Negligence — The Standard of Care" (*Texas Technical Law Review* 1979; 10:351-79).

Medical groups in Washington State moved quickly to seek legislative relief from the rule imposed in the *Helling* decision. They were successful in having a remedial statute enacted in 1975. In a later decision, however, the majority of the bench in the same Supreme Court of Washington State refused stubbornly to find that the state legislature had succeeded in abrogating the *Helling* rule. See *Gates* v. *Jensen,* 92 Wash. 2d 246 (1979).

For a study of the practice of ophthalmologists after the *Helling* case, see J. Wiley, "The Impact of Judicial Decisions on Professional Conduct: An Empirical Study (*Southern California Law Review* 1981; 55:345-96).

Retaliatory Actions in Malpractice Litigation

One of the results of the increasing numbers of medical-malpractice actions in American courts has been more aggressive retaliation by physicians who believe the actions to be unfounded or improperly brought against them. National surveys have not found any large number of unmeritorious claims annually, but there are undoubtedly some actions filed that are improper or unjustified on any reasonable basis. These types of claims are the ones most resented by the medical profession. In this column I will examine some recent aspects of medical retaliatory efforts and an unusual, if not bizarre, counteraction by some patients in Kansas.

The most well-known countermeasure by a physician is a malicious-prosecution suit against the lawyer who sued him and failed to prove a case. Many a doctor has wished that he could get back at the lawyer who may have seemed callous or negligent in pursuing a case in which the doctor later proved blameless. But most doctors let pass the opportunity as time heals the sore wounds of anxiety and pride. Reluctantly, even begrudgingly perhaps, they follow the wise counsel of their own lawyers that a malicious-prosecution case against a lawyer is a very, very difficult cause to sustain and win. In recent years, however, a few physicians have persisted despite these obstacles and paid the cost in personal and professional time, and perhaps most hurtful of all, in the sizable noninsured legal fees necessary to sue their former legal adversaries—virtually all have lost.

A new decision in the Supreme Court of Kansas, however, may indicate some new life for malicious-prosecution cases in medical malpractice.[1] The plaintiff, Dr. Nelson, was originally sued in 1976 along with the Wesley Medical Center, for alleged improper practice as one of the treating physicians in a delivery by caesarean section, a

From the *New England Journal of Medicine*
1981; 304:211-212.

dilation and curettage, and alleged birth injuries to the child resulting in permanent disabilities. The suit involved allegations of huge damages: a plea for $5 million in actual damages and an additional request for $10 million in a punitive award for gross negligence and recklessness.

Such a huge claim can be understood to cause great concern and anxiety to the physicians and medical center who were sued. The patients' case was filed by a Topeka law firm and a firm from Philadelphia and was brought in the Kansas courts.

Early in the case, Dr. Nelson was voluntarily dismissed as a defendant without prejudice to being rejoined later if discovery showed any grounds against him. The case was continued against other physicians and the medical center. Some six months later, after further investigation produced no support for the allegations, a summary judgment (without need for a trial on the merits) was granted for all the defendants, and the case ended. The judge found that the medical procedures concerned matters of so-called "medical judgment" not involving negligence or other misconduct to the mother or child.

Dr. Nelson brought his action for malicious prosecution and an added count for the negligent pursuit of a malpractice case against him. The lower court denied both claims. In a detailed opinion the Kansas highest court reversed the lower court on the first claim, finding valid grounds in the complaint for the malicious-prosecution case. It did, however, agree with the denial of the negligence action. On the latter, it was held that only the lawyers' own losing clients could sue for negligent pursuit of the case; the malicious-prosecution claim was found adequate to satisfy any damage done to the physician himself.

Most important, the Kansas Supreme Court spelled out all the grounds necessary for a malicious-prosecution claim by a physician in the modern era of the late 20th century. First of all, it was held that the voluntary dismissal of Dr. Nelson early in the case was adequate to satisfy the legal prerequisite that the malpractice case be judicially determined and terminated in the doctor's favor. Secondly, the court ruled that lawyers must conduct an adequate and diligent investigation of the facts of the claimed malpractice and cannot rely solely on the patient's unsupported statements. This latter holding was a reversal of former Kansas law, which was a major basis for the difficulty of ever proving a case against an attorney, who could nearly always claim that he had relied in good faith on what his client told him. Thirdly, it was ruled that the plaintiff doctor did not need to plead and prove "special damages," another serious obstacle to malicious-prosecution cases by physicians in the past. English common-law doctrine is still followed in many American jurisdictions; it requires such grievous damages as arrest of the plaintiff in the previous malpractice case or seizure of his property or other serious interference with his person or property. The Kansas Supreme Court rejected this doctrine and held that only the ordinary rule of damages need be followed. The doctor could allege such damages as harm to his professional reputation, expenses incurred in defending himself in the suit, emotional distress as a result of the malpractice action, and loss of income because of the case. Finally, the court held that "malice" on the part of the lawyers in bringing the action must be proved, but that malice was adequately pleaded by the doctor and its proof was a matter of fact for the trial court. It was observed that malice could be found by a jury "from the absence of probable cause." It does seem, however, that the physician must prove that the lawyers brought the case against him "for a wrongful purpose." The court cited the Restatement of Torts (Second), Section 676, for various examples of "improper purpose," including awareness that the claim is not meritorious, intentional hostility toward the doctor, or use of the malpractice claim as a means of forcing settlement of the case on a "nuisance" basis with the insurance company or the defendant's own funds.

This case can now go back for trial, and the plaintiff doctor must prove his allegations. He has, however, already overcome serious barriers preventing medical practitioners from using this retaliatory measure in the United States.

Another case, also quite recently decided, involved a "class action" by two former patients on behalf of all other former patients so situated. It was brought against all the practicing physicians and the defendant hospital in the area of Joliet, Illinois. It is alleged that the defendants had all acted together to deny all medical services to any patients in that area who had brought malpractice cases. After bringing their case, the two plaintiffs and their children sought to take sworn statements (depositions) from 50 physicians in the area and succeeded in gathering six statements.

The federal district court dismissed the case on the various grounds sought by the plaintiffs. This seemed the end of this strange case. However, the prestigious Federal Court of Appeals for the Seventh Circuit, which covers a large portion of the midwest, reversed this decision and granted a basis for the claim as alleging a violation of the federal antitrust laws and the Illinois law of the same character.[2] The situation could be called an economically motivated restraint of trade, a concerted effort of the providers of medical care to retaliate against the patients who have sued them. Of course, the claim remains unproved and must now go to trial; the plaintiffs could recover treble their money damages if the suit is successful.

This is one of a growing number of antitrust cases occurring in the medical field since the U.S. Supreme Court recently indicated that practicing professionals[3] and hospitals, even small hospitals,[4] could be considered clearly covered by the federal jurisdiction under the Sherman Antitrust Act.[5] One sentence of Judge Dumbauld's opinion seems particularly worthy of quoting in regard to this decision. Perhaps with tongue in cheek the judge observed,

> One of the paradoxical aspects of this interesting case is that patients whose low opinion of the professional skill of their physicians impelled them to institute law suits for malpractice now seek . . . to require those physicians to continue to provide medical care for the plaintiff patients.

Of course, it is not only the actual physicians who were sued who, the plaintiffs claim, now will not serve them, but all doctors in the Joliet area. This is a serious charge requiring sober attention. This unfortunate case has now advanced to a very high court, apparently without satisfactory compromise or disposition.

Neither of these types of cases would be necessary if other, more comprehensive preventive measures were available and used effectively. Many states now have screening panels of physicians and lawyers who work to eliminate spurious malpractice cases before they ever get to trial.[6] In California, the plaintiffs' lawyers in malpractice cases must post a certificate of merit with courts before bringing a suit, providing verification for their suits and efforts at pretrial medical evaluation of most types of claims. Florida recently has come up with another means of discouraging lawyers from filing doubtful medical-malpractice claims: the losing party in a malpractice case must pay the full legal expenses of the opposing, successful party.

REFERENCES

1. Nelson v. Miller et al., 227 Kan. 271, 607 P.2d 438 (1980).
2. Williams v. St. Joseph Hospital, 629 F.2d 448 (7 Cir. 1980).

3. Goldfarb v. Virginia Bar Assoc., 421 U.S. 773, 95 Sp.Ct. 2004 (1975).
4. Hosp. Building Co. v. Rex Hospital, 425 U.S. 738, 96 Sp.Ct. 1848 (1976).
5. U.S. v. Amer. Soc. of Anesthesiologists, 473 F.Supp. 147 (S.D.N.Y. 1979).
6. Curran WJ. Screening panels in malpractice cases: some disturbing progress reports. N Engl J Med 1980; 302:954-5.

♦

COMMENTS

The outcome of *Nelson* v. *Miller,* the Kansas case that I described in this column, accelerated the trend toward removing traditional barriers to retaliatory suits by physicians against plaintiffs and lawyers bringing spurious malpractice cases. In recent years, a growing number of suits brought by physicians for malicious prosecution have been successful. For additional important appellate court cases supporting actions against attorneys filing malpractice cases without adequate investigation and without expert medical evidence to support the claim, see *Wong* v. *Tabor,* 422 N.E.2d 1279 (Indiana Ct. App., 1981), and *Mahaffey* v. *McMahon,* 630 S.W.2d 68 (Kentucky, 1982). For law review commentary, see G.P. Johnson, "Attorney Accountability in Kentucky—Liability to Clients and Third Parties" (*Kentucky Law Journal* 1982; 70:790-805), and D.I. Jackson, "Professional Responsibility" (*Indiana Law Review* 1983; 16:265-78).

On the other hand, the Illinois decision, *Williams* v. *St. Joseph Hospital,* has provoked no similar cases against physicians or hospitals on grounds of violations of the antitrust laws. However, I do suggest a review of one of my later columns ("Breaking off the Physician–Patient Relationship: Another Legal Hazard," reprinted in Chapter 5), which examines another aspect of patients' reactions to physicians' refusal to treat those who bring malpractice actions.

The Secretary's Commission on Medical Malpractice: Findings of a National Study

The first comprehensive national investigation of the "crisis" in medical-malpractice litigation in the United States has now been completed and the report has been officially published.[1] In the news release on the report, Health, Education, and Welfare Secretary Weinberger greeted it as an important work of research and study and asserted that the findings and recommendations will "serve as a beginning for further public discussion of the problem of malpractice. . . ."[2] That it undoubtedly will be. However, it may also be a center of severe, quite bitter controversy. It is difficult to satisfy anyone in this field, let alone to achieve mutual agreement on findings and recommendations for action.

The commission itself was broadly representative of provider, legal, insurance, and consumer interests.* There was mutuality of findings and recommendations on many issues, but there were also some very heated dissents.

Dr. Charles A. Hoffman, of West Virginia, president of the AMA, filed a strong dissent to the report in which he asserted, "After studying this final draft of the report, I am regretfully forced to the conclusion that the Commission has failed to accomplish the primary purpose for which it was established." He further charged that despite

From the *New England Journal of Medicine*
1973; 288:1222-1224.

*There were 21 members – 8 legal representatives, 4 M.D.s, 1 D.O., 2 R.N.s, 3 insurance-industry representatives, and 3 consumers. Actually, the legal representation was even more lopsided, since two of the M.D.s, one nurse, and one insurance representative had law degrees as well.

the expenditure of approximately $2 million the commission report is not calculated "to ameliorate the problems" as was the charge given to the commission by the secretary of Health, Education, and Welfare. Dr. Hoffman asserted that many of the recommendations, in his judgment, seem likely to stimulate an increase in claims rather than a decrease.

Since most of the readers of the *Journal* are physicians, these comments by Dr. Hoffman must be taken very seriously. This column and my next will summarize the findings and recommendations of the commission and comment on them in the light of these concerns of the AMA president.

MAGNITUDE OF THE PROBLEM

Most of the factual data of the report on the magnitude of medical malpractice came from the so-called "Closed Claims File" study of all insurance-company files in 1970. Of the 16,000 files actually closed in 1970, 50 percent were closed without any lawsuit brought. In 50 percent of this group, or 25 percent of the whole, some payment was made in settlement to the claimant. In the remaining 50 percent, lawsuits were brought. In 80 percent of this group, no trial ever took place. A settlement was reached, and the claimant was paid some money in 60 percent of these cases. The remaining 20 percent of the lawsuits were resolved in trials by juries. The defense won 80 percent of these cases. The plaintiffs got nothing in these cases. In only 20 percent were verdicts rendered for complaining patients.

The report also considered the frequent allegation, believed by many physicians, that most malpractice claims are baseless and without merit and are only an effort by disgruntled patients and unscrupulous lawyers to shake the tree of insurance dollars. The commission firmly disagreed. It was found that "the vast majority" of malpractice claims are not entirely baseless.

It was also found that "most doctors" have never been sued in malpractice and that in 1970, on the basis of the total of 382,000 doctors, dentists, and hospitals in the United States, only 1 out of every 21 health care providers was the object of a malpractice "claim."

What about money paid out in claims? The statistics again do not give comfort to the crisis proclaimers who seem to think every malpractice award is in the hundreds of thousands of dollars. Among the claims receiving any money at all (only 45 percent of the total claims closed), over half (59.5 percent) received less than $3,000. Only 3 percent of the claims were settled or received court awards over $100,000.

The only place where the commission agreed with the general impressions of the medical profession on the "magnitude of the problem" was in the rising—even the skyrocketing—cost of medical and hospital malpractice liability insurance. During the 1960s average premiums paid by surgeons rose 949.2 percent, those paid by other physicians rose 540.8 percent, those for hospitals rose 262.7 percent, and those for dentists rose 115 percent. It was estimated every hospitalized patient pays 50 cents per day of his bed cost for the hospital's malpractice coverage and that patients pay from 20 cents to 50 cents out of every $10 doctor's bill for the doctor's malpractice insurance policy.

PHYSICIANS' FEARS OF MALPRACTICE SUITS

The commission report is also forthright in its findings in two areas where physicians' high level of fear of being sued has caused reactions in physicians' conduct: the failure to aid in emergency situations, and the use of practices called "defensive medicine." On the first, the commission bluntly found that there is "no factual basis for the commonly-asserted belief that malpractice suits are likely to stem from rendering emergency care at the scene of accidents." In defensive medicine, the commission found that such practices were being carried out, but it could not document their extent. It was also found that these practices increased the cost of medical care to the patient. It was recommended that overutilization of health care resources in the interest of defensive medicine be aggressively attacked by regulatory agencies as improper and abusive to patients. It was also recommended that medical and osteopathic organizations exert "maximum moral suasion" over doctors who avoid their medical responsibilities solely because of a fear of being sued for malpractice. At the hearings held by the commission, examples were frequently cited of physicians who refused to offer their medical services in situations they considered "too risky" to lawsuits. It is ironic that in nearly all, if not all such cases, these examples were offered by physician witnesses, often concerning themselves.

The only area where the commission seems to have agreed that the health care professions needed immunity from vexatious lawsuits is where they answer "Code Blue" calls in hospitals, as in cardiac-arrest cases. It was recommended that the states enact laws providing "qualified immunity" from lawsuits in such situations when the rescuers act "in good faith."

PATIENTS' RIGHTS AND COMPLAINTS

It was recommended that hospitals and other health care facilities adopt statements of patients' rights and also establish patient-grievance mechanisms. To give teeth to this recommendation, the commission recommended that the establishment of such grievance mechanisms be made a condition of receiving Medicare and Medicaid payments from the federal government.

AMELIORATION OR AGGRAVATION?

The above are only some of the 100-odd findings and recommendations of the commission, which functioned for some 18 months and held public hearings all over the country. Does the work of the commission help in ameliorating the malpractice problem, or do its findings and recommendations only further aggravate the issues? We shall see more in my next column.

REFERENCES

1. Department of Health, Education, and Welfare. Report of the Secretary's Commission on Medical Malpractice. Washington, D.C.: Government Printing Office, January 16, 1973. (DHEW publication no. (OS) 73-88.)
2. News release of the Department of Health, Education, and Welfare, April 18, 1973:1.

♦

COMMENTS

This was one of two columns concerned with the work of the malpractice commission. This first essay summarized the report and its recommendations. It also pointed out the continuing differences between physicians and lawyers with regard to both the cause of the problems and the most effective ways of dealing with them.

In the longer view, the most important aspect of the commission's work may well have been not its recommendations but its investigations and its contract-research projects. The research studies, which cost nearly $1 million, were the first large-scale efforts at field research into medical malpractice ever conducted in this country. They prepared the way for later important federally supported research in the field. The research studies of the commission have been collected in an *Appendix: Report of the Secretary's Commission on Medical Malpractice* [Washington, D.C.: Government Printing Office, 1973. (DHEW publication no. (OS) 73-89)].

In the later 1980s, in the face of another looming crisis in medical-malpractice law, a major private foundation has launched an effort to support research in the field. In 1987, the Robert Wood Johnson Foundation announced that it intended to support grants in the range of $200,000 to $300,000 for investigations into basic causes of malpractice and means of preventing it, and for demonstrations and evaluations of the probable effectiveness of legal, insurance, and health care reforms that have been proposed with this end in view.

The Secretary's Commission on Medical Malpractice: An Insider's View

A previous column[1] reported on the major findings of the Secretary's Commission on Medical Malpractice.[2] The report, as noted in the first column, has been severely criticized by the American Medical Association's president, who was a member of the commission. On the other hand, it has been much praised by consumer advocate Ralph Nader. I was also a member, the only full-time medicolegal academic in the group. I suppose that my own views were somewhat more in the middle of the positions of the AMA and the Nader-type consumer representatives on the commission.

Middle grounds can be dangerous, of course, as was learned by the brave 600 at Balaklava. As they charged into that valley of death they were shot at from both sides. In the main, I avoided getting wounded seriously at most of the commission meetings by taking a position out of the range of the largest guns at the table. Position is everything, we are told by all gamesmanship sages. Also, the major advocates were much too busy shooting at each other most of the time to bother too much with a lonely academic.

For example, there were heated arguments at nearly every session over just who or what was a "consumer" of health services. Many of the physicians in practice or working for the drug industry insisted that we were all consumers and that no one person or group is exclusively entitled to represent the public who are hospitalized, or who see a doctor or dentist, or who take prescription or over-the-counter drugs. For some, however, "consumer" is a code word for "poor" or racial minority. This was evident even in the selection of members for appointment. Two of the three consumers on the com-

From the *New England Journal of Medicine*
1973; 289:252-253.

mission were active in consumer movements in black, chicano, and American Indian communities, respectively. These two members filed dissenting statements that should be called to the attention of readers of the *Journal*. In her dissent, Ms. Norma Almanza, formerly of the Pedro Alvizu Campos Clinic in Chicago, wrote of her feelings toward teaching hospitals, where she said the urban poor must go for care:

> I look around Chicago with its various medical schools and though to some outsiders patient care at these teaching hospitals may seem a *nightmare,* to Chicago's poor it is a *reality* . . . I do not wish to see the teaching hospital close its doors, but as a human being I would like to see it become a little more sensitive to its patients as human beings rather than objects of teaching. Maybe here I am naive, but I would like to recommend that teaching institutions offer patients the right to choose whether they want to be seen by students or not.[3]

Ms. Ella L. Strother, a member of the Board of Directors of the National Consumers Health Organization, also wrote a "separate statement" in which she reiterated the major recommendations of health consumer groups: (1) the right of consumers to participate as "equal components in all levels" of the health care system; (2) the right to a patient's bill of rights; and (3) the right to quality comprehensive health care for all Americans. It is noteworthy that Ms. Strother's entire statement had the concurrence of Richard M. Markus, who was the foremost member of plaintiff's personal injury bar on the commission. Mr. Markus is a past president of the American Trial Lawyers Association. Personally, I found all the consumer members valuable contributors to the commission's work.

As one reads the report of the commission, it seems to have come forth with recommendations that pleased both sides and angered both sides. The many dissents and separate statements of the members are evidence of this division.

In my first column I concentrated most of my attention on the findings and recommendations that might be found offensive by some medical groups. Here, I should like to note briefly some of the recommendations that can, if followed, improve the current situation for physicians and health care facilities. First of all, the commission recommended current rate-making practices be reexamined in the insurance industry in regard to malpractice coverage, particularly in such areas as group rates for hospital staffs and county medical societies and level premium rates for hospitals in given geographic areas. Secondly, it recommended that all states adopt legislation to control contingent fees charged by plaintiffs' lawyers. Thirdly, it recommended that all states adopt legislation granting qualified immunity from suit for hospitals and members of rescue teams who answer "Code Blue" signals or otherwise render aid in emergencies in the course of medical treatment by other health care personnel. Lastly, the commission recommended further study of alternative compensation systems for injured patients to replace the current tort system. The major alternatives to be studied would be compulsory arbitration and a total "no-fault" compensation plan.

On the whole, the report seems to me to present a fair picture of the current situation in medical and hospital liability. If the recommendations are not outstandingly imaginative, they are basically sound. After all, I did sign as a concurring member. I learned a great deal at the public hearings. I enjoyed the working sessions of the commission, even those that included the sound and fury of interprofessional battle. For my friends, I can report in conclusion that I have returned and am alive and well in Boston, no worse for the experience.

REFERENCES

1. Curran WJ. The Malpractice Commission Report: controversy unabated; the findings. N Engl J Med 1973; 288:1222-4.
2. Department of Health, Education, and Welfare. Report of the Secretary's Commission on Medical Malpractice. Washington, D.C.: Government Printing Office, January 16, 1973. (DHEW publication no. (OS) 73-88.)
3. *Idem.* Report of the Secretary's Commission on Medical Malpractice. Washington, D.C.: Government Printing Office, January 16, 1973:110-1. (DHEW publication no. (OS) 73-88.)

♦

COMMENTS

This was the second, and much more personal, discussion of my work on the malpractice commission, in which I again pointed out the still unresolved conflicts between the two professional groups represented on the commission: the physicians and the lawyers. The fact is that not even the "consumer members" appointed to all national commissions in Washington in those years were satisfied. Two of these consumers filed dissenting statements, the purpose of which was not so much to voice disagreement with particular findings as to express a "consumer viewpoint" as such. The subject of the inquiry may have been medical malpractice, but the game was still politics as usual.

Many of the members of the commission, especially the physicians, believed strongly that the rise in medical-malpractice claims in the late 1960s and early 1970s represented a serious crisis. The commission did not concur, and this finding angered several physician members. Only a few years later, in 1975, the first genuine crisis did hit the field, but, as it turned out, the problem did not relate to claims, but to the availability and cost of insurance. This crisis is examined in the next two columns reprinted here.

Malpractice Insurance: A Genuine National Crisis

Complaints about an alarming increase in malpractice suits and about the rising cost of malpractice liability insurance can be found in the medical literature of the United States during most of the decades of this century. For example, Louis Regan, of Los Angeles, a defense attorney, wrote in the first edition of his medicolegal textbook in 1943, "During the past twenty years there has been a tremendous increase in unjustified malpractice cases."[1] In his second edition in 1949, Regan complained of "a plague of malpractice suits."[2] In neither edition are any statistics provided to support these allegations.

It was not until 1969 that there was any national review of the subject. In that year, a Congressional committee report, the first on medical malpractice, found that the number of such suits and claims was rising, but only in certain regions of the country, not throughout the nation.[3] Three high-volume areas were named as California, New York, and the District of Columbia. Very sparse statistics were provided even to justify this rather mild confirmation of the scare literature of the late 1960s about rising claims nationwide. In only one area were statistics available to support allegations of a serious problem: the rising cost of malpractice insurance to physicians and hospitals.

Two years later, Secretary Elliot L. Richardson, of the U.S. Department of Health, Education, and Welfare, established a Secretary's Commission on Medical Malpractice. The report of this body again confirmed the scarcity of statistical information about any aspect of the malpractice problem except the high rise in premium charges. Regarding claims, the commission concluded, "Despite the publicity resulting from a few large malpractice cases, a medical malpractice incident is a relatively rare event; claims are even rarer and jury trials

From the *New England Journal of Medicine*
1975; 292:1223-1224.

rarer still."[4] The commission also dispelled the widespread belief that most awards are very high. It found that in 1970, 59.9 percent of all awards nationally were under $3,000 and only 3 percent were over $100,000.

The State of California is nearly always the jurisdiction cited as having the most serious problem with malpractice suits, both now and in years past. What are the facts? A recent study by a select committee of the California Legislature has reported that claims filed against physicians in that state had risen by 40 percent from 1965 to 1974[5] – a nine-year period, it should be noted. Yet in only two years, 1968 through 1970, the Committee found that the group insurance rate for physicians had risen by 400 percent. It is also interesting that the first sentence of this report asserts that this is "the first report ever issued by a state legislative committee on the important subject of medical malpractice." Even in California, the government has been very slow in gathering facts on this subject.

As the above indicates, there may have been some basis for a charge of "crying wolf" too often in the past about malpractice litigation, but it is now clear that the most chronic problem of all, rising insurance premiums and inadequate insurance coverage, has become, in 1975, a genuine national economic crisis. The few companies still writing policies have announced that they are either leaving the field entirely or must have premium rate increases this year and next of inordinate amounts. In a number of states, rate increases for physicians have been requested of 100 percent to nearly 750 percent. (Ohio was the highest, with a request for a 747 percent increase.) Rate-increase requests for hospitals have been as high or higher. Recently, the Argonaut Insurance Company announced rate increases for hospitals in New York from 200 percent to 600 percent. For one institution, however, Jewish Memorial Hospital in New York City, it was alleged in a federal district court that the increase would amount to almost 120 percent in one year. The per-bed rate was to be increased from $112 to $1,425. On April 2, the court issued an injunction against the insurance company, barring it from raising its rates in New York and from canceling its policies in 35 hospitals throughout the state.[6]

A few states like New York and Wisconsin have acted to prevent the insurance companies from canceling all their policies and leaving the doctors and hospitals totally unprotected against claims and suits. Usually, this action has taken the form of forcing all liability-insurance carriers authorized by law to sell any liability insurance of any kind in the state to join a pool to provide malpractice insurance for all the physicians and hospitals. Even more recently, Governor Carey, of New York, and key legislators in Albany have announced their support for a bill to establish a state government–financed public insurance fund for malpractice insurance.[7]

The Ford administration in Washington is examining various methods of federal intervention in the malpractice field. Currently, several bills are being considered in Congress to bring reforms into the field, or to provide federally funded reinsurance to support the private insurance companies staying in the business, at least for a few years longer until more permanent solutions can be found.

One thing is clear: both the states and the federal government are now convinced of the existence of a crisis and the need for action, fast action, this year.

REFERENCES

1. Regan LJ. Doctor and patient and the law. St. Louis: C.V. Mosby, 1943:6.
2. *Idem.* Doctor and patient and the law. 2nd ed. St. Louis: C.V. Mosby, 1949:7.
3. United States Congress, Senate Committee on Government Operations, Subcommittee on Executive Reorganization. Medical malpractice: the patient versus the physician: a study by the Subcommittee on Executive Reorganization. Washington, D.C.: Government Printing Office, 1969.
4. Department of Health, Education, and Welfare. Report of the Secretary's Commission on Medical Malpractice. Washington, D.C.: Government Printing Office, January 16, 1973:12. (DHEW publication no. (OS) 73-88.)
5. Assembly Select Committee on Medical Malpractice. Preliminary report. Sacramento, California State Assembly, June 1974:3.
6. Malpractice policy cancelling is enjoined. New York Times. April 2, 1975:C19.
7. Clines FX. Insurance accord gained on medical malpractice bill in Albany. New York Times. March 20, 1975:C33.

♦

COMMENTS

I believe that I was one of the first commentators to label the crisis of 1975 as more one of insurance premiums and insurance availability than of "skyrocketing claims and suits," as the news media usually had it. The data just did not bear out the insurance industry's assertions about rapidly increased claims levels in these years. In fact, very few claims data were published.

As the next column indicates, the state legislatures were called on to act to make insurance available to physicians and hospitals in their states, preferably at affordable rates. Organized medicine and the hospitals also began to take unofficial steps to solve the insurance problem. In the long run, these efforts have been at least as effective in improving the situation as the official legislative reforms, if not more so. Medical professional groups in various states formed medically controlled and owned, nonprofit insurance companies to sell insurance to physicians at more reasonable rates. Also, large hospitals (or, more frequently, groups of hospitals) and health maintenance organizations moved to establish self-insurance programs under their own control. Most of these programs contained an important element of preventive activity, usually called patient-risk management. In recent years these programs have proved much more effective in preventing and handling claims than the previous, uncoordinated, and largely cosmetic programs of most of the private insurance companies. There is now an organization of professional patient-risk managers at health care institutions. It is affiliated with the American Hospital Association.

The Malpractice Insurance Crisis: Short-Term and Long-Term Solutions

The major medical-malpractice insurance carriers, after asking for and receiving huge premium increases in the last three years, are threatening to drop out of the field entirely after July 1, 1975. Medical societies and other medical professional groups are threatening curtailments of certain high-risk procedures and even all-out strikes or "vacations" in midsummer if something is not done before July 1.

Insurance commissioners and governors are in panic all over the country. Legislative bills that seem patently unconstitutional are being seriously proposed and seriously considered in one state legislative assembly after another. All sorts of pleasant cajoling, tearful pleading, and militant strong-arm tactics are being applied to the insurance carriers to encourage or require them to write malpractice insurance for medical professionals and hospitals.

The problem is being addressed in two parts: short-term solutions and longer-term remedies. In the short term, the states are trying merely to keep some sort of financial protection alive after July 1, 1975. Two immediate actions are being taken. The first is to force the current carriers to stay in the business now and during the next fiscal year. Maryland tried to order St. Paul Fire and Marine Insurance Company to continue to write insurance for its physician policy holders in that state. The Maryland Supreme Court struck down the order as totally without legal support. In Wisconsin, a bill was very hastily passed requiring all casualty carriers in the state, whether they write medical-malpractice insurance or not, to join a pool for required assignment to insure doctors who cannot otherwise

From the *New England Journal of Medicine*
1975; 293:24-25.

get insurance. Other states have passed or are considering such assigned-risk pools.

The other short-term problem is the explosive increase in premium rates. Here, the strong-arm tactics are not as effective. Legislation is being enacted to cut down on insurance pay-outs in awards as an encouragement to the companies to cut rates, or at least to reduce the level of increase. The most popular solution offered here has been the placing of a cap over total recoveries. Much attention is being paid to the law recently passed in Indiana (which has a practicing physician as governor) that places a limitation of $500,000 on any recovery in any single case involving one plaintiff. The individual physician's liability is limited even further to $100,000. The other $400,000 would be recovered under a state-operated fund established by a surcharge of not more than 10 percent on physicians' insurance premiums. As another means of reducing the pay-outs, the Indiana law creates a screening panel of three physicians and a nonvoting presiding lawyer to review all claims and pass on whether they are justified. The opinion of the panel is not binding on the insurance company or the lawyers handling the case, but the opinion is admissible in any court action on the claim.

I am not greatly impressed with the chances that any of these short-term remedies will have an immediate effect on the problem. Awards and settlements in six and seven figures are extremely rare. In 1970, they accounted for only 3 percent of all payments to plaintiffs. Even in this group, the great bulk are within $300,000. Doctors will not be helped much by all this – and in Indiana will receive a further premium increase of up to 10 percent (egregiously too much) for this coverage.

The constitutionality of all this Indiana award limitation is highly doubtful. I cannot see any good argument in its favor that would hold up in court. There is no beneficial trade-off being received by injured plaintiffs to justify taking away the right to recover a larger award or settlement. Lawyers also question seriously the constitutionality of the Indiana all-doctor screening panel. There is no great evidence that "nuisance claims" or unjustified claims make up an important part of the volume of litigation. In fact, two different federal investigations seem to have found otherwise in recent years.

On the federal level, another short-term solution is beginning to receive greater attention. This is Senator Gaylord Nelson's proposal for a federally supported reinsurance program for all claims above $25,000. This is a very realistic proposal and undoubtedly constitutional. It would take the risk of all large suits, not just those over six and seven figures, out of the hands of both primary carriers and reinsurance carriers. Physicians would be charged nothing for this protection. It would be a nationally supported program, similar to existing federal reinsurance programs for catastrophic losses in floods and earthquakes.

In the area of long-term solutions, most of the attention is being given to radical reform in the litigation system. The two most popular remedies, for discussion purposes at least, are arbitration and a no-fault compensation system. Even more popular among physicians is the proposal to eliminate or reduce substantially the contingent-fee method of paying plaintiffs' attorneys' fees. Needless to say, the legal profession is fighting the latter idea with passion and fury. Senator Kennedy, a very powerful figure on health care matters in the Senate, seems to be concentrating his attention on these long-term matters. He has submitted bills on both arbitration and a no-fault system.

Medical societies that are advocating both the short-term and the long-term solutions examined above are aware of backlash reactions, which can demand that the medical profession "clean its own house" as well as ask for reform in insurance and the legal system. The societies have generally supported the idea of improving disciplinary machinery against incompetent doctors. Some have even suggested that the state and local medical societies take over these activities from the state governments. I rather doubt if the latter suggestion will survive legislative scrutiny. In fact, the legislatures are more apt to enact proposals aimed at separating disciplinary responsibility from the present licensing boards, placing the disciplinary power in new public agencies not entirely composed of physicians.

♦

COMMENTS

As predicted in this column, the constitutionality of many of the hasty legislative reforms of medical-malpractice law enacted during this period was challenged in the courts. Most of the first-impression court reviews dealt harshly with the enactments and struck down many of the provisions. These decisions, and the general uncertainty created by extensive judicial questioning of the new legislation, undoubtedly hurt the chances that the programs in question could do much to remedy the problems that had arisen. As time passed, however, and the crisis in malpractice law failed to subside, the courts became more sympathetic to the cause of reform and passed down decisions upholding the validity of many of the most important measures. See the cases and statutes collected in W.J. Curran and E.D. Shapiro, *Law, Medicine, and Forensic Sciences* (3rd ed. Boston: Little, Brown, 1980:517-92). The most important judicial turnabout took place in California when the Supreme Court of that state upheld the constitutionality of a "cap," or limitation, of $250,000 on recovery for noneconomic loss in a medical-malpractice case. See *Fein* v. *Permanente Medical Group,* 211 Cal. Rptr. 368 (1985); see also an article on the pioneering legislation in Indiana: C.S. Hurlbut, "Constitutionality of the Indiana Medical Malpractice Act, Reevaluated" (*Valparaiso Law Review* 1985; 19:493-520).

Several worthwhile articles deal with various aspects of the legislative activity in the middle and later 1970s. See, for example, A.W. Cunningham and R. Lane, "Malpractice: The Illusory Crisis" (*Florida Bar Journal* 1980; 54:114-21); E.D. Shrero, "Patient Compensation Funds: Legislative Response to the Medical Malpractice Crisis" (*American Journal of Law and Medicine* 1979; 5:175-95); and G. Calabresi, "The Problem of Malpractice: Trying to Round out the Circle" (*Toronto Law Journal* 1977; 27:131-41).

In the mid-1980s problems of availability and affordability of medical-malpractice insurance appear to be resurfacing. As with the earlier insurance crisis, no consensus has been reached as to the causes of the problem or potential remedies. For a review of the various theories, compare Department of Justice, *Report of the Tort Policy Working Group on the Causes, Extent and Policy Implications of the Current Crisis in Insurance Availability and Affordability* (Washington, D.C.: Government Printing Office, 1986) with National Association of Attorneys General, *An Analysis of the Causes of the Current Crisis of Unavailability and Unaffordability of Liability Insurance* (Washington, D.C., 1986).

The Role of Lawyers in Medical-Malpractice Claims

The literature of the medical-malpractice crisis has been reaching overkill proportions. Yet the amount of fundamental research is still very, very thin in many areas. The darkest corners are still reserved for insurance practices and the volume and nature of claims. Next is the practice of the lawyers in the field.

Very little notice has been given in the literature to a comprehensive study of how lawyers actually handle malpractice cases. This study was supported by the Secretary's Commission on Medical Malpractice.[1] Because the study was completed very late in the period of operation of the commission itself, it had little or no influence on the commission's findings and recommendations. Owing to this fact, the Department of Health, Education, and Welfare asked me, a member of the commission, to prepare an analysis of the data and to make a report on the subject, taking into account the reform legislation passed in the states in recent years. This report was published by the Health Resources Administration in October 1976.[2]

The national survey of lawyers' practices was conducted from January 1970 to September 1972.[3] A representative sample was drawn from the practicing bar of the country; 809 lawyers were surveyed by mail questionnaire, with an overall response of 78 percent. An additional, more intensive survey, including interviews, was conducted among a group of 169 legal practitioners identified as substantially active in the personal-injury field.

First of all, the national sample showed that medical-malpractice litigation was a very small part of the practice of lawyers of the country. Among privately practicing lawyers (eliminating those employed

From the *New England Journal of Medicine*
1977; 296:24-25.

by government, corporations, etc.) only 4.9 percent handled and closed cases during the 33-month period. Among those who were involved to any degree in either screening or handling cases, the yearly average was extremely low. Plaintiffs' representatives handled only 0.4 case annually whereas defense attorneys handled 4.3. No evidence was found of a large number of specialist attorneys on the plaintiffs' side spending all or nearly all their time on medical-malpractice litigation. If there was a concentration, it was on the defense side. I should point out, however, that among the lawyers in the intensive survey six plaintiffs' practitioners with an average yearly load of 858 formal claims were found. These figures were so unusual that they were excluded from the case-volume calculations so as not to distort the averages. No information was given on who these "extraordinary six" were or where they practiced, though an educated guess would place them in California and would probably also find all or most of them doctor-lawyers.[4] In all probability, these six handle a heavy referral practice evaluating claims for many other plaintiffs' practitioners.

The most important findings of the survey were probably those concerning the role of lawyers in screening claims brought to them by plaintiff patients. In the national survey, it was found that lawyers rejected 88 percent of all claims that they reviewed. Even among the intensive-survey group of personal-injury lawyers, the rejection rate was 71 percent. The most frequently cited reason for rejection – "no perceived liability" – vastly outweighed any other one. The next closest reason, the smallness of the potential recovery, was named only 10 percent of the time. In the interviews of the experienced trial lawyers in the intensive survey, the question was put: "Would you accept a case where the injuries were severe but the perceived liability was very low or nonexistent?" The answer was a resounding no. Only 1 percent indicated they might accept such a claim for investigation, possible negotiation, or trial. It was also found that virtually all (99 percent) of the plaintiffs' attorneys seek out a medical evaluation of all claims.

Both plaintiffs' lawyers and defense counsel in the intensive survey were asked to estimate what percentage of the claims brought involved actual malpractice. In one of the most surprising results, the two groups agreed on a percentage of about one third of the total.

The most common contingent fee was one third of the recovery. In the national survey, only 3 percent of the lawyers on the plaintiffs' side used exclusively an hourly rate of compensation. The survey concluded that the contingent-fee system did not result in exorbitant earnings per hour by plaintiffs' lawyers. The national averages per hour were found to be $63, close to those of the defense bar, which were estimated at $50 per hour. However, among the intensive survey of experienced trial lawyers, these averages were substantially exceeded. My own evaluation of the data indicated that this group earned approximately $250 per hour on cases handled, and the average gross recovery in cases won by them was $81,000, with a median of $25,000. This compared with a national gross recovery of $22,000, with a median of $3,000. It seems clear that well-known, experienced trial lawyers in the country do very well when they win. How often do they win a recovery? More often than most lawyers think: the plaintiffs' attorneys in the survey reported that they achieved some recovery in 79 percent of their cases.

In the literature of medical malpractice, much attention has been paid to such legal doctrines as *res ipsa loquitur* and informed consent. Among the practicing plaintiffs' lawyers these doctrines were not found very influential in evaluation of claims. Much more important were such matters as the availability of expert witnesses and the rules for discovery of evidence. The only formal legal doctrine of great importance was the statute of limitations.

In the few years that have passed since the survey was conducted, the character of personal-injury law practice has changed in some important characteristics. No-fault insurance laws for automobile-caused injuries have been passed in many states. These programs have cut severely into the practice of most lawyers handling such litigation. There seems no doubt that the slack in this area has been taken up in part by an increase in the handling of product liability cases and, to a lesser extent, medical malpractice and other health facility–related claims.

The other important change has been the passage of malpractice reform legislation. A number of states have added screening panels to eliminate unjustified claims. A few have revised the laws on the statute of limitations, *res ipsa loquitur,* informed consent, and the use of expert witnesses. There seems to be very little evidence that these states acted on the basis of reliable data on how malpractice claims are actually handled in their jurisdictions. If they had been so based, the approaches might have been very different. It is expected that many more states will enact further reform legislation, taking into account, one hopes, the results of this research, augmented by findings of further surveys conducted in the states by special state-level commissions set up in legislation passed over the last two years.[5]

REFERENCES

1. Report of the Secretary's Commission on Medical Malpractice. Washington, D.C.: Government Printing Office, 1973. (DHEW publication no. (OS) 73-88.)
2. Curran WJ. How lawyers handle medical malpractice cases: an analysis of an important medicolegal study. Washington, D.C.: Government Printing Office, 1976. (DHEW publication no. (HRA) 76-3152.)
3. Dietz S, Baird OB, Berul L. The medical malpractice legal system. Appendix, Report of the Secretary's Commission on Medical Malpractice. Washington, D.C.: Government Printing Office, 1973. (DHEW publication no. (OS) 73-88.)
4. Curran WJ. Cross-professional education in law and medicine: the promise and the conflict. J Legal Educ 1971; 24:42-71.
5. *Idem.* Malpractice crisis: the flood of legislation. N Engl J Med 1975; 293:1182-3.

COMMENTS

It is puzzling how little research has been done on the lawyers' role in malpractice litigation, including the claims-prevention and screening roles of both plaintiff and defense attorneys. So far as I know, no further studies on this subject have been published in the years since this column appeared.

In practice, the current situation is as follows: The preventive role has largely been taken over by hospital-based malpractice risk-management programs. These programs have grown considerably during the 1980s. Most of the screening – i.e., the identification of meritorious cases and rejection of the clearly spurious or nonmeritorious – is still done by lawyers, but in several states official and unofficial "screening panels" have also been set up. However, the official panels have not been as effective as had been hoped. Some of them have been struck down as unconstitutional by state supreme courts, and others have run into administrative difficulties. Nevertheless, the concept of screening panels composed of both physicians and lawyers is a good one. The role of such panels is examined in the column reprinted next in this chapter.

Screening Panels in Malpractice Litigation

Among the major reforms in recent years in the field of medical malpractice has been the establishment of interprofessional screening panels designed to review and eliminate frivolous and unsupportable claims. Before the insurance crisis of 1975, only a few states had experimented with review panels.[1] Most of the panels were informal, and their decisions nonbinding. Twenty-one states now have screening systems of various types. Most can make binding decisions, at least to the degree of requiring plaintiffs to present their cases to the panels before a court trial can be obtained. The panel's determination is not controlling, but its finding is usually admissible as evidence in any later trial.

The U.S. Department of Justice thought so much of the screening-panel system and its alleged success that in early 1979 a bill was prepared for the Congress that would have required all 50 states to establish screening panels and other medical-malpractice reforms. In the past year, however, the Justice Department has apparently had second thoughts about the wisdom of proposing national legislation at this time, and the bill has been quietly delayed or shelved.

One of the major reasons for the change of policy at the national level has been the growing number of disturbing reports of failures and ineptitude in the state screening panels. The latest comprehensive report in the *National Law Journal* labels the programs as ineffective, ill conceived, and badly administered.[2]

The screening panels were supported by medical groups and malpractice-defense lawyers as a means of reducing the number of claims. There was considerable disagreement about the number of frivolous claims in any state; statistics of the insurance industry did not support the impression that there were large numbers of unsup-

From the *New England Journal of Medicine*
1980; 302:954-955.

portable allegations and lawsuits. Nevertheless, the screening-panel system was thought to be a useful experiment that could help. Even some plaintiffs' lawyers believed that the panels could achieve beneficial results for some claimants by encouraging early settlement of claims that the panels found meritorious.

The *National Law Review*'s survey seems to indicate that defense lawyers and insurance carriers in the field have now joined the plaintiffs' lawyers in their disenchantment with the screening panels.

Most of the state systems have been bogged down with serious challenges to the constitutional validity of their operations. Some court challenges have virtually ended the effectiveness of the programs. In other states, court challenges and administrative difficulties have caused substantial delays in the processing of cases. In Florida, a state with many claims, 72 lower-court cases have raised questions, as yet unsettled, about the system's operation. The Florida Supreme Court heard arguments in January 1980 that challenged the system's legal validity. In Maryland, 315 of 350 claims filed for preliminary review since the program was established in 1976 are still pending. The worst administrative tangle seems to be in Pennsylvania. There has been serious difficulty in obtaining cooperation in filling the medical positions on the panels. As a result, only 14 of nearly 3000 cases have been processed through full hearings in the four years of the system's functioning.

In states where the panels have been operating more effectively, there have been complaints that their work has not been worth the delay and expense of the systems. In some states, the unfavorable findings of the panels have not discouraged plaintiffs' lawyers from going to trial in cases that they believe they can win before a jury. The associate counsel for the American Insurance Association is quoted as having found that the screening panels have failed to achieve their main objective, the deterrence of court trials of nonmeritorious claims, in at least half the states adopting the system.[2]

Not all the sources surveyed were critical of the screening panels. Some believed that many of the systems are achieving good results and that it is too early to judge the reform measures a failure. The administrative problems may well be solved, particularly after the questions of constitutional validity are settled by the highest courts of the states. The variety of systems in the states is bewildering. States where problems have occurred should be allowed to test and adopt better methods.

One state where the panels seem to be working well is Massachusetts. The medical community is cooperating fully with the panels, and lawyers are meeting the tight scheduling of case review, usually two to three weeks after the claims are formally entered in court. In addition, the parties generally comply with the findings and in most cases do not proceed against defendants if the claims are found to be unsupported. Perhaps the fact that the Massachusetts screening panels, called "tribunals," are headed by experienced judges from trial court (superior court) has given them a credibility and smoothness of operation not achieved in states where the panels are composed of physicians, practicing lawyers, and lay people. The early settlement of claims found meritorious has not been achieved frequently enough to satisfy most plaintiffs' lawyers, however.

Most nonmeritorious claims are not being pressed forward to trial in Massachusetts because a bond must be filed before trial and the bond is lost if the plaintiff loses. The posting of a bond in such cases also discourages the practice of indiscriminately "suing everyone in sight" in a malpractice case in the hope that, at a later stage, evidence may be found against one or another physician, surgeon, anesthesiologist, nurse, administrator, or other person allegedly involved in the treatment of the patient. The plaintiff's lawyer, in Massachusetts at least, must have a serious reason based on solid evidence to go forward against multiple medical defendants.

In some states, the panels have been accused of improper bias toward physicians and hospitals. The statistics have tended to support such allegations, especially in states where the systems have been informal and the panels composed largely of doctors. The Massachusetts system has avoided this criticism also. Even though the panels have generally applied strict standards in finding an adequate basis to go to trial against a defendant, the Massachusetts tribunals have found as many claims meritorious as they have found unsupported. From their inception in January 1976 until the end of July 1978, the panels handled 916 cases. In the cases heard and disposed of, 261 were found to have insufficient evidence against a party, and an equal number were found sufficient to proceed to a trial in court. There were 53 split decisions, 184 cases still pending, 100 claims dismissed before a screening-panel hearing was held, and 57 that required no hearing. In the 261 cases found to be unsupported, only 72 plaintiffs posted bonds indicating that they intended nevertheless to go forward with lawsuits. The trend seems to have continued into 1979. According to correspondence from the Massachusetts Malpractice Joint Underwriting Association, which provides insurance for most physicians and hospitals in the state, their cases before the panels in 1979 were again divided almost evenly between meritorious and nonmeritorious claims (Thistle FC, claim manager, Medical Malpractice Joint Underwriting Association of Massachusetts: personal communication). Of 267 cases, 127 (48 percent) were found for the plaintiff and 140 (52 percent) for the defendant. There was a slight increase in the percentage of cases (44 cases, or 31 percent) in which bonds were posted by losing parties, indicating an intent to proceed to a trial despite the tribunal's findings against them.

It is my judgment that the disturbing reports about failures in the screening-panel systems in some states may be outweighed by the successes in others, and that the more effective mechanisms should be given further time to prove their worth. It is too early either to scuttle the whole idea or to impose a single, federally legislated mechanism on all the states. The states should continue to be, as in Justice Holmes' formulation, experimental laboratories for social reform. They should be allowed to continue to test reforms in trial litigation and the processes of justice within their own court systems.

REFERENCES

1. Documentary Supplement. Medical-legal screening panels as an alternative approach to medical malpractice claims. William and Mary Law Rev 1972; 13:695-723.
2. Margolick DM. Mediation isn't cure for patients' claims. National Law Rev. February 4, 1980.

COMMENTS

At least 33 states have enacted statutes providing for some form of prelitigation screening of malpractice claims. The effectiveness of the panels that perform this function has never been conclusively assessed, and their feasibility and practicality continue to be debated. The published investigations have been limited to individual state reviews. For example, see J.D. Ossyra, "The Massachusetts Malpractice Plaintiff's New Hurdles: The Expanding Role of the Medical Malpractice Tribunal" (*American Journal of Law and Medicine* 1983; 8:481-508); G.T. Dance, "Medical Malpractice: Prelitigation Screening Panels in Idaho" (*Idaho Law Review* 1983; 19:31-46); W.H. Daughtrey, Jr., and C.H. Smith, "Medical Malpractice Review Panels in Virginia" (*University of Richmond Law Review* 1985; 19:273-99); and Student Comment, "The Illinois Medical Malpractice Review Panel Provision: A Constitutional Analysis" (*Loyola University Chicago Law Journal* 1986; 17:275-301). For recent developments see Student Note, "The Utah Medical Malpractice Prelitigation Panel" (*Utah Law Review* 1986:199-212).

Medical Malpractice since the Crisis of 1975: Some Good News and Some Bad

The insurance system in the United States for protection of physicians and hospitals against financial loss due to malpractice claims almost collapsed in 1975. Many private insurance carriers withdrew from the field, and the remaining companies increased their premiums in one year from 100 to 750 percent.[1] The impact on many practitioners was catastrophic. Radical restructuring of the malpractice system, with extensive tort-law reforms, was sought from the state legislatures, and nearly all responded.

Among the most important reforms was the adoption of arbitration systems and pretrial screening panels designed to direct the handling of claims away from the courts and to eliminate frivolous and clearly nonmeritorious complaints. Many states imposed a financial limitation, usually $500,000, on the total award and moderated the so-called collateral-source rule in order to prevent plaintiffs from recovering, as part of their legal damages, medical and other expenses already recovered from other insurance policies. Reforms of the requirements for informed consent, expert testimony, and the burden of proof were also enacted. The reforms were designed to make malpractice trials fairer and more evenly balanced between the parties in litigation. In 1975 it seemed clear that court decisions had altered the basic law to an extent that made it very difficult for physicians to defend themselves effectively with reasonable medical evidence. The legal reforms of that year were intended to modify these decisions and to reduce the liability of physicians and hospitals, within feasible limits.

From the *New England Journal of Medicine*
1983; 309:1107-1108.

What has been the impact of all these legislative efforts at reform? Has the availability of malpractice insurance improved across the country? Have premium rates become more favorable? Have claims and awards gone up or down since 1975?

Insurance coverage is clearly more readily available to all practitioners through the establishment of insurance pooling arrangements, called joint underwriting agreements. These systems have also helped to eliminate the practice in many insurance companies of canceling the coverage of any physician who has had even a single claim filed against him or her in a policy year.

The most difficult information to obtain, and to interpret when available, has been the actual claim and lawsuit experience on a nationwide basis. The federal government financed a study by the Rand Corporation, and its report, in rather brief summary form (48 pages of text in a pamphlet), has recently been published.[2] Data were examined on closed insurance claims in 1970, before the crisis and reform period, and from 1975 through 1978. Apparently, more recent information was not available. The 1970 survey involved data from 26 insurance companies, accounting for some 90 percent of the national market. The review of closed claims for the later period covered all insurers in the country writing over $1 million in premiums.

The Rand report states that the frequency of claims nationwide declined in the three years after 1975. The rates of decline were striking. In the first year the decline was 27 percent (from 24,240 claims closed to 17,683). In the next year there was a further 12 percent decline (down to 15,556 closed claims). In 1978, the last year surveyed, there was an increase of 11 percent (to 17,238), but the totals continued to be far below the figure for 1975. In the previous five years (1970 through 1974) the reported median average growth in claims frequency had been between 20 and 30 percent per year; thus, the upward trend had clearly been at least temporarily reversed in the later 1970s. This is the good news. The bad news comes in regard to what the report calls the "severity" of claims, meaning the amount of payment received by a claimant either in a settlement or as a court award. There were no detailed data available for use as a base line for 1970, but it can be noted that only 3 percent of closed claims in that year exceeded $100,000. From 1975 to 1978, however, the median severity increased at a rate of 30 percent. Differences in severity from state to state and within states from year to year fluctuated greatly because of the small numbers of claims paid in many states. In 1976, for example, there were 35 states with a total of less than 100 paid claims per state.

The report is properly cautious in drawing conclusions from the data. However, a few interesting observations are made. It is suggested, for example, that in the states (17 in number) where a financial limitation was placed on awards and in those (16 in number) where the collateral-source rule was repealed or modified, the severity, but not the frequency, of awards was reduced substantially. No other substantive legal reform — and there were many across the country — was found to have any statistical relation to reductions in either the frequency or severity of claims. Most surprising, perhaps, is the fact that the establishment of screening panels to eliminate spurious or nonmeritorious claims seems to have had no comparative effect in reducing the total number of claims. Also, the limitations imposed on contingent fees for plaintiffs' lawyers were not found to affect either the frequency or severity of claims.

Some commentators have assumed that the density of lawyers in the population, which varies from place to place, has a direct effect on the frequency of claims made against doctors, which is intensified when automobile-accident suits have been reduced by a no-fault administrative system of handling claims. The Rand study found no support for this assumption.

With or without a state no-fault system for automobile-accident claims, lawyer density had no significant effect on the frequency of malpractice claims in any state. However, the study found that lawyer density did have a positive effect on the severity of claims.

The density of physicians in the population was also studied. It was found that physician density over the past two decades did seem to correlate positively with the frequency of claims but not with their severity — the opposite of the findings on lawyer density. In fact, the report suggests that an increase of 100 physicians per capita in a state was associated with an increase of 3.6 claims per capita per annum. Thus, it is observed that the 40 percent increase in the numbers of physicians practicing in this country from 1960 to 1978 may account for a 24 percent increase in the frequency of claims over these years.

The Rand report is unique in emphasizing the overall effects of urbanization of the population of the various states as the most likely explanation for differences in the frequency and severity of claims. It is in the urban centers that both lawyers and physicians are clustered. It is also clear that awards are higher in urban courthouses than in rural ones, largely because of the higher cost of living and the varied life styles of urban dwellers in general. Thus, the number of claims per 100,000 population in 1976 is reported as a low of 1.24 in Maine and a high of 22.99 in Washington, D.C. I find this observation reasonable, but even the sparse "examples" actually provided by the Rand report (no complete state data are included) produce some puzzling state-by-state comparisons. The number of claims closed in 1976 per 100 physicians was 0.47 in Maine but 9.08 in Idaho, a comparably rural state. In fact, the experience in Idaho was worse than that in California, the supposed mecca of malpractice suits, where the corresponding frequency in 1976 was 8.81. The Rand report concludes, however, that urbanization is "the single most powerful predictor" of both frequency and severity, even after controlling for a higher density of lawyers and physicians in urban states. The report also observes that more complex medical facilities, higher per capita income, and higher welfare and unemployment-benefit rates in the urban states were not significantly related to these regional differences.

Overall, the Rand study admittedly produced only one finding that can be compared with the precrisis years – i.e., that the frequency of claims decreased considerably in the three years after 1975. The report does not venture a prediction that this reduction indicates a long-term downward trend. In terms of the causes for the reduction, the study offers many more negative than positive conclusions. All those impressive tort-law reforms enacted in state after state[3] are reported as apparently not having affected the reduction in claims frequency – the goal toward which most reforms were directed.

Even with the Rand report in hand, however, we can probably expect more bad news. Many joint underwriting groups and other insurers across the country have been requesting substantial premium increases in recent years, apparently because of increased claims activity. I will cite Massachusetts as an example, since the information is so current. In 1976 the screening-panel system reviewed only 11 malpractice claims. In 1977, 58 claims were reviewed. Predominantly, these claims were found against the patient. By 1982 the total number of claims had risen to 402, and 65 percent were found to be meritorious in favor of the patient. The joint underwriting group in

Massachusetts has requested that the state insurance commissioner approve a rate increase of 162 percent for 1984.[4] These figures do not encourage physicians to believe that the crisis in the medical-malpractice field is behind them.

REFERENCES

1. Curran WJ. Malpractice insurance: a genuine national crisis. N Engl J Med 1975; 292:1223-4.
2. Danzon PM. The frequency and severity of medical malpractice claims. Santa Monica, Calif.: Rand Corporation, 1983.
3. Curran WJ. Malpractice crisis: the flood of legislation. N Engl J Med 1975; 293:1182-3.
4. Insurer asks big jump in malpractice rate. Boston Globe. July 14, 1983:20.

♦

COMMENTS

This Rand report has become the classic study of the effect of medical-malpractice reforms on litigation in the field. For a later review of this general area by the same investigator, see P.M. Danzon, "The Frequency and Severity of Medical Malpractice Claims: New Evidence" (*Law and Contemporary Problems* 1986; 49:57-84).

The middle and later 1980s have produced another crisis in the medical-malpractice field. The most serious issue continues to be the radical increase in premium rates, but there is now more evidence than there was in the mid-1970s of rising claims rates and higher total pay-outs to plaintiffs in settlements and awards. The medical and legal literature has called attention to the problems and to proposed reforms. See particularly F.P. Grad, "Medical Malpractice and the Crisis of Insurance Availability: The Waning Options" (*Case Western Reserve Law Review* 1987; 36:1058-98); D.A. Saichek, "A Summary of the New Statutes Governing Medical Malpractice" (*Wisconsin Bar Bulletin* 1986; 59:811-25); A.B. Steiglitz and M.I. Gomez, "Medical Malpractice Reform: It's a Major Departure" (*American Bar Association* 1985; 71:39-41); B.R. Furrow, "Malpractice Revisited: Of Medical Errors, Social Transformation, and Tort-Law Standards" (*Nebraska Law Review* 1984; 63:810-34); D.H. Mills, "Malpractice Reform Legislation: The Seventeen Percent Solutions" (*Legal Aspects of Medical Care* 1984; 12(7):1-2); and E.K. Adams and S. Zuckerman, "Variations in the Growth and Incidence of Medical Malpractice Claims" (*Journal of Health Politics, Policies, and Law* 1984; 9:475-88).

Multimillion-Dollar Verdicts in Malpractice: Causes and Consequences

New England has not been an area where very large verdicts have been common in medical malpractice cases. Widespread publicity was therefore to be expected when the Supreme Court of Connecticut recently upheld as proper and justified a jury verdict of $3.6 million.[1]

The defendant was a local general hospital with a psychiatric ward in which a 23-year-old psychotic patient harmed herself severely in a seclusion room, having been unattended for nearly four hours. The jury had not found negligence against the plaintiff's psychiatrist but returned its verdict only against the hospital. The defendant claimed that the verdict was obviously excessive, being four times as large as any ever returned in the state, and that "its size alone [was] indicative of prejudice, passion, bias, sympathy and total misunderstanding of the law and the facts on the part of the jury."

The trial judge had not only denied a motion to set aside the verdict as excessive but had also remarked that the evidence would have supported "a substantially higher verdict."

The trial judge's comments were certainly unusual in the relatively conservative judicial precincts of Connecticut. Most general discussion of the case will tend to note only the size of the verdict, not the circumstances of the case. As the entire, complex trial record is examined, however, the full picture of an aggravated, tragic situation is revealed. The features leading to a verdict so high can be summarized as follows: negligent failure to safeguard a very sick patient; a blatant effort by the hospital to rewrite, alter, and disguise the patient's record; serious neurologic injury and disability with conscious

From the *New England Journal of Medicine*
1980; 303:143-144.

pain and suffering; and the requirement for lifelong medical and nursing care for a young plaintiff with a life expectancy of 41 years after the trial. Although it may not be part of the legal precedent for which the case will later be cited, one could also note the high technical quality of the plaintiff's expert witnesses in both medical and economic areas, the use of a 20-minute videotaped motion picture starkly displaying the plaintiff's condition and requirements for daily nursing care (the plaintiff could not testify personally because of her condition), and the professional competence of her counsel in preparing and presenting the case at trial.

The plaintiff had been admitted on January 14, 1976, in an agitated, confused condition diagnosed as schizophrenia. She was later placed in seclusion, and a steel-frame bed and other furniture were removed for the sake of safety. After three days, the bed was returned to the room without authorization from the plaintiff's psychiatrist. During the hospital stay, restraints were often necessary. On January 21, the doctor ordered "antipsychotic medication," but the nursing staff failed to record the order until the following day. At that time, the hospital pharmacy had run out of the medication. The doctor was not notified and the patient was not given antipsychotic medication over the next few days; her condition worsened and she spoke of voices telling her "to hurt herself." On the morning of January 24, the patient was observed to be awake between 7:30 and 8:00 a.m. No one on the nursing staff spoke with her. No one entered the locked room from 6:15 a.m. until slightly after 10:00 a.m., when she was discovered with her head wedged between the steel side rails of the bed as she was kneeling on the floor. She was then unconscious with no pulse or respiration. The patient was revived but had permanent brain damage. At the time of the trial she was in a semicomatose condition and cared for in a skilled-nursing facility.

The hospital attempted to characterize the failures of observation and supervision as merely poor professional judgment. It was also argued that the bizarre manner of self-destruction used by the psychotic patient was unforeseeable by the nursing staff and could not have been prevented. The Supreme Court had little trouble dismissing both defenses. "Poor judgment" was held not a defense if it was proved to be professional negligence. One of the plaintiff's expert medical witnesses described the conduct of the staff as "not a question of judgment but rather a sheer matter of responsibility." On the issue of foreseeability, the court pointed out that the hospital needed only to anticipate and guard against the general type of injury, i.e., self-imposed harm within the seclusion room. There was no necessity to foresee the exact action taken. Two classic papers on the law of foreseeability published a quarter of a century earlier were cited as controlling on the issues.[2,3] Ironically, one was written by a law professor at a nearby Connecticut law school—Fleming James of Yale. (As a former tort-law teacher who used these papers as sacred gospel in instructing first-year law students, I was pleased with these relevant citations by Justice Parskey.)

The court pointed out that the amount of a verdict is particularly within the province of the trier of fact and will not be disturbed unless plainly exorbitant. Justice Parskey summarized the evidence of the injuries and the need for lifelong medical and nursing care. Up to the date of the trial, the medical and hospital bills were $317,000. Annual future bills were estimated by plaintiff's witnesses at $91,900. The chairperson of the Department of Economics at the University of Hartford testified and projected the cost of professional care over the plaintiff's expected life, discounted for present value, as in excess of $6 million. Another witness estimated the plaintiff's loss of earning capacity, also discounted to present value, as $220,000. To these figures the jury could add general damages for the plaintiff's conscious pain and suffering. The defendant's counsel did not offer contradictory evidence on these factors.

It may be judged, after a review of the above evidence and circumstances, that a large verdict was supported in this instance. For the future, however, the key may be that the barrier against a large multimillion-dollar award was breached. Although the first big cases, the pioneer findings, continued to be uncommon in later years, they became the grist for the insurance-company underwriters and their always pessimistic predictions; the malpractice premiums will now take another quantum leap upward. The so-called reforms of the mid-1970s in malpractice law, including arbitrary limits on awards for damages, have not fared well under challenges based on constitutional law, as predicted at that time in this column.[4] The answer will probably be found more readily in improved patient care and well-planned risk management and claims processing than in poorly developed legal reforms.

REFERENCES

1. Pisel v. Stamford Hospital. Conn Law J 1980; 41(43):14-23.
2. Prosser WL. Palsgraf revisited. Michigan Law Rev 1953; 52:1-40.
3. James F. Scope of duty in negligence cases. Northwestern Law Rev 1953; 47:196-220.
4. Curran WJ. The malpractice insurance crisis: short-term and long-term solutions. N Engl J Med 1975; 293:24-5.

♦

COMMENTS

Verdicts of over $1 million have become more frequent in metropolitan areas all over the country. For an early comment on the effect of very high verdicts on malpractice premiums, see B. Winter, "Medical Malpractice: Will Jumbo Awards Spark Another Insurance Crisis?" (*American Bar Association Journal* 1982; 68:1545-7). See also Student Note, "Medical Malpractice Damage Awards: The Need for a Dual Approach" (*Fordham Urban Law Review* 1983; 11:973-1000).

The legislative response in many states has been to enact statutory limits on awards, usually affecting only the so-called noneconomic aspects of the award, or damages for "pain and suffering." In 1986 alone, 13 states enacted statutory limitations on malpractice awards. The constitutionality of these limitations is still unsettled. The California decision upholding such a statute—*Fein* v. *Permanente Medical Group,* 211 Cal. Rptr. 368 (1985)—seemed to indicate a trend in favor of such reforms, but later decisions have continued to strike down some of the statutes as improperly restricting the jury's right to award full damages. See, for example, *Boyd* v. *Bubala,* 647 F.Supp. 781 (W. District of Virginia, 1986). See also a student note summarizing constitutional arguments on both sides of the issue: "The Constitutionality of Recent Efforts to Limit Personal Injury Damages Following the 1984–1985 MICRA Decision" (*Western State University Law Review* 1986; 13:595-613).

One of the disadvantages of statutory limits is the effect of monetary inflation. The limit upheld in the *Fein* case in California was $250,000. Later enactments in the middle and later 1980s have been in the $300,000 to $450,000 range.

2 ♦ Hospitals: The New Legal Doctrines

Hospital Liability for the Quality of Patient Care

Hospital personnel have been brought up for many years on the principle that "hospitals do not practice medicine." The law courts have in the past agreed with this proposition, asserting that only physicians can be licensed by law to practice medicine and, therefore, that hospitals can neither practice medicine nor control the actions of physicians. This proposition applies as well to dentists and nurses and other health professionals who are legally licensed. The hospital can no more perform these services than those of physicians, at least from the point of view of a legal authority under license.

But the law is changing. A number of courts have rejected the implications of this dichotomy. In one of the most important decisions in hospital law in many years,[1] the Colorado Supreme Court held a community hospital liable for the negligence of a registered, professional nurse in administering an injection to a postoperative patient. The court refused to hold the surgeon liable for the nurse's negligence on the mere fact that he had ordered the medication. He was not even present in the hospital when the nurse administered the injection, struck the sciatic nerve, and caused a permanent foot drop in the seven-year-old plaintiff. The court held the hospital liable because it was the employer of the nurse and had actually assigned the nurse to the particular service and had supervised the nurse in her duties. The principle of law under which the hospital was held liable is commonly known as *respondeat superior*—that is, let the employer answer for the negligence of a servant or agent. The court rejected the argument that the nurse's actions were professional in nature and therefore not answerable by the hospital. Justice Groves concluded,

From the *New England Journal of Medicine*
1969; 280:316-317.

> If we were to rule that *respondeat superior* does not apply because the hospital is not licensed as a nurse, then it would seem to follow that an airline should not be liable for the negligence of its pilot because the airline is not licensed to fly an aircraft. . . . The hospital [in this case] was the employer of the nurse [who committed the act]. Only it had the right to hire or fire her. Only it could assign the nurse to certain hours, certain areas and certain patients. There was no choice in the doctor [defendant] or the plaintiffs as to the identity of the nurse who would serve [the child plaintiff]. In this day and age a hospital should be responsible for the acts of its nurses within the scope of their employment, irrespective of whether they are acting "administratively" or "professionally."[1]

The *Bernardi* case is also important for a number of other holdings: the court asserted that the plaintiff is entitled to receive by court-ordered discovery a copy of the hospital's "incident report" regarding the injury to the patient. The hospital could not prevent the plaintiff from obtaining a copy because of the fact that it might be useful to the defendant hospital's attorneys in preparing their case for court. It was held that the primary purpose of the incident report is to report the facts of untoward injuries and losses to the hospital administration. As such, they are hospital records and are subject to discovery and examination by a suing party.

Another important part of the *Bernardi* case was the rejection of a "release of liability" signed by the plaintiff's parents upon the admission of the patient. The Colorado Supreme Court ignored this language in a preoperative consent form signed by the parents and gave it no effect whatever in relieving the hospital of liability. A hospital is completely within its rights in requiring that a patient or his parents consent to an operative procedure after being properly informed of the nature and purpose of the procedure. However, the hospital cannot couple with this a complete release of liability on the part of the hospital for any negligence or other legal wrongdoing. The patient or family clearly does not realize the meaning of the term "release" and has no reasonable basis for granting it under the circumstances. The court, therefore, refused to enforce any such blanket release of liability.

REFERENCE

1. Bernardi v. Colorado Comm. Hosp. Assoc., 166 Colo. 280, 443 P.2d 708 (1968).

COMMENTS

This early column from the late 1960s is a good introduction to the new doctrines in hospital law. I chose it for this book because the Colorado Supreme Court was one of the first high courts in this country to recognize hospitals as "enterprises," which, like airlines and manufacturing concerns, must be held responsible for the actions of their professional employees, even if these employees are separately licensed by the state within their professions. The Colorado court rejected the old excuse that "hospitals do not practice nursing" or "do not practice medicine" and therefore cannot control the conduct of such professionals. The court also rejected old distinctions in nursing between "administrative actions" (for which the hospital was liable) and "professional actions" (for which the professional alone was liable).

The *Bernardi* case laid the foundation for later considerations of a doctrine of "corporate liability" as described in the next column. It should be made clear, however, that the finding in the *Bernardi* case and decisions following its reasoning that were made in other states were limited to employer–employee liability for the negligent actions of professional nurses and physicians. These early decisions did not apply to independently practicing physicians who charged direct fees for services to hospitalized patients. Actually, the reasoning in *Bernardi* could have been extended to cover these practitioners as well. For patients as consumers of hospital services, the differences were not apparent, and hospitals could exert as much control (regarding quality assurance) against independent physicians as against employee doctors.

The decision most often cited as having anticipated the concept of making hospitals corporately liable for both medical and nursing services is *Darling* v. *Charleston Community Memorial Hospital,* 33 Ill. 2d 326 (1965). As in *Bernardi,* the Illinois court held the hospital liable for failing to provide an adequate level of nursing care. However, the court also held the hospital liable for the negligent actions of an independent medical practitioner. The legal basis cited by the high court in Illinois for its decision was the hospital's own responsibility to see that, when appropriate, independent practitioners consult medical specialists and act on their recommendations. In later Illinois decisions, it has also been pointed out that the physician in the *Darling* case was not selected by the patient or the patient's parents. The physician was provided by the hospital as part of its emergency ward services, even though he charged that patient independently for his professional services. For an analysis of the effects of the *Darling* opinion, see J. Rapp, "Darling and Its Progeny: A Radical Approach to Hospital Liability" (*Illinois Bar Journal* 1972; 60:833-53). For a recent review, see H.W. Claussen, "Hospital Liability for Independent Contractors: Where Do We Go from Here?" (*Arkansas Law Review* 1987; 40:469-503).

A Further Solution to the Malpractice Problem: Corporate Liability of Hospitals

> I have reached the conclusion that the hospital is liable with great reluctance because I am sure that the Sisters of Mercy have done everything within their power to run a proper institution. But they, like every other governing board, are corporately responsible for the conduct of their medical staff.
>
> *Moore* v. *Carson–Tahoe Hospital*

There has developed in the United States a quiet revolution in malpractice liability, little noticed in the medical literature. It is the movement to assign responsibility for all types of professional malpractice, including acts of independently practicing physicians, to the hospital corporation itself.

The establishment of this type of corporate legal liability has been slow to develop in the medical-care field, although it has become the most common form of legal responsibility in nearly all other aspects of "enterprise liability" in American law during this century.

The movement to a form of corporate responsibility for all malpractice in hospitals carries distinct advantages for both patients and physicians. For injured patients, it means that there would be only one party, the hospital, from whom redress would be sought. For the physician, it would mean that the hospital would carry the insurance and pay the premiums for physician-related malpractice problems. For the public, it would mean increased incentive in hospitals to improve the quality of patient care and to install and support effective programs to manage the risk of malpractice.

From the *New England Journal of Medicine*
1984; 310:704-705.

Two major factors are generally cited as having impeded the development of hospital corporate liability. First, the great majority of hospitals were charitable enterprises and were, up to recent years, immune from suits regarding injury to patients within their walls. The leading decision establishing immunity occurred in 1876 and involved the Massachusetts General Hospital.[1] Second, physicians, whether salaried or independently practicing, were considered to act entirely independently of supervision or control by the hospitals.[2] Both these conditions have changed considerably. Charitable corporate immunity has been removed or severely reduced in nearly all states in the country. There is also no doubt that the modern hospital and its organized medical staff have become much more involved in the monitoring of physician performance, in terms of both quality and cost, than they were even 10 years ago.

In a recent article, Southwick points to two legal theories as merging to support this new movement.[3] These he describes as an increased application of *respondeat superior,* the obligation to answer for the wrongs of hospital employees and agents, and an expanded concept of institutional or corporate negligence, the direct obligation of the hospital to patients for a proper level of hospital management and operation, including the enforcement of an acceptable level of professional medical care.

Southwick clearly views this development as highly salutary for hospitals, professional staffs, and patients. He abhors the present situation in which lengthy litigation, involving high costs and personal trauma, is necessary "to fix blame on particular individuals" for injuries to patients. He sees the new doctrine as eliminating the present adversarial relationship between the hospital and the treating physician in many medical-malpractice cases.

Approximately 80 percent of all malpractice claims arise out of events occurring within hospital walls.[4,5] A large part of the remaining claims relate to prehospitalization treatment or posthospitalization complications. Furthermore, serious injury claims, those involving over $100,000 in settlement or court award, are nearly all hospital-based or related. Concentration of liability in hospitals would therefore cover the bulk of malpractice vulnerability. Insurance policies issued on behalf of hospitals could also be expanded to include claims arising outside the hospital for physicians who are members of the hospital medical staff. Efforts from time to time among medical-professional organizations to develop no-fault medical-liability insurance plans to replace the current fault system are also said to be encouraged by the movement toward hospital corporate responsibility.

Legal commentary has not been universally favorable to this movement.[6,7] In the most recent article, Cohoon criticizes the same decisions praised by Southwick.[1] The main argument he offers is that hospital governing boards cannot assume this new degree of responsibility because they are composed mainly of lay people who are "incapable of passing judgment on the quality of medical treatment rendered by trained physicians." He also predicts that the imposing of this expanded liability on hospitals will lead to increased costs for health care because of higher hospital-insurance premiums.

My own view is that Southwick is closer to being correct in his assessment of the legal development and the reasons for it than Cohoon is. The American courts have always favored doctrines that result in simplification of rules on the liability of an enterprise for injuries to the public it serves. Simplification leads to reducing the need for lengthy and complex litigation. Contrary to Cohoon's point, this simplification also usually results in lower costs of insurance, since the administrative costs of investigation and trial are substantially reduced. Economies of scale are achieved by concentrating insurance coverage in the corporate structure rather than individualizing costs and claims reserves around each practicing physician, which is further complicated by the different premium rates for the various medical specialties. This complex rate structure would no longer be necessary if coverage were provided at the hospital level.

Cohoon's argument about the lack of technical medical capacity in hospital governing boards is also apt to impress the courts very little in the late 20th century, though perhaps it did impress them a century ago. His point has been rejected for virtually all other corporate structures in this country.

Corporate boards of directors are obliged to set general policies for their enterprises and to ensure continued financial stability. They need not possess in their own members the scientific or technical capacity to direct day-to-day operations. This is the job of the administrative officers, not the governing board. In a modern hospital, the operation of the institution is the duty of its administrative personnel and its organized medical staff, all of whom are responsible to the governing board for their actions.

The movement in the courts toward hospital corporate responsibility for medical malpractice is strongly under way. However, the case law at present has not gone quite as far as Southwick argues it should. In most of the major cases, some administrative responsibility of the hospital board can be found to have been breached. A clear-cut no-fault doctrine has not as yet been imposed on hospital corporations. Physicians still exercise independent medical judgments about patient care. The change that is developing should concern malpractice insurance coverage and financial responsibility rather than issues of control over patient care decisions.

Malpractice claims have become so serious a problem for physicians, and malpractice insurance premiums are rising so high in proportion to physicians' practice income, that leaving the situation as it is has become untenable.[8] Hospital-based programs to control and manage the risk of malpractice are growing across the country and are proving quite useful. Along with the movement toward broader corporate responsibility in the hospitals, these risk-management programs can help considerably in coping with the new crisis in medical-malpractice suits. This combined effort should be watched carefully by physicians. It is not without its problems, but it has promise in a field where reforms thought to be effective have been failing all too often.

REFERENCES

1. McDonald v. Massachusetts General Hospital, 120 Mass. 432 (1876).
2. McConnell v. Williams, 361 Pa. 355 (1949).
3. Southwick AF. Hospital liability: two theories have been merged. J Legal Med 1982; 4:1-50.
4. Legal review. Hosp Risk Manage 1983; 5:148-50.
5. Secretary's Commission on Medical Malpractice. Magnitude and impact of the medical malpractice problem. Washington, D.C.: Department of Health, Education, and Welfare, 1973:5-9.
6. Slawkowski JR. Do the courts understand the realities of hospital practices? St Louis Univ Law J 1978; 22:452-60.
7. Cohoon JB. Piercing the doctrine of corporate hospital liability. San Diego Law Rev 1983; 17:383-401.
8. Curran WJ. Medical malpractice claims since the crisis of 1975: some good news and some bad. N Engl J Med 1983; 309:1107-8.

COMMENTS

This column is a quite recent update of the arguments for and against a doctrine of "corporate liability" for American hospitals.

As pointed out in the essay, the courts have not uniformly taken the ultimate step of making hospitals legally liable for the negligence of all independently practicing physicians who treat patients within the walls of the hospital merely because these physicians are acting within the hospital environment. In each of the key cases, the courts have been able to find some negligence by the hospital's administration, either in admitting the physician to the staff or in monitoring the physician's later performance. See, for example, a review of decisions by J.E. Butler, Jr., and S.S. Lazzlo, "Hospital Liability for Physician Negligence in Georgia: A Realistic Approach" (*Mercer Law Review* 1987; 37:701-23).

The standards of the Joint Commission on Accreditation of Health Care Institutions concerning the quality of patient care reflect a shift away from the philosophy that hospitals are not legally responsible for the quality of care provided by independent medical practitioners. In 1987, the commission proposed new standards of patient-injury risk management in response to legislative enactments in several states, notably Florida, Rhode Island, California, and Massachusetts. On the interrelation of quality-assurance programs and patient-injury risk management, see J.E. Orlikoff and G.B. Lanham, "Why Risk Management and Quality Assurance Should Be Integrated" (*Hospitals* 1981; 55(11):54-9). See also A.P. Seilicki, Jr., "Risk Management Philosophy and Techniques: An Overview" (*Topics in Health Care Financing* 1983; 9(4):1-4).

Hospital Charity for the Poor: The Legal Obligation

In previous columns I have called attention to the class-action suits being brought by public-service law firms and other groups on behalf of consumers, including medical patients.[1] Among the most active of the legal groups have been the neighborhood law offices supported by the Office of Economic Opportunity. The primary concern, or primary client population, for these offices has been the poor. In the medical field, these Office of Economic Opportunity lawyers have concentrated a great deal of their efforts on class-action suits against nonprofit hospitals in various parts of the country for their failure to provide a "reasonable amount" of free medical care, or care at lower charges than normal, to the poor in their communities. In these cases brought in such places as New Orleans, the District of Columbia, Miami, Florida, New York, and rural Colorado, the claim has been made that this obligation is owed under the Hill–Burton Hospital Survey and Construction Act of 1946 by all hospitals and other health care facilities that have received construction grants under the program, regardless of the amount of the grant or when it was made over the past 26 years.

The common practice in the cases, such as in *Cook* v. *Ochsner Memorial Hospital,* entered in New Orleans in 1970, has been to join as defendants all nonprofit voluntary hospitals in the entire area. In this case the allegation is that all the hospitals are ignoring their legal obligation under the federal act and are engaged in a pattern and practice of "dumping" both elective and emergency cases of indigent patients into the Charity Hospital, a public institution in New Orleans.

From the *New England Journal of Medicine*
1972; 287:498-499.

The theory of a continuing obligation without regard to time or the extent of the original Hill–Burton grant is supported by a well-known Fourth Federal Circuit Court of Appeals case, *Simkins* v. *Moses B. Cone Memorial Hospital*.[2] In that case the court required the hospitals to comply with the federal constitutional mandate of nondiscrimination and nonsegregation regarding hospital patients and physician staff privileges.

In the midst of all this pending litigation, the U.S. Department of Health, Education, and Welfare reacted on April 18, 1972, by issuing proposed regulations under the Hill–Burton Act purportedly clarifying the obligation of nonprofit hospitals to provide "charity care" under the law.[3]

To the everlasting shock of many in the health care field, the federal agency seemed to be in full agreement with the contentions of the plaintiffs in the class actions. Under the new regulations, the obligation of the hospitals was made unlimited in time and extending to all parts of the institution, regardless of the scope of the construction grant. State agencies would be required to establish levels of charity care on an institution-by-institution basis, taking into account the financial status of the institution, the types of services rendered, the need for charitable care in the area, and the extent of charity care jointly provided by other institutions. This type of requirement might not have been so unpalatable to the hospitals if the regulations had not also provided a level of "presumptive compliance." Under this, the institution would be presumed to render a reasonable level of charitable care if it provided uncompensated care to the extent of 25 percent of its net income or 5 percent of its operating costs, whichever was greater. Furthermore, bad debts of patients and Medicare and Medicaid reimbursement would be excluded from operating costs or charity care in these calculations. To obtain credit for a charity case, the hospital would in practice be forced to determine that the patient was in this indigent class before admission, and would be required to budget in advance for its reasonable level of such care.

The response of the health care institutions to these regulations was loud, clear, and nearly hysterical. In the first days after the regulations appeared in the *Federal Register,* the Department of Health, Education, and Welfare received over 200 responses, nearly all unfavorable. The American Hospital Association indicated its intent to protest "very vigorously" and asked for a 90-day delay in the effective date of the regulations in order to answer. The department granted only a 30-day extension.

According to a communication to institutional members from Madison B. Brown, M.D., acting executive president, a fact-finding survey by the American Hospital Association issued on June 5, 1972, indicated that only 14 percent of its member institutions would meet the presumptive standard. It was also asserted that 93 percent of the institutions would be forced to raise charges to nongovernment patients by more than 4 percent to finance the proposed obligation.

In communications to the federal government, hospitals and other medical groups, including the AMA, protested that the proposed requirements went substantially beyond any Congressional intent to finance care for the poor by the private sector of the economy, either in 1946 or in 1972. Furthermore, it was alleged that the legal obligation of the institutions to the government under the Hill–Burton Act ended in 20 years.

It has been indicated that the Department of Health, Education, and Welfare may well heed the protestations of the hospitals and modify the proposed regulations substantially. It is indicated that the obligation of the hospitals will be limited to 20 years or the period of repayment of the construction loan. Furthermore, the "presumptive compliance" will be limited to 3 percent of operating cost or 10 percent of the original construction grant, whichever is lower. Many of the hospitals will be particularly pleased to see the last mentioned change adopted since it would tie the obligation to at least some relation to the construction grant itself rather than a free-standing general obligation. Also, it is indicated that the government may have in mind an alternative method of compliance — that of an "open-door policy" toward all patients regardless of ability to pay. Moreover, the classification of indigency could be made after discharge and even after a bill for services had been sent as long as the case had not been turned over to a collection agency for recovery. Other procedural modifications may be made in the system of compliance.

If these changes are made, the new standards may be made more acceptable to the health care community. There are indications, however, that the litigants in the class actions may not be satisfied with either the April 18 regulations or any modification in favor of the hospitals. In at least one of the suits injunctive relief may be sought in the courts to prevent the enforcement of the new program. The fight for a new definition of American medical charity may not yet be over.

REFERENCES

1. Curran WJ. The "class-action" approach to protecting health-care consumers – the right to psychiatric treatment. N Engl J Med 1972; 286:26.
2. 323 F.2d 959 (4 Cir. 1963).
3. Medical services for persons unable to pay: nondiscrimination. Fed Regist 1972; 37:7632-4.

♦

COMMENTS

The obligation of most hospitals to provide an adequate level of uncompensated care for the poor under the Hill–Burton law will terminate in the late 1980s. The increasingly frequent purchases of charitable hospitals by for-profit hospital groups (or chains) have also aggravated this situation since the purchases end the hospitals' charitable obligations. See D.O. Nutter, "Access to Care and the Evolution of Corporate, For-Profit Medicine" (*New England Journal of Medicine* 1984; 311:917-9); G. Dallek, "The Loss of Hospitals for the Poor" (*Health Services Research* 1983; 18:593-7); J. Feder, J. Hadley, and R. Mullner, "Poor People and Poor Hospitals: Implications for Public Policy (*Journal of Health Politics, Policy, and Law* 1984; 9:237-50); R.R. Bovbjerg and W.G. Kopit, "Coverage and Care for the Medically Indigent: Public and Private Options" (*Indiana Law Review* 1986; 19:857-917); and Student Note, "New Regulations for Hill–Burton Hospitals: Can the Poor Still Afford to See the Doctor?" (*Syracuse Law Review* 1987; 37:1219-41).

The Power and Authority of Hospital Medical Staffs

The internal organization of most American hospitals is an uneasy union of medical care delivery by physicians and the administration of a medical care facility by the hospital's governing board. For most patients, the key functionary is the attending physician, who has an independent contractual relation to the patient. In the traditional view of hospital organization and management, the health care facility exists to further and support this relation.

In recent years, the orthodox position has been breaking down. The famous *Darling* case in Illinois in 1965 was the first major legal ruling that challenged this system and declared that the hospital itself had a responsibility, even though shared with the medical staff, to the patients for the quality of their medical care.[1] This position has been restated as the policy of the American Hospital Association in its *Patient's Bill of Rights*.

The clash in the application of this new principle comes when a disagreement arises between the organized medical staff and the governing body of the hospital. Which group prevails? How is an impasse resolved?

This issue has rarely, if ever, been faced in court, strange as that may seem in today's litigious society. In late 1976 it came to the Supreme Court of South Dakota, an unlikely forum for resolving major health-law problems.[2]

The hospital was the St. John Regional Medical Center. In 1972, the hospital's board of directors wanted to strengthen its authority over patient care and the organization of the medical staff by a number of measures. One would allow the administrator of the hospital to suspend temporarily the clinical privileges of a staff physician when suspension was found necessary in the interest of patient care. An-

From the *New England Journal of Medicine*
1977; 296:264-265.

other measure would require approval by the board of appointments of all officers of the medical staff. These changes were in conflict with the medical-staff bylaws. The medical staff refused to amend the bylaws to conform to the changes desired by the board. In the face of the impasse, the governing board unilaterally amended the medical-staff bylaws to comply with the new plan. The medical staff went to court seeking a declaratory judgment that the action of the board was illegal. The Supreme Court of South Dakota upheld a lower-court determination that agreed with the medical staff's contention. It was held that the provisions of the bylaws were equally binding on the board and the medical staff and could be amended only in accordance with the provisions of the bylaws themselves. The bylaws required that all amendments be adopted by a two-thirds majority of the medical staff and then be approved by the governing board before becoming effective.

The theory of the court was that the medical-staff bylaws constituted a binding contract between the incorporated hospital and the medical staff. The hospital had argued that the power to resolve a conflict between the hospital and its medical staff must lie with the governing board. It was pointed out that recent malpractice cases had placed heavy responsibility on the governing boards to police the quality of care in their institutions, including much tighter regulation of physicians' clinical privileges in the hospital. It was also alleged that the changes were needed to avoid an impending loss of accreditation. Lastly, it was argued that the medical staff was not a legal entity and did not have standing to bring the legal action being considered.

The Supreme Court of South Dakota held that the medical staff was a legal entity. It was found to be an "unincorporated association" of the physicians holding staff privileges at the hospital. Ironically, the legal basis for the "association" was the very same set of bylaws that was the real bone of contention in the lawsuit.

There are other ironies in the history of the situation in South Dakota. The current hospital was formed in 1947 from two former hospitals, the Sprague Hospital and the Tschetter Hospital, each operated by a medical-group organization. The Franciscan Sisters of Chicago had been called in, according to the court, to form the new hospital for the group at the Sprague Hospital. Before the new facility was completed, the group from the Tschetter Hospital decided to join the new hospital center. The Franciscan Order proposed to the physicians from both groups a set of medical-staff bylaws taken in toto from McKechrine's textbook, *Hospital Organization and Management,* a common source of model provisions for hospital and medical-staff bylaws in this country at that time. It was this set of bylaws that was adopted in 1947.

The case has many implications. It is considered a disturbing precedent that is contrary to the modern trend in hospital administration.[3] On the other hand, it is an important victory for the independence of medical-staff responsibility for medical care. The problem now is to devise effective mechanisms for resolving hospital disputes. The impasse in this case consumed nearly four years of effort—and a rehearing has been requested that may prolong the conflict. It seems clear that the court is saying that hospitals will have to continue to live with the uneasy union that they themselves have helped to create.

REFERENCES

1. Darling v. Charleston Community Memorial Hospital, 33 Ill.2d 326 (1965); *cert denied,* 383 U.S. 946 (1966).
2. St. John's Hospital Medical Staff v. St. John Regional Medical Center, Inc., Docket no. 11746, Supreme Court of South Dakota, Sept. 3, 1976 [Mimeographed advance opinion].
3. Few winners in Huron affair. Hospitals 1976; 50(21):77-80.

♦

COMMENTS

The case reviewed in this column, *St. John Regional Medical Center,* is still the landmark court decision regarding relations between hospitals and their organized medical staffs. Nevertheless, many observers in the field of hospital management still believe that the case was wrongly decided. As pointed out in the column, the decision is commonly described as resisting the current tendency to shift power toward hospitals and third-party payers and away from practicing physicians. See, generally, A.F. Southwick, *The Law of Hospitals and Health Care Administration* (2nd ed. Ann Arbor, Mich.: Health Administration Press, 1988).

The American Hospital Association and the American Medical Association have published a report designed to facilitate the settlement of disputes in hospitals. The report was prepared by a joint task force of lawyers representing both organizations. The document attempts to clarify the roles of the hospital administration and the organized medical staff. On the whole, the report accepts the position of the court in the *St. John* case as correct in describing the amendment of medical-staff bylaws as a joint responsibility of the medical staff and the hospital governing board. The disciplining of impaired and unqualified physicians is described as a "shared responsibility," but responsibility for conducting investigations and making recommendations for action is placed on the medical staff. Fiscal matters are described as the responsibility of the hospital's administration, but the report suggests consultation on decisions with the leadership of the medical staff. The report describes its objective as providing a framework for resolving disputes, not on a legal basis, but on the basis of a "prudent management arrangement" in the best interest of all parties, in order to avoid or minimize conflict in the hospital. See *Report of the Joint Task Force on Hospital–Medical Staff Relationships* (Chicago: American Hospital Association, 1985).

Hospital-Staff Privileges: Can Medical Staffs Exclude Uncooperative Applicants?

The California Supreme Court continues to puzzle many medical-law commentators with a succession of controversial decisions. If appellate judges are expected most of the time to provide cool reason and clear logic in analysis and results, then the California high court falls short in the medical area more often than it seems to score points for justice and equity.

A careful review of California medical decisions is a studied and deliberate effort on my part for the *Journal*. Except for the U.S. Supreme Court, the California high court is probably the most influential judicial body in this country.

I limit my evaluation here to appellate cases requiring a depth of investigation and understanding of medical and hospital practice and the effect of particular rulings on that practice. In many other areas that touch on medical litigation, I find no major fault with the California opinions. However, when values of a legal or judicial nature clash with ethical or practice values in medicine, this court seems to impose the legalistic value without adequate regard for the effect on medical practice and values. The best-known examples of this tendency have been in such decisions as *Tarasoff*[1] (disclosure of confidential patient information), *Cobbs* v. *Grant*[2] (informed consent), *Landeros* v. *Flood*[3] (liability for injuries to a battered child), and most recently *Truman* v. *Thomas*[4] (liability for not aggressively persuading a patient to have a Pap smear) and *Miller* v. *Eisenhower Medical Center*[5] (admission to the medical staff of a private hospital). Some of

From the *New England Journal of Medicine*
1981; 304:589-591.

these cases have been examined in other columns in this series. Here we will concentrate on the last case that I have named.

The issue in the *Eisenhower* case was initial admission to the medical staff of a private hospital. The applicant had been denied admission on several occasions. The hospital followed its bylaws and permitted two separate appeals to internal review committees before the hospital board finally confirmed the rejection. This decision was apparently the end of the long affair, but one year and 17 days later the applicant filed suit to require the hospital to admit him forthwith to the staff.

A trial court heard the suit and dismissed it, holding that the requirements for membership were rational and not arbitrary or contrary to public policy. This criterion was the traditional standard for reviewing a private organization's membership matters. The court found that the hospital had followed its bylaws and had had substantial evidence to support its findings. The applicant had been afforded a fair hearing and proper procedure.

Evidence gathered by the hospital, including letters received from physicians whose names were provided by the applicant himself, indicated that the applicant was known to have problems in relations with many other physicians with whom he had worked and had had trouble in another hospital where he was a staff member. He was alleged to be a controversial person with an impetuous nature. Examples of his previous actions were provided. At his first hearing, the applicant was asked about the termination of his internship at Cook County Hospital, Chicago, some eight years before he had come to California and made his first applications to the staff. He answered that he had left because of a "disagreement of some kind" but could not recall the details of the incident and was surprised to be asked because he had not been warned that he would be questioned on this matter. Letters from the Cook County Hospital indicated that the applicant had been asked to leave after seven months of a rotating internship on which he had received a "poor" (D) rating for physical examination, attitude toward patients, cooperation with other personnel, personality, and appearance.

There was also evidence that the applicant had performed poorly in conducting an emergency room service at a nearby hospital, and that when a new group had purchased the hospital, they had refused to enter the contract of purchase until the applicant was removed from charge of the emergency service.

A majority of the California Supreme Court (5 to 2) reversed the trial court's determination. It found that the above evidence, of which I have presented only highlights, was not enough to support the finding under the hospital bylaws that this physician had not been proved to have "ability to work with others" with sufficient adequacy to assure the medical staff and trustees of the hospital that "any patient treated by him would be given a high quality of medical care." The court also ruled that the year's delay did not work against the applicant to the extent of denying the appeal. It further held that the hospital could not consider his "lack of veracity" regarding termination of his internship because he did not have "fair notice" of the question.

A bylaw such as that used by the hospital in this case has often been highly recommended as an important and necessary addition to the written standards for medical-staff membership, both initial and continuing. In the past, hospitals have often used such a general criterion but have had their determinations challenged because the requirement for good professional relations, ability and willingness to serve on hospital committees, ability to work with the nursing staff, and other requirements for cooperation in a modern hospital environment were not spelled out in the articulated standards of the institution.

The supreme court imposed a high test of compliance with the bylaw. It held that the hospital must show that the applicant's inability to work with others in the hospital setting would pose a "realistic and specific threat" to the quality of care. By examining the counterarguments at the hearings, largely by opposing counsel for the hospital and the applicant, the majority strangely held that there were "conflicting views" in the medical staff and the hospital on the meaning of the standards. Despite the evidence that was produced concerning the applicant's past conduct, the majority ordered that the hospital grant the applicant membership on the staff—or, in the alternative, reopen the matter for rehearing "in the light of this opinion." Unless the hospital merely accepts the order, the controversy over this physician's admission will thus continue into a 10th year and more hearings.

There was a scathing dissent by Justice Mosk, joined by Justice Clark. The dissenters pointed out that this was the first time that such strict and detailed judicial review had been applied by a high court in this country for initial admission to a private hospital's medical staff. Other decisions had uniformly allowed private institutions considerable freedom from "external intervention" in their determinations in the absence of a finding of unfair procedures, improper discrimination, or arbitrary and capricious action. Justice Mosk asserted that the trial court's decision on the merits was "clearly correct."

Justice Mosk brought out and described damaging evidence concerning the applicant that was not mentioned by the majority. He noted a recent comment in a California law review: "It is difficult to understand how a hospital can adhere to modern concepts of hospital administration if it cannot consider the ability of its staff members to cooperate."[6]

The distressing aspect of this decision is the unwillingness of the majority of the California court to allow the hospital to exercise its proper function of weighing the evidence and interpreting the anticipated effect of admitting this physician to the staff. The weighing of this evidence required a deliberate judgment, a prediction, about the ability of a particular professional who had never served on the staff before to cooperate with, and not adversely disrupt, the complex human and technological operation of a modern hospital, whose objective is the high-quality, safe administration of patient care.

It must be remembered that this case involved a question of initial admission to the medical staff, not the exclusion of a physician already on the staff who had gained through service a right to answer only specific, relevant charges relating to in-hospital conduct. In the latter circumstance, I strongly support a physician's right to a tight evidential hearing, with exclusion allowed only on strong and direct grounds. Here, however, the entire medical staff, the review committees, and the board were exercising a preventive responsibility. They could only review the character and personality of the applicant and indirect evidence of experiences in other settings bearing on work relations in their hospital. They could only draw inferences about his abilities to function in their institution. They did just that. The board made its ruling citing the bylaw that itself was held by the Supreme Court of California to be an adequate and proper standard. There were ample hearings. There is little else that the board of the hospital could have done to make their inferences more concrete or to estimate a "specific threat" to patient care and safety. No hospital could meet a higher requirement at the time of initial admission to its staff.

REFERENCES

1. Tarasoff v. Regents of Univ. of Calif., 529 P.2d 533, *rehearing denied and re-affirmed*, 551 P.2d 334 (1976).
2. 104 Cal. Rptr. 505 (1972).
3. 131 Cal. Rptr. 69 (1976).
4. 165 Cal. Rptr. 308 (1980).
5. 166 Cal. Rptr. 826 (1980).
6. Hospital staff privileges: the need for legislation. Stanford Law Rev 1965; 17:900-16.

♦

COMMENTS

The California decision reviewed above was particularly poorly reasoned in its pronouncements on the authority of hospitals to refuse staff privileges to unqualified, disruptive, or uncooperative physicians. The decision has not been followed in other states. Some jurisdictions, notably Massachusetts and Illinois, take a strong position against reviewing decisions made by the governing boards of private hospitals regarding initial applications to the medical staff. A recent Massachusetts decision held that a physician denied membership on the staff had no rights against the hospital and was thus not even entitled to demand that the hospital's medical staff follow its own bylaws, which required a hearing on all new applications for membership. It was held that only the state's attorney general could require that the hospital's medical staff follow its bylaws. See *Bello* v. *South Shore Hospital,* 384 Mass. 770 (1981). See also *Jain* v. *Northwest Community Hospital,* 67 Ill. App. 3d 911 (1978); *Scappatura* v. *Baptist Hospital,* 120 Ariz. 204 (1978); *Bricker* v. *Sceva Speare Memorial Hospital,* 111 N.H. 276 (1974).

Other jurisdictions do, however, allow judicial review of initial application to hospital medical staffs and require the observance of certain aspects, both procedural and substantive, of "due process of law" in such reviews. See the leading decisions: *Silver* v. *Castle Memorial Hospital,* 53 Hawaii 475 (1972), cert. denied, 409 U.S. 1048 (1973); *Greisman* v. *Newcomb Hospital,* 40 N.J. 3889 (1963). For an analysis of the procedural due-process issue, see "Procedural Due Process Rights of Physicians Applying for Hospital

Staff Privileges" (*Loyola University Chicago Law Review* 1986; 17:453-80).

On preparing and revising medical-staff bylaws, see some useful suggestions in two publications by the leading professional organizations: *By-Laws: A Guide for Hospital Medical Staffs* (Chicago: American Medical Association, 1984) and *The Medical Staff Bylaws Handbook* (Chicago: American Hospital Publishing, 1987). See also N. Hershey, "Revising Medical Staff Bylaws: An Organizational Challenge" (*Law, Medicine and Health Care* 1987; 15:137-43).

Hospital Contracts for Anesthesia Services: Antitrust Consequences

Hospitals throughout the United States have long been making various types of exclusive service arrangements with physicians and other suppliers of goods and services. These arrangements have generally been encouraged by the health-planning agencies when hospital costs have been reduced or the quality of services has been improved. In recent years, however, the heavy shadow of the antitrust laws has fallen over these practices. The shadow took on substance last year when the federal court of appeals found an exclusive arrangement for anesthesiology services in a New Orleans hospital to be an illegal tying agreement – a per se violation of the federal antitrust laws.

The court of appeals decision sent a strong shock through the ranks of a number of hospital-based medical specialties. The broad implications of the case, if the decision survived challenge in the Supreme Court, were thought by many observers to be among the most devastating of all applications of the antitrust laws to the health care field in the history of this country.

Those favoring the development of exclusive-service arrangements can now be reencouraged, although within limits, to continue the practice. The Supreme Court, in *Jefferson Parish Hospital District* v. *Hyde,*[1] reversed the court of appeals decision with a unanimity rare in such matters, not a single justice dissenting from the overall decision. (There was a majority opinion by Justice Stevens, with separate concurring opinions filed by Justices Brennan and O'Connor.)

Most important, all the justices agreed that the type of arrangement in question should not have been considered a per se violation of the antitrust laws. Had the Supreme Court agreed with the lower

From the *New England Journal of Medicine*
1984; 311:243-244.

court on this point, the hospital could not even have defended its position. The mere existence of the exclusive contract would have been illegal. On the contrary, the Supreme Court applied the so-called rule of reason, which allows the hospital to produce evidence of the reasonableness of such arrangements in medical–hospital relations. Under this more liberal test, the hospital was able to convince the justices — all of them — that the arrangement in this situation was justified and did not unduly restrict competition in hospital and medical care in the New Orleans area.

Justice Stevens began his opinion by finding that the contract in question was indeed a tying agreement, since all patients who underwent surgery at the hospital were required to receive their anesthesia from one of the four anesthesiologists in the group contracting exclusively with the hospital. These four physicians were the only anesthesiologists on the hospital's medical staff. Under the contract, the group promised that these physicians would not practice at any other hospital. The plaintiff, Dr. Hyde, a board-certified anesthesiologist, applied for membership on the hospital's staff. He alleged that he was refused admission solely on the grounds of the hospital's exclusive agreement with the group. On the basis of this refusal, Dr. Hyde brought his lawsuit.

The hospital was one of some 20 hospitals in the New Orleans metropolitan area. About 70 percent of the patients going to general hospitals were found to use hospitals other than East Jefferson Hospital. The court of appeals found that the 30 percent market share of the hospital was enough, because of its geographic location in the East Bank of the parish, to give it a monopoly that enabled it to coerce patients to accept the tying arrangement. The Supreme Court disagreed. The justices were not convinced that the limited market share of the hospital was strong enough to force patients to accept services they did not want. Furthermore, the Court pointed out that every patient undergoing surgery needed anesthesia and that no evidence had been submitted that any patient received unnecessary services. There was also no evidence in the record that any patient admitted to the East Jefferson Hospital could not have gone to another hospital that would have given the patient a wider choice of anesthesiologists. In a particularly telling comment, Justice Stevens pointed out that the patient's choice of anesthesiologists is always limited to the practitioners who have been admitted to the hospital's medical staff. The plaintiff was not challenging the "unquestioned right" of this or any other hospital to exercise some control over the number of doctors on its staff. At the time of this suit, there were four anesthesiologists, all members of the group, from among whom patients and surgeons could choose. If the plaintiff were admitted to the staff, the number would be increased from four to five. The Court could see no compelling difference in such a limited change, since all the other restraints on patients' freedom to select a specific anesthesiologist would still remain. These circumstances within the health care field were enough for the majority of the bench to join in Justice Stevens' opinion and to dismiss the case against the hospital.

It remained for the three justices concurring in Justice O'Connor's opinion to point to the defendant's indicated reasons for adopting an exclusive contract for its anesthesia department. Justice O'Connor asserted that there were several grounds for finding that the tying agreement improved patient care and promoted more efficient hospital operation. The contract with the group assured the hospital of having all the anesthesiology services needed by the hospital available at all times on a 24-hour basis, with flexibility of scheduling and efficiency in the use of equipment. The arrangement allowed the hospital an effective method of monitoring the quality of the service and its contribution to patient care. Justice O'Connor also pointed out that the trial court had found that such exclusive arrangements were employed by anesthesia departments in the majority of hospitals in the New Orleans area and "in the health-care industry generally" because of the proved benefits of such practices for patients and hospitals alike.

The end result of this case is that "reasonableness" prevails in arrangements between hospitals and medical services. Care should be taken, however, against construing this decision as a complete withdrawal of antitrust interest in the exclusivity of service arrangements in the health care industry. The existence of a larger operation and greater control of the marketplace may subject such contracts to deeper scrutiny. In a footnote to his opinion, Justice Stevens called attention to the district court's finding that this case "would be different" if the group in question had exclusive contracts in several of the hospitals in the relevant market.[2] Also, the contract with the East Jefferson Hospital was probably assumed to be open to renegotiation and to the competition of other groups for the contract at the end of each term of five years. The Court further noted that circumstances might have been different had the effect of this contract been to monopolize the services of all or nearly all the qualified anesthesiologists in the market area, thus depriving other competing hospitals of needed practitioners. Lastly, in his concluding paragraph, Justice Stevens made an enigmatic remark, otherwise unexplained, to the effect that the type of exclusive arrangement in this case might "raise questions of medical ethics" even though it did not have the unreasonable impact on patients' purchasing power that would make it illegal. Does this remark imply that all medical contracts involving exclusivity are ethically suspect? Such a position has not been seriously advocated in this country for decades, and the policy has rarely been a part of professional medical ethical standards in other countries in this century. With all these qualifications noted by the justices, we undoubtedly have not heard the last of the questions to be raised about exclusive hospital–medical service arrangements.

REFERENCES

1. Jefferson Parish Hospital District no. 2 v. Hyde. US Law Week 1984; 52:4385.
2. Footnote 7. The quoted statement was at p. 541 in the District Court opinion, 513 F.Supp. 532, 541 (1981).

♦

COMMENTS

The *Hyde* decision provoked considerable commentary in medical and law journals, most of it favorable both to the Court's finding in the case and to its reasoning on antitrust law. See K.B. Jones, "Hyde Decision Affirms Current Practice" (*Pennsylvania Medicine* 1984; 87(5):22-4); T.J. Reed, "High Court Relaxes Exclusive Contract Antitrust Rules in Hyde" (*Hospitals* 1984; 58(11):74-9); W.J. Lynk, "Restraint of Trade through Hospital Exclusive Contracts: An Economic Appraisal of the Legal Theory" (*Journal of Health Politics, Policy and Law* 1984; 9:269-79); and R.C. Bern, "*Jefferson Parish Hospital* v. *Hyde:* Return to Reality in Economic Analysis in Trying Cases" (*University of Missouri, Kansas City Law Review* 1985; 53:145-73).

Health Planning, Blue Cross Organizations, and the Antitrust Laws

The Supreme Court is not known for hasty decision making. Rapid review is generally reserved for matters of national crisis in which determination cannot be delayed. The medicolegal field, or health care law, has rarely presented issues demanding such pressing attention. In fact, in earlier years, much of this field was left to the states and regarded as particularly within the sensitivities of local law and custom.

It was, therefore, a new experience for the nation's highest court to deal with an important medicolegal case in very rapid order. It is obvious that the reason for the expeditious treatment was the fact that the case concerned a novel application of the federal antitrust laws to another area of national policy—health care planning.

The case, *National Gerimedical Hospital* v. *Blue Cross of Kansas City,*[1] was argued before the Court on April 29, 1981. Only six weeks later, on June 15, 1981, the justices issued a full opinion by a unanimous bench (nine to zero), providing a complete reversal of the decisions of both federal courts that had heard the case below. It was clear that the Court had no doubt at all about the policy it wanted to express, and that it did not want that expression to be carried over until the fall session of 1981.

Much of the health care–planning field, along with the lawyers for Blue Cross–Blue Shield and other health insurance groups, were taken by surprise, not only by the rapidity of the Court's handling of the matter but also by its substantive decision in reversing the lower courts, which had held so firmly that the actions of the health planners and the Blue Cross organization were exempt from the federal antitrust law.

From the *New England Journal of Medicine*
1981; 305:1194-1195.

The lower courts had held that there was incompatibility between the objectives of the National Health Planning and Resources Development Act of 1974 and the free-competition policy of the antitrust laws. The Health Planning Act was designed to encourage cooperative use of facilities and to curtail further hospital construction and expansion that was found by the planners to be unnecessary. The lower courts went on to hold that the congressional intent, supported by some references to the history of the act, was that such activities were not subject to the antitrust laws, whether the activities were by official health-planning agencies or private organizations cooperating voluntarily with the planners.

Health planners had heaved sighs of great relief, especially when the court of appeals disposed of the case quickly, agreeing with and adopting most of what the district court had said about a "blanket exemption" from the antitrust laws for official planners, cooperating hospitals and health-care providers, and health insurers such as Blue Cross–Blue Shield. Any disagreement with this policy was considered a serious threat to health planning and multi-institutional cooperation.

The Supreme Court was not convinced. It found that support for an implied exemption was not strong in the Planning Act or its history. The Court obviously considered the free-competition requirements of the federal antitrust laws to be firmly rooted in the national public policy of Congress, not to be violated without clear evidence and specific intent. It was particularly bothered by the sweeping language and blanket exemption thrown around so many actors in the health care field by the lower courts' opinions. A much narrower focus might have helped to meet the objectives of the health planners.

Further understanding of the case may be aided by a brief summary of the actions taken by the parties. National Gerimedical was in the process of constructing a new private, acute care hospital in the Kansas City, Missouri, area. It applied to Blue Cross of Kansas City to become a fully participating member hospital. Blue Cross refused to admit the hospital on the grounds that it had not applied for and not been granted a certificate of need for a new hospital from the local metropolitan area health-systems agency (Mid-America HSA). National Gerimedical had not applied because it was known publicly that the HSA had determined that the Kansas City area was "overbedded" and that it would not consider any further petitions for acute-care hospitals. The action of Blue Cross was voluntary on its part and did not result from any official order directed to it by the HSA. Blue Cross was following what it considered good policy in supporting the objective of curtailing further hospital construction.

National Gerimedical considered the refusal of Blue Cross as effectively blocking it out of the Kansas City hospital market, preventing it from competing with the existing hospitals for patients. It therefore brought an antitrust suit against Blue Cross and the Mid-America HSA, alleging a wrongful refusal to deal with the hospital and allow it to operate on a competitive basis. The lower courts dismissed this suit on the grounds indicated earlier—that the entire field was exempted on a blanket basis from the Sherman Antitrust Act.

The Supreme Court dealt with the case on a much narrower basis. It concentrated on the Blue Cross action, not on the entire range of health-planning activities. It found that the refusal of Blue Cross to admit the petitioning hospital was "neither compelled nor approved by any governmental, regulatory body." It also found that the HSA in question was not operating under state law because, at the time of this refusal, the state of Missouri did not have a state regulatory agency with authority to review hospital construction and to delegate any functions to local HSAs. It was pointed out that the evidence in the case revealed no formal request by the HSA that Blue Cross refuse to admit the petitioning hospital to its plan. These were the crucial findings. The Court went on to say that the record was not strong for a broad exemption of anticompetitive cooperation under the Planning Act. The antitrust laws, on the other hand, were found to constitute a fundamental national economic policy. The case was remanded to the lower court for further proceedings under the suit.

This case should not be viewed as a complete defeat for cooperative health planning. It is a good object lesson for health planners and the health care industry to be careful with its national mandate and to act under official rulings rather than voluntary agreements. The federal planners took some serious risks in trying to use voluntary, private groups, the comprehensive planning agencies, and then the HSAs to carry out functions requiring state-law recognition. My own writing in this field a number of years ago warned against this weakness in the earlier law, a failure to provide a link to state law.[2] The revised federal act was an attempt to remedy weaknesses in the earlier law, but the concept of the private agencies for health planning was retained, since it allowed greater federal control. Nevertheless, state action was necessary to make the rulings of the HSAs effective within their states.[3]

Blue Cross of Kansas City was caught in the middle. It certainly believed it was following local and national policy in the interest of cost containment for health care consumers. The Supreme Court itself, in the conclusion of the opinion, admitted to this by observing, "Although respondents [Blue Cross] may well have acted here with only the highest of motives in seeking to implement the plans of the local HSA, they cannot defeat petitioner's antitrust claim by an assertion of immunity from the requirements of the Sherman Act."

Health planners like to use drawing boards. It is back to the boards now for the planners and the providers, but the actions will need to be more formal and more under the color of state law and agency rulings than in the past. There may be little time to waste. The new administration in Washington is taking a fresh look at the effectiveness of the HSAs and may pull the blanket of federal law even further off the cooperative planning functions, leaving the field to the states for action and implementation.

REFERENCES

1. National Gerimedical Hospital and Gerontology Center vs. Blue Cross of Kansas City. US Law Week 1981; 49:4672-7.
2. Curran WJ. Health planning agencies: a legal crisis? Am J Public Health 1970; 60:359-60.
3. *Idem.* Present at the creation: health planning and the inevitable reorganization. Health Care Manage Rev 1976; 1:33-43.

♦

COMMENTS

The *National Gerimedical* decision was an important early instance of the U.S. Supreme Court's interpreting the Sherman Antitrust Act as applying to cooperative activities of hospitals in cases in which the effect of the cooperation was to reduce competition and rationalize the use of hospital and medical resources. Useful comments on the case were made in the law reviews. See J.B. Chase, "Antitrust Implications of Health Planning" (*American Journal of Law and Medicine*

1982; 8:321-48); and G.B. Agrawal, "Antitrust: Implied Repeal of the Antitrust Laws by the National Health Planning Act" (*Tulane Law Review* 1981; 56:749-63).

Malpractice Arbitration in Hospitals and Health Insurance Systems

Several of the malpractice-law reform measures enacted by state legislatures in the past few years have included methods for arbitration of claims. The National Center for Health Services Research has published a useful report on the present statutory provisions of the 50 states.[1] Under an arbitration agreement, the parties agree to submit their dispute (a malpractice claim) to an impartial arbitrator or a panel of arbitrators for resolution. The regular court system is not used. The hearing before the arbitrator is less formal than before a court; the technical rules of evidence law do not apply. The decision of the arbitrator or panel is binding on the parties under these modern statutes – that is, no party can resort to a trial court to litigate the claim all over again. Arbitration should be distinguished from the use of "malpractice screening panels" that have been adopted in many states. The screening mechanisms are not binding. At most, the results can be admitted as evidence in a later trial, and such admission has been found unconstitutional in some states as a compromise of the right of jury trial.

Physicians generally favor arbitration of malpractice claims. They seem to think that the informal setting and the use of trained arbitrators will give them a fairer hearing than a lay jury. Many lawyers and insurance experts also favor arbitration, but not for the same reason. They usually stress the fact that arbitration is a much faster, more efficient, and less expensive method of settlement than the court system, where delays in trial and legal investigational costs mount up very quickly. Some consumer groups oppose arbitration as too favorable to the defense. The new report[1] indi-

From the *New England Journal of Medicine*
1977; 296:1045-1046.

cates that malpractice claims can be arbitrated with binding effect in 35 states.

One of the most serious problems in this complex subject of malpractice arbitration is whether agreements to arbitrate can be made a condition of entering into a prepaid health insurance plan or health maintenance organization (HMO) plan or, even more seriously, can be made a condition of a patient's entry into a hospital. Two very recent decisions in California provide different, though perhaps not conflicting, rulings on these issues. In *Madden* v. *Kaiser Foundation Hospitals*[2] the Supreme Court of California held that a provision in a Kaiser HMO plan requiring subscribers to submit malpractice claims to arbitration was entirely valid. It was not held to be an illegal "adhesion contract," and it was held not to violate the subscriber's right to a jury trial. The interesting point in the case was that the health insurance contract was actually negotiated for the subscriber-plaintiff, a state employee, by the State Employment Retirement System (SERS), which acted in a fashion similar to that of a labor union negotiating on behalf of its members. The action of the SERS was found to be an effective representation of the state employer's interests, even though the subscriber claimed he was unaware of the arbitration agreement.

Only a few months later, an intermediate appellate court in California, in *Wheeler* v. *St. Joseph Hospital,*[3] held that a hospital could not enforce a patient's alleged agreement at admission to arbitrate a malpractice claim. The patient was admitted for angiography and catheterization studies for coronary insufficiency. It is not indicated that the admission was an emergency. Among the admission papers were paragraphs headed "Conditions of Admission." Under this heading was a provision called "Arbitration Option," which provided that the patient would agree to binding arbitration of any malpractice claim unless he put his initials in the space provided, thus indicating his refusal to agree to the arbitration system. Also, the same paragraph indicated that the patient could refuse to participate in the arbitration if he gave written notice to the hospital within 30 days of his discharge. The patient neither initialed the form nor gave the specified 30 days' revocation notice. After the plaintiff-patient sued the hospital, the defense placed before the court the "Arbitration Option" and requested that the arbitration be ordered. The lower court so ordered, and the parties went to arbitration before a panel of a physician, a lawyer, and a businessman. The panel's finding was that no malpractice had occurred, and it dismissed the claim.

The plaintiff went back to court and petitioned that the finding be vacated and a trial be held. The wife of the plaintiff (who was rendered quadriplegic after a brain infarction and could communicate only by blinking) alleged that the plaintiff had not read any of the admission forms and had merely signed them; the wife was present at the admission. She also said that no one at the hospital had told them about the arbitration option then or at any time and that they had not been given a copy of the admission forms.

The upper court, in a split decision (two to one), held that the agreement to arbitrate was an illegal "adhesion" forced on the patient and could not be enforced against him. The court stressed the circumstances of the case and the method used by the hospital as not offering the patient an effective choice about the agreement. No effort was made to inform him of the "option" and to allow him time to decide. The court distinguished the *Madden* case as one in which the parties were of basically equal strength, bargaining at arm's length over employee benefits. The presiding justice of the court dissented vigorously, asserting that the decision would add "a new and crippling dimension to the concept of arbitration." The case may well be appealed to the California Supreme Court.

No matter what the outcome of an appeal, it does seem reasonable that hospitals and other health care facilities take effective steps to inform patients about "arbitration options" and all other matters that the hospitals seek to have patients decide at the time of admission. The time of admission is always a distressing experience for patients and their families. Care must be taken not to impose on patients conditions that may not be in their best interests, or that may not be adequately understood, no matter what their actual "decision" may be at the time.

REFERENCES

1. American Arbitration Association. Statutory provisions for binding arbitration of medical malpractice claims. Bethesda, Md.: National Center for Health Services Research, October 1976. (DHEW publication no. (HRA) 77-3165.)
2. 131 Cal. Rptr. 882 (1976).
3. 133 Cal. Rptr. 775 (1977).

COMMENTS

In the years since this column was published, arbitration programs for medical malpractice have not spread very far beyond the health maintenance organizations and other group medical practices in which they were found in the 1970s.

In the legislative reform movements of the 1980s, relatively little notice has been taken of arbitration as a major alternative to lawsuits. As a means of avoiding the tort system, no-fault plans using informal or contractual mechanisms seem to have more general support.

Despite the strong dissent of one of the three judges, the *Wheeler* case was not appealed to the California Supreme Court. Instead, the hospitals sought to change their practices in order to avoid the outcome of this litigation. For an informative article on the functioning of malpractice arbitration conducted by the most experienced group in the field, the American Arbitration Association, see I. Ladimer, J.C. Solomon, and M. Mulvihill, "Experience in Medical Malpractice Arbitration" (*Journal of Legal Medicine* 1981; 2:433-69). On the practical aspects of the operation of a system in one large state, see J.C. Aslanian-Bedikian, "Arbitrating a Medical Malpractice Claim" (*Michigan Bar Journal* 1983; 62:788-92). For a more recent attempt to support the more widespread use of arbitration in medical-malpractice disputes, see R.M. Powsner and F. Hamermash, "Medical Malpractice Crisis the Second Time Around: Why Not Try Arbitration?" (*Journal of Legal Medicine* 1987; 8:283-304).

An End to Federal Regulation: The Good, the Bad, and the Unnecessary

The Reagan administration in Washington is vigorously dismantling federal regulatory programs. Old-time political opponents of even the most traditional and seemingly secure public control and surveillance programs are, at long, long last, having their day. The regulators are being shoved out into the cold, and their many rules, regulations, and statutes are being fed into the shredders in preparation for public burning.

There is probably some good in all such purging. There are always identifiable excesses and unnecessary regulatory growths cultivated in the name of the greater public good. However, the danger with purging and pruning is that the enthusiasm about cutting often gets carried too far. The good often dies with the bad.

There is a difference between this administration and the recent, more pragmatic conservative administrations of Presidents Ford and Nixon. This administration seems much more doctrinaire and determined to reduce governmental controls in all areas, not only in selected areas of obsolescence. As the President said repeatedly during the election campaign, "The government *is* the problem." Therefore, the pruning itself is the objective. The idea is to reduce the forest, not merely to cut some branches from unhealthy trees.

In the medical and health areas, it is being widely assumed that health-planning regulation at the local level in federally supported health-systems agencies, federal hospital-construction controls, and many types of therapeutic drug and appliance regulation will end next

From the *New England Journal of Medicine*
1982; 306:653-654.

year. There will be support across political lines for some of these reductions in control programs. Many will welcome sensible reform in health-planning regulation or in control of construction and equipment purchases in the health care industry. These programs have grown in a decade or so from a few branches providing needed emphasis on rationality and priority setting to a forest and then a jungle of confusing pronouncements.

But there is some important regulatory effort that should be saved from the ax. The Food and Drug Administration (FDA) has never been overstaffed and has rarely, if ever, overstepped its mandate of consumer protection. Heavy cuts should not be made there. Since 1962, with the Drug Amendments Act of that year, the FDA has carried an uneasy responsibility as a scientific evaluator of the efficacy of therapeutic drugs, not merely performing a policing function over their safety and the truth of their labeling. This duty has been carried out faithfully and should have the medical community's continued support.

Some other endangered regulatory species among the newer and less secure federal programs are also worth saving. The national regulations on nursing homes and related extended health care facilities are not very old. There may be legitimate complaints about some of the detail in the programs. However, recent proposals would gut the needed—very needed—mandatory guidelines for this program under Medicaid. A task force of the federal Health Care Financing Administration has recommended pruning that would all but kill the federal role in this field. Accreditation of nursing homes would end, and voluntary industry certification would be accepted. Federal standards regarding broad aspects of construction and patients' safety, medical supervision, operational sanitation, infection control, and even patients' rights and welfare would be repealed as unnecessary. If any industry in this country requires close supervision, I submit that it is the nursing home industry. Even the best nursing home operators need federal controls, if for no other reason than to protect them from the unfair competition of the vicious exploiters of the old and the chronically ill who are attracted to this industry.

The other important newer type of endangered species that I would mention is control of environmental hazards. Here the regulatory target is much more elusive than poorly run or exploitive nursing homes. In addition, the impact of the regulations is much more widespread among business enterprises. Heavy industry—very big business—is affected by environmental controls. The costs of a healthy environment and reasonably clean air and water are often expensive additions to already high developmental and production costs in the largest and most important industries. Closely related to the general environmental-hazard control programs, and equally widespread in its impact on industry, has been the federally operated occupational safety and health program. All these programs are under heavy attack at present. A 50 percent reduction in support for the Environmental Protection Agency has been proposed for next year. The Council on Environmental Quality has already had a two-thirds reduction in its operational budget. This is a purge of widespread proportions in agencies that do not deserve it. Both the Environmental Protection Agency and the Occupational Safety and Health Administration have made superb efforts in recent years to minimize the detail of industrial surveillance and bring common sense to the language of federal regulations.

Conservative politicians and traditional economists are now favored species in Washington. Both advocate using cost-effectiveness tests on regulations that can affect free (uncontrolled) competition in industry. I have never been sure what is measured in these tests. One part of the exercise seems to be to calculate how much it costs the industry to install the safety or health standards or group of standards. This seems fairly straightforward, although it is often difficult to have confidence in the figures used by the controlled industry when uniform accounting principles are not used and base-line, preregulation data are not available. But it is the other side, the effectiveness side, that I often find has no definition or boundaries. When the effectiveness can be measured easily, as in measuring the greater purity of the air inside a factory, this exercise is worthwhile. But measuring effectiveness in terms of the personal health of workers or the air of a metropolitan area affected by many sources of pollution is another matter. Even when the exercise can be completed and the cost calculated for a given measure of effectiveness, who decides what costs are too high to be tolerated?

Nevertheless, let it be said that cost-effectiveness measures could offer a better way to decide on the pruning of federal regulations than the current wave of indiscriminate purging, which could leave most of us feeling very unprotected in many areas of health, safety, and the environment.

♦

COMMENTS

In its later years, the administration of President Reagan continued its program of reduction in federal regulatory programs, especially those affecting major industries. An exception was made, however, in the case of the federal Food and Drug Administration, as a result in part of a series of much publicized public crises concerning consumer protection, including incidents in which packages containing pain medicines and other over-the-counter drugs were tampered with and caused several deaths. In addition to these traditional areas, the FDA was also involved in the investigation of the effects on food of the nuclear plant disaster at Chernobyl in the Soviet Union. The FDA's representatives conducted on-site investigations of food suppliers in such heavily hit European nations as Finland and Italy. For a review of the FDA's activities in the Reagan years, see F.E. Young, "FDA's Philosophy of Regulation in the 1980's" (*Food, Drug and Cosmetic Law Journal* 1987; 42:157-61).

Medical Judgment and Medical Ethics in Cost-Containment Programs: A Supreme Court Review

Physicians are participating in the administration of medical and nursing home care under Medicare and Medicaid. Much of the control over the Medicaid program is vested in the state governments under a complex array of federal statutes and regulations.

The question before the U.S. Supreme Court in an important appeal from the Second Circuit Court of Appeals was whether the federal Constitution's requirements of "due process of law" apply to medical determinations of the physical and mental status of nursing home patients. The legal action was brought in New York by a group of patients protesting their transfer from skilled nursing facilities to lower levels of care.

The type of facility in which nursing care is given is obviously of great concern to sick elderly patients and their families. The New York Medicaid program did protect the rights of nursing home patients under a utilization-review system. However, the patients who brought the action argued that they should be provided with the more extensive procedural safeguards of the federal Constitution. The Supreme Court did not agree with this viewpoint. The majority (there were two dissenters) refused to find the functions of the medical panels and the decisions of individual medical reviewers to be "state action," thus invoking the application of the Fourteenth Amendment. The Court's analysis was heavily technical, and the discussion of the New York program rather dry and intricate, but all this judicial examination was relevant to the administration of the greatly overcrowded

From the *New England Journal of Medicine*
1983; 308:435-436.

federal court dockets. The justices were obviously trying to avoid the need to impose further federal requirements on the state Medicaid programs, as well as to prevent controversies over decisions on patient transfers from further clogging the federal courts. In this case, *Blum* v. *Yaretsky,*[1] the Court followed its recent trend in the hospital-law field and elsewhere by refusing to extend the meaning of "state action" to cover another area of local decision making. Had this case gone the other way, we could have seen huge numbers of hospital and nursing home patients contesting in the federal courts transfers downward in the system and providers contesting transfers upward, or even decisions to continue care at any level, covered under the state insurance program.

For the medical readers of the *Journal,* however, I did not choose to comment on this case merely for its relevance to court administration and crowded federal dockets. I was particularly struck by the majority's insistence that the reason for its finding was that this case involved medical judgment uncontrolled by the state. Justice Rehnquist specifically stated: "Those decisions [to discharge or transfer] ultimately turn on medical judgments made by private parties according to professional standards that are not established by the State." In his concluding sentences, Justice Rehnquist referred to the fact that physicians in these situations act in accordance with canons of ethics established within their own professional groups rather than under rules of conduct dictated and imposed by the state. Thus, the determination of physicians of "medically appropriate" care and placement in various types of facilities is an independent medical decision.

The two dissenters, Justices Brennan and Marshall, hotly disagreed with the majority's characterization of the doctor's role in Medicaid. They cited the sentences quoted above from the majority and then said flatly, "The Court is wrong." They pointed out that the standards applied by the utilization-review panels and the individual doctors were developed and implemented by the state of New York. Also, it was indicated that "virtually every action by a [nursing home] operator is subject to State oversight." The dissenting justices observed that classifications of nursing home care at various levels were "legislative constructs," not medical standards at all.

The dissenters were convinced that the purposes of the physician's actions were related primarily to cost containment. They indicated that if the doctor's decisions had been clinical in nature, such as prescribing drugs, they would have agreed with the majority. However, they argued, decisions on levels of care "have far less to do with the exercise of independent professional judgment than they do with the *State's* desire to save money" (emphasis in original).

In this case the goals of the medical assessment of nursing home patients did relate to cost containment. However, the physicians were actually applying clinical skills in examining and reporting on the physical and mental status of the patients. The majority of the Supreme Court found that the activity of the doctors was primarily clinical in nature. What was the relevance of the reference to canons of ethics? In the main, it seemed to support the independence of the judgment of the physicians – a confidence displayed by the Court in its assumption that the physicians would act with personal integrity and only on behalf of the best interests of each patient.

One can predict that physicians will be more involved in cost-containment efforts in the future than they have been in the past. As long as these efforts are essentially clinical, the Supreme Court seems willing to leave them outside the scope of "state action" and thus not regularly subject to the requirements of the Fourteenth Amendment and federal judicial review. The majority of the Court did not, however, provide any guidance in drawing what could become a very thin line between activities that can be described as primarily clinical and others that could reasonably be considered exercises of socioeconomic judgment, such as application of cost-effectiveness analysis[2,3] and allocation of public resources.[4] Physicians' judgments in these areas, even though they may involve medical knowledge and experience, have not traditionally been governed by any of the existing canons of professional medical ethics.[5] Should the decisions of physicians on behalf of the state in areas such as these be considered beyond the reach of federal due process of law?

REFERENCES

1. Blum v. Yaretsky, 102 S.Ct.2777 (1982).
2. Weinstein MC, Stason WB. Foundations of cost-effectiveness analysis for health and medical practices. N Engl J Med 1977; 296:716-21.
3. Shepard DS, Thompson MS. First principles of cost-effectiveness analysis in health. Public Health Rep 1979; 94:535-43.
4. Hiatt HH. Protecting the medical commons: who is responsible? N Engl J Med 1975; 293:235-41.

5. Curran WJ. The freedom of medical practice, sterilization, and economic medical philosophy. N Engl J Med 1978; 298:32-3.

COMMENTS

For a comprehensive review of legal aspects of programs designed to contain the costs of medical care, see a symposium in the *Case Western Reserve Law Review* (1987; 36:605-1233). See also K.W. Wing and C.J. Craige, "Health Care Regulation: Dilemma of a Partially Developed Public Policy" (*North Carolina Law Review* 1979; 57:1165-86); S.F. Jencks and A. Dobson, "Strategies for Reforming Medicare's Physician Payments: Physician Diagnosis-Related Groups and Other Approaches" (*New England Journal of Medicine* 1985; 312:1492-9). See also U. Reinhardt, "Economics, Ethics, and the American Health Care System, or Why Some People Can't Get Decent Care" (*New Physician* 1985; 34:20-8, 42). For a revealing discussion of the deleterious effects of cost-containment programs on the quality of care, research, and training, see a recent report by the public-service group Medicine in the Public Interest, "Health-Care Cost Containment Movement: A Reconsideration" (Boston: Medicine in the Public Interest, 1988).

3 • Forensic Medicine and the Law

THE STATUS OF FORENSIC PATHOLOGY IN THE UNITED STATES

The condition of forensic pathology has never been strong in the United States. It has been a specialty of virtually handfuls of dedicated people over the nearly 200 years of the American republic. By contrast, the field of *legal medicine* (a broader field than forensic pathology, but including this subspecialty) has been strong and vigorous in continental Europe for over 400 years. In 1876 Chaillé reviewed the field of legal medicine in the United States and could not name a single leading practitioner of forensic pathology and legal medicine in the United States.[1] In the late 1920s and early 1930s, the National Research Council produced four important reports on the development of medical examiner systems.[2-5] Only three programs, in New York City, Newark, New Jersey, and Boston, were found to be adequate, and none of these were without important weaknesses.

There are many reasons for the lack of development in forensic pathology and legal medicine in this country. Among the most important deterrents is the lack of recognition and support in the legal system of this country for impartial medical investigation, expert medical testimony, and forensic science generally.

Some very important new light has been cast upon this field by the recent publication of three papers produced for the Pathology Training Committee of the National Institute of General Medical Sciences.[6-8] The papers, written by three of the country's most eminent forensic pathologists, Drs. James L. Luke, William Sturner, and Charles S. Petty, were intended to provide the Pathology Training Committee, headed by Dr. Alan R. Moritz, himself

From the *New England Journal of Medicine*
1970; 283:1033-1034.

highly qualified in forensic pathology, with a general picture of the status of the field and of its training and research needs. The papers answer this request in superb fashion. They are the best expression in precise and clear terms of the needs of this field that this writer has ever seen.

Regarding the current status of the field, the papers point out that some 164 specialists are currently certified by the American Board of Pathology in this subspecialty. However, Dr. Luke estimates that only between 30 and 40 qualified, full-time forensic pathologists are at present in actual practice in the country, and these are clustered in a few large metropolitan areas. It is probably a conservative estimate to say that two thirds of the American people live in jurisdictions without *any kind* of solid program in forensic pathology covering their communities.

As these papers point out, the great tragedy for the American people in not having these services is felt not only in the criminal field, with the growing violence in the country, but also in all public health and community health areas. All these endeavors suffer greatly from inadequate and inaccurate death and cause-of-death investigation.

The papers discuss very well the vast need for increased manpower in the field. Over 60 percent of the currently available positions for forensic pathologists in this country are unfilled. There are at present some 15 approved residency training programs in forensic pathology in the country. Only one, that associated with the Chief Medical Examiner's Office in Baltimore, has been able consistently to fill its traineeships annually. It is noteworthy that this is the only program supported by the National Institutes of Health for research training in forensic pathology. An excellent and practical outline for a one-year residency training program in forensic pathology is proposed. In addition to what might be expected in fundamental skills of scene investigation, autopsy performance, and forensic reporting, the program would include advanced work in neuropathology, toxicology, anthropology, and serology, along with interdisciplinary training in forensic-science laboratory work and law as related to the medical examiner's work.

The articles by Luke, Sturner, and Petty provide the basis for an expanded program of support for the field of forensic pathology by the National Institutes of Health. I certainly hope that such a program can be given a high priority in the years ahead. Forensic pathology has waited, perhaps too long, and perhaps too patiently, for its time to come.

REFERENCES

1. Chaillé SE. Origin and progress of medical jurisprudence, 1776-1876: a centennial address. Reprinted from the Transactions of the Medical Congress, Philadelphia, September 1876. Philadelphia: Collins, 1876.
2. Schultz OT, Morgan EM. The coroner and the medical examiner. Washington, D.C.: National Academy of Sciences, National Research Council, 1928. (Bulletin no. 64.)
3. Weinmann GE. A survey of the law concerning dead human bodies. Washington, D.C.: National Academy of Sciences, National Research Council, 1929. (Bulletin no. 73.)
4. *Idem.* A compendium of the statute law concerning coroners and medical examiners in the United States. Washington, D.C.: National Academy of Sciences, National Research Council, 1931. (Bulletin no. 83.)
5. Schultz O. The possibilities and need for the development of legal medicine in the United States: with a supplement on university departments in the field of criminology. Washington, D.C.: National Academy of Sciences, National Research Council, 1932. (Bulletin no. 87.)
6. Luke JL. The status of forensic pathology in the United States today. Forensic Sci Gaz 1970; 1(3):3-8.
7. Sturner W. Suggested guidelines for training in forensic pathology. Forensic Sci Gaz 1970; 1(3):8-10.
8. Petty CS. Source material regarding training in forensic pathology. Forensic Sci Gaz 1970; 1(3):10-3.

♦

COMMENTS

This was the first of a series of strongly worded critiques that I wrote in the early 1970s deploring the poor conditions in forensic pathology and what I called the public medicolegal death-investigation systems in the United States. Several other columns in this chapter also illustrate the problems of presenting high-quality forensic evidence to the American courts during this period.

The medicolegal field owes a substantial debt to forensic pathologists of the early decades of this century for the part they played in keeping an academic interest in legal medicine alive in the medical schools. None of this group had legal training. Their contact with law was mainly through exposure to the unashamedly brutal and consistently anti-intellectual law-enforcement and criminal-court system then prevailing in a few large cities of the country. The demands for their services were so great and the budgets so low that they did little if any research. Yet, this small group persevered and tried to maintain contact with the academic programs in legal medicine on the continent of Europe, where a rich tradition supported effective programs in most of the metropolitan centers.

Forensic pathology is not my field, and my own career was devoted to expanding medicolegal interest beyond this one area; nevertheless, I considered it my obligation as law–medicine columnist for the *New England Journal of Medicine* to call attention to the sorry state of affairs in this most traditional of forensic medical environments. My efforts in this direction did not invariably win me friends. The field at that time was so weak that close scrutiny by outsiders was resented and without the support of respected figures in forensic pathology, such as Alan Moritz and Charles Petty, I would not have been able to criticize the conditions of the public programs as openly as I did.

I am glad to be able to report that the campaign waged in the 1970s for improvements in the public medicolegal systems responsible for investigations into deaths was highly successful. The movement was greatly aided by the Johnson administration's federal programs of support for improved criminal-justice systems at state and metropolitan levels.

At present, the majority of the states have coordinated forensic-pathology programs, and a large number of metropolitan areas operate comprehensive death-investigation systems. As of 1987, a total of 32 accredited residency programs in forensic pathology have been established across the country, and 350 board-certified forensic pathologists are registered with the American Board of Pathology.

For a review of the programs of the 1970s, see *Death Investigation: An Analysis of Laws and Practices in the United States* (Rockville, Md.: Department of Health, Education, and Welfare, 1978. DHEW publication no. (HSA) 78-5252). See also K.S. Field, *Assessment of Personnel of the Forensic Science Profession* (Rockville, Md.: Forensic Science Foundation, 1975).

For a recent review of the operation of public systems of death investigation, see C.S. Petty and W.J. Curran, "Operational Aspects of Public Medicolegal Death Investigations" in W.J. Curran, A.L. McGarry, and C.S. Petty, eds., *Modern Legal Medicine, Psychiatry, and Forensic Science* (Philadelphia: F.A. Davis Co., 1980). For a survey of the situation in Canada, see C. Granger, *Canadian Coroner Law: A Legal Survey of Coroner and Medical Examiner Systems in Canada* (Toronto: Caswell, 1984).

Medicolegal Investigational Systems: New Demands for the 1970s

In the United States today, medicolegal investigation of deaths is poorly handled in well over 60 percent of American legal jurisdictions. Part of the shame, the scandal, of this condition lies in the fact that it has existed for so long. It has improved but little during this entire century. Yet longstanding problems tend not to be remedied for that very reason: they have been around for so long that officialdom and the man in the street alike see no pressing need to cope with them.

If there was a fault in the recently released reports on the status of forensic pathology in this country that were reported upon in a recent *Journal* column,[1] it was a lack of urgency, a lack of new "relevance" in the statement of needs of the field. I believe that there are new problems in this country in the 1970s vastly more powerful in their demands on our society and its legal system than in the past that call for improvement in our methods of investigation of medicolegal deaths.

These four new problems of the 1970s may be briefly described as follows:

The increase in violent death. Our current times have become violent times. From 1960 to 1969, violent crimes increased in the United States 104 percent. Most of this rise has been since 1963. During these years, the general population grew only 11 percent. The murder rate showed a similar precipitous rise in the later years of the 1960s. I believe that we can expect this trend to greater violence to continue. It places a great strain on poor medicolegal systems, as certain spectacular cases in recent years have shown. Good medico-

From the *New England Journal of Medicine*
1971; 284:30-31.

legal systems can absorb a larger caseload of violent crimes. Inadequate or corrupt coroner or medical-examiner systems collapse entirely in the face of such public pressure.

The greater difficulty of determining cause of death in drug usage and drug abuse cases and other cases. There has been a huge increase in drug abuse in the United States in recent years. Particularly disturbing has been the rise in drug abuse among teen-agers. These young people not merely are becoming addicted but also are killing themselves by a variety of methods: they are overdosing themselves to a lethal degree; they are administering the drugs carelessly and killing themselves accidentally; they are experimenting wildly with all sorts of combinations of drugs and paraphernalia to get more and better kicks; and they are killing themselves in all sorts of ways while under the influence of drugs.

Furthermore, this is only one of the new areas of death in the 1970s that require more effective public investigation. Others are related to the therapeutic use of drugs, to suicide, to new environmental hazards, and to many other circumstances. These fields of investigation require new technologies and new disciplines in the medicolegal field.

The polarization of political activity and the resort to violence in protest movements. Some readers may wonder how this factor is related to medicolegal systems. It is closely related. Public outcry is greatest at protest movements when violence and death occur, on either side, among the protesters or among the police or other law-enforcement personnel. There is an immediate demand for proper, independent investigation. When the police are involved and may be charged with overreacting, with brutality, or even with murder, they cannot themselves conduct the investigation. Independent, highly qualified, professional medicolegal systems are required to deal with these issues. We cannot have Warren commissions to conduct ad hoc reviews of every political killing. The 1970s demand a new approach in medicolegal work. The investigations of the killings of the two Kennedy brothers, the Watts riot inquests in California, where police were accused of killing 21 black persons in the course of the disturbance, and the killings of Black Panthers by the Chicago police all illustrate the need for such programs.

The growing distrust and hostility toward the American system of justice and law enforcement. The last factor I point to is a growing distrust of American law and order by young people and minorities in this country. Much of this distrust and hostility is misguided, and much of it is exaggerated by radical groups and the press. However, there is a basis for distrust in some of our methods and institutions. We must improve them, or they will be torn down around us.

Yet it is not impossible to construct highly qualified, professionally respected, independent medicolegal systems in this country. A fine model meeting all these criteria is the Office of the Chief Medical Examiner in New York City, headed by Dr. Milton Helpern. This office enjoys an excellent reputation in all quarters of the city and with the professional groups of the area. Recently, a member of the Young Lords, a militant group of Puerto Rican youths in the city, was found dead in a jail cell. A report was circulated widely in the press and on television that the deceased had been beaten to death in the cell. Dr. Helpern's investigation proved conclusively that there was no evidence to support such a conclusion and that all medicolegal evidence was consistent with suicide. The official report was accepted in the community because of the reputation of the office and its scientific and medical soundness. Substantial further unrest and possible large-scale violence was thus averted. In contrast, a similar incident took place in Augusta, Georgia, last May. A mentally retarded juvenile offender was alleged to have been beaten to death in a county jail. The official investigation was delayed, and rioting occurred. From 500 to 1000 National Guardsmen were called out to stem the disturbance. In the course of the incidents, five black persons were shot to death by the police. A local coroner declared all the deaths to be due to gunshot wounds in the back. Despite the importance of this allegation, no autopsies were ordered. When questions were raised about this failure, the officials replied that each autopsy cost $100 and they could not do autopsies in all cases.

This absurd reply from Augusta should ring in the ears of all of us. No matter what "the experts" in medicine or law may say, it is the ultimate responsibility of the political system to decide whether the public can and will pay for this protection, which we claim is vital to our survival in civil peace. We who are interested in improved medicolegal investigational programs can only persevere in our arguments and have hope in the process of democratic government.

REFERENCE

1. Curran WJ. The status of forensic pathology in the United States. N Engl J Med 1970; 283:1033-4.

♦

COMMENTS

This column was much more an expression of my personal philosophy about public medicolegal systems investigating deaths than the first essay appearing in this chapter. The four "new problems" of the 1970s described here were the key issues around which forensic-pathology services were built up and expanded during these turbulent years; and, as of the 1980s, the investigation of violent and drug-related deaths continues to attract the most publicity of all the various functions that such programs perform. Especially when there are overtones of political protest or racial discrimination, investigations of deaths in police custody are the most sensitive of all investigations conducted by these medicolegal offices.

This column singled out for considerable praise the conduct of the Office of the Chief Medical Examiner in New York City under the venerable Dr. Milton Helpern. For the more than two decades in which Dr. Helpern was its head, that office was the unquestioned leader of the field across the country. At that time it was already located in its own building, on the grounds of the New York University School of Medicine.

After Dr. Helpern's death, however, the quality of the program in New York City declined, city budgets were reduced, and personal disputes erupted among the office's professional staff. As a result, in 1985 the problems of the office were publicly exposed in a series of front-page articles in the *New York Times,* in which the fall from grace of the once-proud flagship of the country's public medicolegal systems was described in florid detail. The *New York Times* rarely engages in investigative reporting in the metropolitan area, but it went after this story with a vengeance. The newspaper charged that the office was poorly organized and administered and that it had tried to "cover up" police brutality in the arrest and custody of black youths in the city. (See the newspaper articles beginning on January 27, 1985, on page 1: B. Shenon, "Chief Medical Examiner's Reports in Police Custody Cases Disputed.") The later articles, all on page 1, appeared on January 28, 29, and 30. The last article in the series was accompanied by an editorial asserting that the newspaper stories had painted "a portrait of a once world-renowned agency fallen into terrible disorder."

The chief medical examiner, Dr. Eliot Gross, made a vigorous public defense of his administration and charged that budgetary cuts had hurt the effectiveness of the program. A rival newspaper in New York City expressed opposition to the attack on Dr. Gross and his agency. (See G. Hawtin, J. Wells, and R. Pierson, "Bizarre Case of Dr. Gross' Accuser: What the Times Didn't Print." *New York Post,* Feb. 1, 1985:1). The *Times* stories provoked several public reviews of the office by state and federal authorities. The results corroborated some of the allegations of poor standards in the office, but uncovered no wrongdoing by Dr. Gross in the course of his forensic investigations.

Public charges have been leveled against some other medical examiners' offices across the country in recent years. However, in the later 1980s the great majority of state and metropolitan systems have managed to operate without public controversy under difficult conditions and often with restricted budgets reducing their effectiveness.

THE FORENSIC INVESTIGATION OF THE DEATH OF JOSEF MENGELE

An important report has been published in a highly respected American journal of forensic pathology summarizing the conclusions of an international group of forensic scientists who gathered in São Paulo, Brazil, in June 1985 to help identify a man who had died in a swimming accident some five years earlier.[1] The man was buried under the name "Wolfgang Gerhard," but he was believed to be Dr. Josef Mengele, the most hunted remaining war criminal of World War II – the "Angel of Death" of Auschwitz, who was personally responsible for thousands of deaths, many under the guise of scientific biomedical experiments.[2]

The story of the search for Josef Mengele is as strange and contradictory as it is sensational. The news reports of mid 1985 gave the impression that Mengele had always been one of the most notorious of the war criminals and had been sought continuously and relentlessly since the war's end in 1945. On the contrary, Mengele was not one of the most hunted figures among the Nazi fugitives immediately after the war. The victorious allies had concentrated on the most obvious of the leaders and administrators of the Nazi party, the military, and the government, even when it was the physicians' turn to be tried, in late 1946. (The indictments were handed down on October 25, 1946.[3]) The chief defendant among 23 indicted physicians was Karl Brandt, the head of the national health and medical services and a personal protégé of Adolf Hitler. The trials against the medical leaders and administrators focused primarily on the deaths and mutilations due to experimental programs on behalf of the armed forces and on the prewar and wartime euthanasia program. Among the other

From the *New England Journal of Medicine*
1986; 315:1071-1073.

defendants were several leading physicians in the Schutzstaffel (S.S.) of the Nazi Party who were responsible for administering the concentration camps. The most prominent was Karl Gebhardt, chief physician of the S.S., personal physician to the head of the S.S., Heinrich Himmler, and astonishing as it now seems, president of the wartime German Red Cross. Both Brandt and Gebhardt were among the seven physicians who received the death penalty for their crimes.

The medical defendants generally claimed one of two types of defense: (1) that they were merely acting under orders from higher authority, and (2) that the experimental activities were proper and justified as necessary scientific inquiries designed to aid the war effort. Much of the experimental work cited in the trials did relate to war activities, such as research on high-altitude exposure, sea-water exposure, incendiary-bomb explosion, and epidemic conditions such as jaundice, typhus, and malaria.[4] The first defense was uniformly disallowed throughout the trials but could be considered in mitigation of punishment in individual cases. The second defense caused the most searching legal and ethical inquiries of the entire "Medical Case." As a result, the prosecution produced the famous Nürnberg Code, a set of 10 principles of accepted practice in experimentation in humans, especially as applied to persons under constraint or imprisonment.[5,6] The first and most important of the principles was the requirement of free, informed consent of the experimental subject. The code produced at Nürnberg became the principal legal and ethical standard for all clinical investigations on a worldwide basis in the postwar years.[7] Not one of the defendants at Nürnberg was found to have complied with those principles.

Josef Mengele's name was not mentioned during the war-crimes trials. It was omitted for two reasons: first, he was not one of the high-level leaders of the Nazi party or the government structure; and second, his experimental efforts were of his own design and not related to an overall strategy or national conspiracy, as was alleged of the activities of virtually all the defendants. In my opinion, a trial of Mengele, with its narrower focus, would have presented great difficulties of proof in those early months of investigation after the war, when proof against even the major figures was not easily produced. By no means, however, were Mengele's crimes any less in number or heinousness. I have read the official records of the Medical Case against the 23 defendants and many other official and unofficial accounts of the medical atrocities in the concentration camps. None were worse than Mengele's. The undisputed accounts of his activities at Auschwitz are a revolting litany of depravity, torture, and death. Mengele is most often remembered by survivors as the swaggering, immaculately dressed captain of the S.S. who stood beside the railway cars after their arrival at the camp to select victims for his experiments.[8,9] Those he did not choose went immediately to their deaths in the gas chambers. Those he selected died more slowly at his hands in his laboratory. On several occasions, as he stood by the arriving freight cars of Jewish, Polish, Hungarian, and other discarded and condemned peoples of the Nazi-held territories in Eastern Europe, he took out his pistol and shot to death someone who offended him. Particular targets of his experimental zeal were twins and dwarfs. They died frightful, horrible deaths at his hands in senseless, purposeless experiments notable only for the precise detail with which they were recorded. In his laboratory were displayed openly the trophies of his crimes against humanity: human tissue and organs hung on the walls after being taken from victims, often before their deaths. One laboratory wall was described as almost totally covered with eyes taken from victims' bodies. (In his memoirs, Simon Wiesenthal called his chapter on Mengele, "The Man Who Collected Blue Eyes."[10])

Mengele made his escape from Auschwitz and disappeared into the chaos of a shattered Germany. He obtained his passage to South America in 1949 or 1950 and lived in Argentina under an assumed name until the mid 1950s, when he apparently became convinced that he would never even be sought, let alone returned to West Germany or Israel for trial. He took out identity papers in his own name and even traveled to Switzerland to see his only son, Rolf. He returned to Argentina and was in regular contact with the family business in West Germany until he became greatly frightened by the Israeli capture of Adolf Eichmann on the streets of Buenos Aires.[11] Mengele undoubtedly learned that the Israeli intelligence force had been seeking both Eichmann and himself in Argentina. The highly publicized Eichmann trial called attention to Mengele and his wartime atrocities, and he became, from the 1960s onward, a hunted man throughout South America. He fled from Argentina to Paraguay and then to Brazil, where he apparently settled in São Paulo in late 1961. He lived at different times with two families under the names Peter Hochbichlet and Wolfgang Gerhard. He died in an apparent drowning accident at

Bertioga Beach, a resort area some 40 miles north of São Paulo, on February 7, 1979.

Persistent reports of his death circulated in West Germany, Paraguay, and other countries over the next few years. West German police conducted rather leisurely investigations, surprising in their lack of urgency despite rewards for Mengele's capture amounting by then to over $3 million. In May of 1985, in Mengele's home city of Günzburg, police questioned a retired executive of the Mengele family business and discovered documents that seemed to show that Mengele was living in São Paulo.

The West German police notified federal law-enforcement authorities in São Paulo, who immediately investigated and discovered the family with which Mengele was said to have been living. The family quickly admitted that the man known as Gerhard was actually Josef Mengele. The police found that Mengele's son, Rolf, had come from West Germany to visit Gerhard twice. (The son had used his own name and passport both times.) The last visit was only a few days after the drowning accident in 1979. Contacted in West Germany, the son admitted to his part in keeping his father hidden in Brazil for nearly 20 years.

The Brazilian police were apparently convinced by the evidence they collected that Gerhard was the notorious Josef Mengele, and they released stories to that effect to the world press in early June 1985. Many groups, however, especially in Israel, expressed doubt about the accuracy of the report. The Brazilian police decided to exhume the body and offer undisputed proof of its identity. Confidence in the exhumation process was shaken at first when news photographs in the local and international press showed huge crowds of onlookers at the grave site and one of the official medical examiners holding the detached skull taken from the grave (the photograph is reprinted in Gerald Astor's recent book[2]).

Confidence was fully restored, however, when it was learned that the medicolegal investigation would be conducted under the direction of Dr. Rubens Brasil Maluf, the director of the Institute of Legal Medicine of the State of São Paulo, a highly respected independent investigatory agency in Brazil. A multidisciplinary team of Brazilian experts was formed, along with a group of forensic experts from West Germany and the United States to act as observers and advisers to the Brazilian team. The author of the report of the investigation, Wilmes

Roberto G. Teixeira, M.D., Ph.D., was a member of the Brazilian team and the coordinator of the foreign-observer group.

A preliminary report released in São Paulo on June 21, 1985, concluded that in the opinion of the Brazilian team, supported by the foreign observers, the skeletal remains were those of Josef Mengele "within reasonable medical certainty."[2] The conclusion was carefully worded. It is in accordance with the Anglo-American common law requirements for medical proof in a court of law and with accepted principles of law in Brazil and West Germany.

The report now published in the American journal supports the earlier conclusion, although it is still called a "preliminary forensic anthropological report."[1] The paper summarizes very well the findings of the handwriting and photographic experts and the work of a group who conducted a "psychological autopsy" of the deceased, as well as the very thorough efforts of the forensic anthropologists.

The handwriting experts examined documents, letters, and notes recovered from the house where "Gerhard" was living and compared them with materials known to have been written by Mengele previously. The experts, including the American observers, concluded that the Gerhard samples were definitely written by Mengele. West German photographic experts compared earlier photographs of Mengele taken in Germany with a number of photographs of Gerhard taken during the years he lived in Brazil and concluded, on the basis of 24 individual points of similarity, that Gerhard and Mengele were the same person. The anthropologic examination followed traditional, recognized procedures to determine the sex, age, race, and stature of the skeletal remains, which were cleaned, anatomically reconstructed, and subjected to thorough radiography. The sex was determined by examination of the pelvis, skull, femurs, humerus, and sternum. The age was determined to be "over 50" by examination of the pubic articular surfaces. Mengele's birth date, 1911, would have made him much older in 1979, however. Further examination of the remaining teeth raised the possible age to a range of 65 to 70. One of the foreign experts, Dr. Ellis R. Kerley, was asked to conduct a further microscopical investigation of cross-sections of the femur and tibia, and he set the age at 69 plus or minus 5 years. The race was determined to be Caucasoid by review of postcranial bones, examination of the femur and tibia, and review of the remaining hair. The stature was also found to be compatible with the known height of Mengele: approximately 1.7 m plus or minus 2.99 cm.

More precise identification of the remains as those of Mengele was aided by S.S. records of a dental chart and a history of a serious motorcycle accident, which had incapacitated Mengele for over a month with a fracture of the right hip bone. Particularly telling was a space between the upper central-incisor teeth. The teeth were now missing, but the space was easily established as being in the same place on Mengele's dental chart and in several photographs of "Gerhard." Evidence of the old hip fracture was found, along with later arthritic changes in the spine and the bones of the hands.

Two experts, Dr. Richard Helmer and Dr. Wilmes R.G. Teixeira, used photographic methods imaginatively and convincingly to reconstruct likenesses of Mengele from the skull, in profile and full-face; these likenesses are reproduced in Teixeira's report.[1] Teixeira summarizes the most telling anatomical evidence in his own photographic-anatomical reconstruction: (1) In the profile view, the fitting of the buccal rimae and the eye pupil exactly at the center of the orbital cavity; and (2) in the frontal view, the junction of the upper central incisors of the denture of "Gerhard" fitted perfectly into the space of the diastema, and most important, the pupils of each eye in the photograph were "millimetrically located" at the center of the orbital cavities. (These features are shown in a series of 16 figures, 9 in profile and 7 in full frontal view.[1]) Teixeira concludes that in the absence of fingerprints, which were not available, the photographic drawings and facial reconstructions and superimpositions "must be considered highly corroborative, almost conclusive evidence for personal identification" of the remains as those of Josef Mengele.[1]

After some 40 years, the identity of Josef Mengele and his death in Brazil in 1979 would seem to have been established clearly by fully adequate forensic scientific evidence. The unprecedented international, interdisciplinary effort was well worthwhile to bring to a close this chapter in the grim story of the crimes against humanity committed by so many in the concentration camps of Europe four decades ago.

REFERENCES

1. Teixeira WRG. The Mengele report. Am J Forensic Med Pathol 1985; 6:279-83.
2. Astor G. The last Nazi: the life and times of Dr. Joseph Mengele. New York: DI Fine, 1985:268, 271-2.

3. Trials of war criminals before the Nuremberg Military Tribunals: the medical case (October, 1946–April, 1949). Vol. 2. Washington, D.C.: Government Printing Office, 1949:171.
4. Mitscherlich A, Mielke F. Doctors of infamy: the story of the Nazi medical crimes. New York: Henry Schulman, 1949.
5. Ivy AC. The history and ethics of the use of human subjects in medical experiments. Science 1948; 108:1-5.
6. Curran WJ. Legal codes in scientific research involving human subjects. Lex Sci 1966; 3:65-73.
7. Beecher HK. Experimentation in man. JAMA 1959; 169:461-78.
8. Delbo C. None of us will return. New York: Grove Press, 1968.
9. Nomberg-Przytyk S. Auschwitz: true tales from a grotesque land. Chapel Hill, N.C.: University of North Carolina Press, 1985.
10. Wechsberg J, ed. The murderers among us: the Wiesenthal memoirs. New York: McGraw-Hill, 1967.
11. Harel I. The house on Garibaldi Street. New York: Viking Press, 1975.

COMMENTS

This column describes an international medicolegal investigation using the most advanced of scientific methods. Such highly organized operations are rarely put together to investigate a single death. As later columns in this chapter indicate, the expense of large interdisciplinary teams gathered from among top experts in several countries is usually feasible only in investigations of mass disasters involving hundreds of deaths.

There is no doubt that the Brazilian law-enforcement officials knew that the Mengele investigation could not be handled only as a local matter. This awareness was sharpened when it became clear that Israeli groups were skeptical about the early, premature publicity identifying Gerhard as Mengele. In order to bring the highest possible degree of credibility to the findings, an independent, international investigation was essential, and the plan that was finally put into operation will serve as a model for the organization of future medicolegal investigations of this kind.

Presidential Inability to Function: The Medicolegal Issues

There has been a substantial amount of commentary about the Twenty-fifth Amendment to the Constitution since President Reagan's colon operation for removal of a cancerous growth, a villous adenoma. Much of the analysis has been confusing and overly speculative. The letter sent to the Senate and the House by President Reagan, in which he transferred power to Vice-President Bush, did nothing to reduce the confusion and speculation. In fact, the letter provided an interpretation of Section 3 of the amendment that is not supported by the history of the amendment's adoption by the Congress. In this column, I would like to review some of the medicolegal aspects of this important change in our Constitution.

Sections 3 and 4 of the Twenty-fifth Amendment were intended to deal with different types of temporary inability to function in the presidential office, a crisis in government that was not adequately addressed in the original Constitution. The provisions of Section 3 of the amendment describe a procedure for coping with the least critical political scenario—one in which the President, when ill, would voluntarily invoke the devolution of powers to the Vice-President as "acting President" and, when recovered, would regain those powers voluntarily. Eisenhower's heart attack in 1955 was a model situation for the application of this section.[1,2] The debates in Congress over the amendment actually began shortly after that event.

In his letter to Congress at the time of his surgery, President Reagan asserted that after a consultation with his legal advisers, he was "mindful" of the "uncertainties" of the application of Section 3 to such a "brief and temporary period of incapacity."[3] The President

From the *New England Journal of Medicine*
1986; 314:300-301.

also said that he did not personally believe that the section applied to the immediate situation. On the contrary, the debates and the testimony of witnesses before Congressional committees indicate that the members of Congress were well aware of the potential use of the amendment under such circumstances. Moreover, in one of the most authoritative law review articles written about the amendment at the time of its adoption, Professor Richard Longaker specifically mentioned "temporary designation of the Vice-President as Acting President while a President is under anesthesia."[4] Longaker observed that this type of event was at the opposite end of a spectrum from a "temporary," voluntary designation that could be expected to be quite long or permanent because, for example, of a devolution of powers to the Vice-President when the President was in the later stages of a terminal illness. In fact, the implication that can be drawn from Longaker's article was that voluntary designation under Section 3 was probably most likely to occur in the simple (and politically least disruptive) situation of a period of anesthesia for a non-life-threatening operative procedure in which the President had substantial advance notice of his illness and had time to prepare the legal and political ground for the designation. Thus, the article suggested that Presidents Eisenhower and Johnson might have used the section during their respective operations (ileocolostomy and cholecystectomy), but that it was doubtful, for various reasons, that it would have been invoked during President Wilson's stroke or President Eisenhower's recovery after his cardiac infarction. In 1970, in the second edition of my medicolegal textbook, I adopted the Longaker position in my own analysis of the amendment.[5]

President Reagan has had two opportunities during his presidency to invoke the provisions of the amendment and has not done so either time. One was his recent operation. The other was the recovery period after the attempt by John Hinckley to assassinate him. The sudden attack by Hinckley, which resulted in unconsciousness and emergency surgery because of a bullet lodged close to the heart, obviously did not allow a voluntary devolution of power. As it happened, the recovery period after this event was remarkably short. Had the recovery period been more prolonged, however, and the President's condition more critical, the issue of invoking either Section 3 or Section 4 could well have been raised. Assassination attempts present complex and sensitive problems. The would-be assassin is, after all, likely to be acting to create a governmental crisis. If the suspicion were raised that an assassination attempt was part of a wide-ranging political conspiracy, there could be reluctance to move too quickly to devolve powers because of a fear that such a move might inflame the conspirators to take additional action.

Section 4 of the amendment is much more controversial than Section 3, and its provisions were the primary focus of the many years of consideration of the amendment in Congress before it was finally ratified in 1967. This section deals with the situation in which a President is unwilling or unable to devolve powers to a Vice-President and some action must be taken to remove the President from office. Like Section 3, Section 4 treats all removals as temporary, with the reason for devolution always based on a serious mental disorder, physical disability, or both. At the heart of the problem of applying such an involuntary removal was the designing of a mechanism to resolve dispute over the actual clinical condition and prognosis of an ailing President. The dispute over the President's condition would, in all likelihood, occur among such powerful figures in the government as the President, the Vice-President, the President's personal staff, Cabinet officers, and members of Congress. Who could resolve such a conflict peaceably? An early suggestion was to create an "inability commission" of respected medical experts, either as a standing body or as an ad hoc group named during a specific crisis. It was also suggested that the commission could include, along with medical experts, officials such as the chief justice of the United States and selected Cabinet officers such as the secretary of state. This proposal was weakened, but not abandoned, in 1958, when Chief Justice Earl Warren sent a letter to Congress in which he advised against involving any member of the Supreme Court in such a commission.[4] Ironically, the chief justice did not follow his own good advice in the 1960s, when he allowed himself to be appointed chairman of the commission investigating President Kennedy's assassination. As pointed out earlier, assassinations and assassination attempts probably create the most egregious crises involving the chief executive in this country.

The suggestion to create an inability commission was probably also weakened by the lack of experience at the federal level in the United States with centralized, nationally appointed medical or medicolegal standing commissions that have the authority to examine sensitive issues of mental or physical capacity, to deal with suspicious deaths, or to investigate sources of danger to human life. Many other countries do have national medicolegal commissions that deal with various issues of this nature, but the United States has neither centralized any of these issues at the national level nor developed any national framework for medicolegal investigation. At the time of President Kennedy's assassination, there were no federal laws that covered removal of his body from Texas or provided federal jurisdiction for criminal investigation and medicolegal postmortem examination. Since that time, Congress has made assassination, attempted assassination, and kidnapping of a President, Vice-President, President-elect, or Vice-President-elect a federal crime.[6,7]

When the issue of nonvoluntary devolution of presidential power was finally settled in Section 4, a much more complex mechanism was installed. However, contrary to common belief, the idea of an "inability commission" was not abandoned completely. Under Section 4, the initiative for action rests with the Vice-President. In order to remove the President, however, the Vice-President needs to have the concurrence of a majority of the President's Cabinet officers or a majority of "such other body as the Congress may provide." This latter phrase was intended to allow the Congress to establish an "inability commission" composed as the Congress saw fit. Congress has not yet established such a commission, although Section 4 gives it the responsibility to settle this issue in the event of a dispute.

I can suggest a scenario that I have not seen in any commentary on the amendment. In a highly publicized and heated confrontation between a President and a Vice-President with whom the President has had a serious political or personal disagreement, the President's Cabinet might be very reluctant to choose sides openly. To act against the President, or even to allow a "vote" to be taken among them, might be politically dangerous if the President recovered and regained the presidential powers (again, Section 4 allows only a temporary removal and an "acting" presidency). Under these circumstances, the Congress might be asked by the Vice-President and the Cabinet to establish an ad hoc commission composed largely of respected, politically nonpartisan medical experts, to decide the medical question of the President's level of dysfunction, if any, and the prognosis. The Congress could hardly resist such a request in view of the impasse that would exist in the executive branch if the President were to continue in office under a serious cloud concerning his capacity to function.

These issues and many other procedural and substantive problems of interpretation will undoubtedly continue to surround the application of Sections 3 and 4 of the Twenty-fifth Amendment, a part of the constitution that has not yet been invoked during any presidential term of office.

REFERENCES

1. Brownell H. Presidential disability. Yale Law J 1958; 68:190-220.
2. Feerick JD. Proposed amendment on presidential inability and vice-presidential vacancy. Am Bar Assoc J 1965; 51:915-7.
3. Text of President's letter. New York Times. July 14, 1985:1.
4. Longaker RP. Presidential continuity: the Twenty-fifth Amendment. Univ Calif Los Angeles Law Rev 1966; 13:532-63.
5. Curran WJ, Shapiro ED. Law, medicine and forensic science. 2nd ed. Boston: Little, Brown, 1970:214-6.
6. Public Law 89-141, amended by Public Law 97-285 and Public Law 97-308.
7. Forkosch MD. Presidential murder — the constitutionality of a statute making it a federal crime. Southwest Law Rev 1965; 19:229-38.

♦

COMMENTS

This relatively recent essay reflects an academic interest of mine in the development of the Twenty-fifth Amendment to the Constitution. As far as I know, no other medicolegal scholar has shown an interest in this subject. It seems to me that medicolegal specialists on both the legal and the medical sides of the interface between the disciplines should take a greater interest in this area. The political nature of the subject seems to have discouraged forensic medical inquiries. For a recent law-review analysis, see W.F. Brown and A.R. Cinquegrana, "The Realities of Presidential Succession: The Emperor Has No Clones" (*Georgia Law Journal* 1987; 75:1389-453). See also a recent book exploring presidential illnesses and the Twenty-fifth Amendment: K.R. Crispell and C.F. Gomez, *Hidden Illnesses in the White House* (Durham, N.C.: Duke University Press, 1988).

Medical Quacks and Murder with Words

A report was recently published[1] of a very unusual murder case[2] of special interest to physicians. It involves the first recorded murder conviction of a medical quack, who is alleged to have allowed an eight-year-old child to die of cancer while he fed her his fraudulent concoctions.

The case might never have been entered, let alone won before a jury, if it had not come into the hands of a lawyer later made the chief of the first "medicolegal section" ever established in a criminal-prosecuting agency in the United States. This unique section was established in the Los Angeles County District Attorney's Office in 1963 under Chief Deputy District Attorney John W. Minor.[3] One of the reasons behind the establishment of the section was this medical-quack murder case.

Mr. Minor asserts that the case, *People of California* v. *Phillips,* is the first successful prosecution of murder by words alone. The case rested on two key legal issues: the felony-murder rule and "proximate cause." Under the felony-murder rule, a defendant is guilty of murder if he kills a person while committing another felony, even if he does not intend to kill. He is guilty of murder even if he merely hastens death, even by only a few weeks. This was the theory of the prosecution. Phillips's defrauding of the Eppings had as one of its results the early death of their child. The prosecution contended that Phillips intervened just after the child's condition, embryonal rhabdomyosarcoma, was diagnosed. At that time it was entirely confined to the eye. An operation at the time might have saved her life or, it was contended, would have prolonged it beyond the time that she actually died. The parents were informed of the findings and were advised that an exenteration was necessary immediately. The Eppings consented to

From the *New England Journal of Medicine*
1964; 270:728.

the procedure, but before it could be performed they happened to talk with some other parents at the hospital, who told them that Dr. Phillips, a chiropractor, had cured their son of a brain tumor without surgery. The Eppings called Dr. Phillips, described the situation and asked if he could help. He is alleged by the prosecution to have replied, "Yes, absolutely!" The parents withdrew their daughter from the hospital and put her under Phillips' care. He treated her for some three weeks, during which the tumor grew considerably. The Eppings discharged Phillips when the tumor grew to the size of a tennis ball. They apparently did not again seek medical care but turned to Christian Science. The child died two months after Phillips was discharged from the case.

Is Phillips a murderer, even under the sometimes harsh murder-felony rule? Was his action a "proximate cause" of her death? How strong is the medical evidence to support the theory of the prosecution? The parents were not entirely uneducated; what is their responsibility?

The doctrine of "proximate cause" is one of the most baffling issues in American law. Many a physician finds in court that causation is the most important question upon which his testimony is desired. And yet the doctor often finds that what he means by "cause" is not what the lawyer means. Sometimes, the medical cause, or etiology, is broader than the interests of the court. At other times it is narrower. Under the law, more than one cause can be called "proximate" enough to result in legal liability. Aggravation of a preexisting condition also gives rise to legal liability, at least to the extent of the aggravation.

This matter of causation is no easier for law students to learn than for the physician to accommodate to in the courtroom. It is one of the major stumbling blocks of the first-year law-school course in torts, the law of civil damage suits.

Dr. Phillips was convicted of second-degree murder and faces a prison sentence of five years to life. The case is now on appeal, and very serious legal questions are involved that will not be settled for some months. No matter what the outcome of the case, however, it is notable in all its circumstances. It is evidence of a trend toward a more vigorous enforcement program against medical quacks. There have been two national conferences in the past few years devoted to this subject. Also, the *Phillips* case is part of a strong legal effort to protect children from a variety of harms in childhood. Some of these programs raise problems of reporting to authorities by attending physicians and pathologists. Currently, the "battered-child" reporting laws are receiving attention in this regard. But what obligations exist to report on actions such as those of Dr. Phillips if they come to the attention of a pathologist only at the time of the child's death? And what obligation is imposed on an attending physician or pathologist to report neglect or refusal of medical care by a parent? This is the other side of the coin of the "battered-child" cases. The Phillips case gives reason to raise these issues. They will be discussed more fully in later columns.

REFERENCES

1. Minor JW. Phillips case — new dimension in murder. J Forensic Sci 1964; 9(1): 1-10.
2. People of California v. Phillips, Superior Court of Los Angeles, No. 255480 (1962).
3. Biennial Report, 1961-1962 and 1962-1963, County of Los Angeles District Attorney, pp. 18, 19.

♦

COMMENTS

I have always considered the medicolegal issues raised in this essay as among the most interesting and provocative of any about which I have written for the *Journal*.

The California Supreme Court reversed the conviction of the chiropractor on his first appeal. In the face of a vigorous dissent the majority of the court held that the murder-felony rule could not be applied because the underlying felony, grand theft, was not generally considered to be a crime dangerous to human life; *People* v. *Phillips,* 51 Cal. Rptr. 225 (1966). On retrial the defendant was again convicted of second-degree murder. In this case the conviction was upheld on appeal by an appellate court that found that the murder conviction could stand because the defendant had maliciously "caused" the child's death by effectively discouraging or preventing her parents from seeking medical attention for her; *People* v. *Phillips,* 15 Cal. Rptr. 720 (1969), *cert. denied,* 396 U.S. 1021 (1970).

The attorneys engaged by both sides in this historic conflict of medicolegal standpoints had a part in making it noteworthy. John Minor, the imaginative and energetic prosecutor, who headed the pioneering medicolegal section in the District Attorney's Office in Los Angeles, is mentioned by name in the column, and the defense counsel was also nationally prominent. He was Melvin Belli, one of the most flamboyant trial attorneys in American history. Belli made his reputation primarily as a civil trial lawyer specializing in personal-injury litigation, including medical-malpractice suits. The *Phillips* case was one of his first efforts in the criminal field. Perhaps even more notorious, and just as unsuccessful, was his defense of Jack Ruby in his trial for the murder of Lee Harvey Oswald, the alleged assassin of President John F. Kennedy.

In more recent years, medicolegal opposition to the hawking of worthless cures for hopelessly sick children has been directed against the much publicized cancer drug laetrile. The first case to come to public attention was that of Chad Green, a child from Massachusetts who had leukemia. See J. Brant and J. Graceffa, "Rutherford, Privitera, and Chad Green: Laetrile's Setbacks in the Courts" (*Journal of American Social Law and Medicine* 1980; 6:151-71).

Several state legislative enactments and more than one court action have attempted to prevent action by the Food and Drug Administration to stop interstate shipment of laetrile as a worthless therapeutic compound. The legal arguments made to continue distribution and treatment with the compound were twofold: (1) it was a harmless natural substance, and (2) its use gave comfort and hope to desperate, hopelessly sick people for whom no cure was available. I have reviewed the laetrile controversy in another column reprinted in this collection ("Laetrile for the Terminally Ill: The Supreme Court Stops the Nonsense," Chapter 5).

The Inquest at Chappaquiddick into the Death of Mary Jo Kopechne: The Medical-Examiner System in Massachusetts

The long-delayed inquest into the death of Miss Mary Jo Kopechne on Martha's Vineyard on July 18, 1969, has now taken place. Also, the decision of the Pennsylvania Court denying the petition for an exhumation and autopsy has been passed down. Therefore, it seems appropriate to examine some of the medicolegal aspects of the case and its relevance to the administration of the medical-examiner system in Massachusetts.

No other case in modern times has been the occasion of so much local and national criticism of the Massachusetts system as has resulted from this heavily publicized tragedy.

In the first few days and weeks after the death, the major adverse comment was focused upon the failure to order and to conduct an autopsy. This soon spread to a general critique of the medical-examiner system, the method of political appointment by the governor, the lack of specific qualifications for medical examiners other than possession of a medical degree, the confusion of authority between the district attorney and the physician examiner, and the lack of a "chief" state medical examiner.

The attacks made upon the Massachusetts system were particularly ironic because in the past the Bay State system, the first in the United States in 1877, has usually been considered exemplary, particularly in comparison to coroners' offices operating in many other states.

From the *New England Journal of Medicine* 1970; 282:556-557.

From the legal standpoint, the Kopechne case has already produced some useful new interpretations of the basic law in this field. The opinion of the Massachusetts Supreme Judicial Court regarding the procedure for the inquest resulted, for the first time in our long history, in a fundamental examination of the rights of parties and witnesses called at such hearings. The court specifically engaged in a "general reappraisal of inquest procedure in the interest of making it conform more closely with certain constitutional views" of the U.S. Supreme Court regarding procedural safeguards.[1] The Justices required that this and all future inquests described as "investigational" rather than "accusatory" be closed to the public and the press, that witnesses be allowed to be accompanied and advised by legal counsel, and that the inquest documents, including the transcript of testimony, be impounded and not released unless ordered by the superior court after a decision is made concerning prosecution. The actual conduct of the hearing, including whether or not the attorneys for witnesses would be allowed to cross-examine other witnesses or to call their own additional witnesses, however, was left to the discretion of the district-court judge presiding at the particular inquest.

All the criteria laid down by the court, except the last, probably will find strong support among practicing attorneys. The failure to lay down more specific rules on examination of witnesses, however, leaves much power in the hands of local judges, with little guidance from the highest bench. It must be remembered that these municipal-level courts are not generally conducted with the formality and adherence to rules of evidence found at the superior-court level. Because of this, the judges need more guidance on procedure than would be required in the higher courts. The Supreme Judicial Court would seem to have been unwilling to suggest drastic changes in the inquest procedures, which have always been informal in nature, going back historically to coroners' inquests in the Massachusetts Bay Colony and to the ancient investigatory powers of coroners in England.

Massachusetts is not the only state in recent times to have its procedures for inquests challenged. In California strong attacks have been made on the refusal of coroners to allow cross-examination of witnesses in cases arising out of the Watts riots in 1965.[2]

The other important legal ruling in the Kopechne case was the refusal of the Court of Common Pleas in Luzerne County, Pennsylvania, to grant a petition to exhume Miss Kopechne's body and to order an autopsy. The court reaffirmed the general rule of all American jurisdictions that "The law will not reach into the grave in search of facts except in the rarest of cases, and not even then unless it is clearly necessary and there is reasonable probability that such a violation of the sepulchre will establish that which is sought."[3] The thoughtful opinion of Judge Brominski, which analyzes the medicolegal opinions offered on both sides in this hotly contested case, is well worth reading in full by anyone interested in this field.

Governor Francis Sargent has now reactivated a special commission to investigate the medical-examiner system that was first established in 1968 by former Governor John Volpe before he resigned to join the Nixon administration in Washington.[4] This commission is composed of three medical examiners, representatives of the Massachusetts Medical Society, the Massachusetts Bar Association, the Attorney General's and the District Attorney's offices, a university professor of pathology, and two appointments at large. The two at-large members are a newspaperman and a representative of the State Funeral Directors Association. The author of this column in the *Journal* has been appointed by Governor Sargent as special legal counsel to aid the commission in its investigation and to arrange public hearings of the commission.

It can be hoped that this commission will be able to examine this extremely important investigational system in Massachusetts. It has not been reexamined in a comprehensive way since its creation nearly one hundred years ago.

Finally, it might be pointed out that just this past year another New England state, Connecticut, amended its law to establish a chief medical examiner of the state, and a commission on medicolegal investigations. A bill to establish a chief medical examiner has already been introduced in Massachusetts as a result of the Kopechne case.

REFERENCES

1. Kennedy v. Justice of the District Ct of Dukes Cty, 252 NE 2d 201, at p 207 (1969).
2. Adler JN. Coroners inquests: the impact of Watts. UCLA Law Rev 1968; 15:97.
3. In re Kopechne, Court of Common Pleas of Luzerne Cty, Pa, no. 1114 of 1969, mimeographed opinion, p 4.
4. Executive Order no. 62, signed by Governor John A. Volpe, September 26, 1968.

COMMENTS

This commentary reviewed the system of medicolegal death investigation in Massachusetts, the first state in the United States to replace coroners with medical examiners. The *Kopechne* case received wide publicity because of the involvement of Senator Edward M. Kennedy, but it also illustrated the ineffectiveness and poor organization of the death-investigation program. At that time, the local medical examiners, all appointed directly by the governor, functioned entirely independently, with no state supervision or coordination. There were no special qualifications for the appointments and no on-the-job training.

It was not until 1978 that reform legislation was passed establishing an organized system under a chief medical examiner and a state commission on medicolegal investigation. I am glad to be able to report that at present all six New England states have adopted organized systems in which the chief medical examiners are required to be qualified forensic pathologists. For the current situation in Massachusetts, see S. Seligson, "The Medical Examiner System" (*Massachusetts Medicine* 1987; 2(2):30-6).

Medicine, Medicolegal Programs, and the Press: A Reassessment

Physicians generally tolerate the press and other mass media rather badly. They guard their patients' and their own privacy and confidentiality with a zealot-like intensity, even when the interest of the public in the matter may be very high. Usually, this ethical posture is quite justified, but it has its limitations. Physicians giving medical treatment to public figures have sometimes imposed too impenetrable a barrier around their patients – a white-gauze curtain – to the extent of actually distorting the true picture of the situation. Witness the protective screen of physicians around Presidents Woodrow Wilson and Franklin Roosevelt. This tradition was only broken and a new standard of disclosure and truthfulness established in more modern times by Dr. Paul Dudley White in caring for President Dwight Eisenhower in his heart attack and subsequent rehabilitation. At the time many physicians criticized Dr. White for the frequency of his medical bulletins and their often embarrassingly complete detail.

One area of medicine in which such reticence with the press has never been practicable is legal medicine. The arena of the forensic doctor has always been very public. The interest of the press, and now of television news, has always been very high in medicolegal cases. The specialist in legal medicine would not last long in his work if he did not cooperate with the representatives of the mass media in getting the legitimate story of a medicolegal investigation to the public in reasonable time and in reasonable detail. It was President Harry Truman who displayed the sign on his desk that people who could not "stand the heat" of the presidency should

From the *New England Journal of Medicine*
1977; 297:483-484.

stay out of that particular kitchen. In legal medicine, it could be said that physicians who cannot "stand the press" should not even begin such a medical career.

The publicity that constantly surrounds the forensic physician, especially if he is a publicly appointed, impartial expert whose reports are the primary authority on particular cases, can have its bad effects. The flattering attention can breed overconfidence and overreaching by the entrenched medical expert who becomes too sure of his own conclusions. It is almost inevitable that the press and popular writers will glamorize the forensic specialist who is "good copy" and tag him with the title of a medical Sherlock Holmes, the community's genius of scientific detection.

The limelight may be enjoyed from time to time, but the medicolegal practitioner often has paid a heavy price for it. The public display has been resented by other physicians formed in the more traditional mold. Medical faculties have found it difficult to evaluate professional and scientific merit and accomplishment in forensic medical science. The result has been that publicly active medicolegal practitioners have often become isolated from other medical fields. Some of the most famous of medicolegal figures in Europe and America have suffered this fate. They have satisfied the public need for impartial investigation and opinion, but have functioned in professional isolation, have contributed little to fundamental or applied research, and have rarely left trained associates to carry on their work after they have retired from the scene.

The importance of highly competent and impartial medicolegal work has never been greater than it is now in the mid 1970s. The general public is suspicious of government and of paid experts. Yet the control of information is greater today than ever before. There is a need for the medical profession and medical faculties to support effective forensic scientific programs of both service and research.

The medical community generally needs to reassess its attitude, and its practices, toward the press and other mass media. Newspapers and television have developed trained journalists on medical and medicolegal matters who are handling these subjects responsibly and effectively. Physicians can and should cooperate with the press in legitimate matters of public interest and concern. The forensic physician should be able to work with the press, but also maintain an independence of judgment and professional ties with his colleagues in practice and the universities. There are some excellent models of such medicolegal relations in America and Europe in recent years to prove that such an association is possible.

The media also have something to learn. Journalists tend to be too easily satisfied with a medicolegal report if it is prompt and reasonably clear in language. They do not look for inconsistencies or question opinions unsupported by factual observations and findings. They often fail to distinguish scientific determinations from reports based largely or entirely upon hearsay and other secondary sources. They often add credibility to an otherwise inconclusive and flimsy evaluation, or to an interim report never intended to close the investigation, to get a story published quickly.

Reporters should perhaps also take more time from the everyday coverage of the latest murder or rape or other violence to advocate better medicolegal services in their communities. Most medicolegal programs in this country are overworked and understaffed. They cannot keep up with routine requirements, all of them urgent, let alone do research and reflect upon their actions. Medicolegal programs could have done more effective research on problems that often came to them quite early in their development, such as child battering, sudden infant death syndrome, and many other types of environmental and industrial hazards, but most of the practitioners have been too busy to gather their experiences into logical patterns and to alert other researchers to follow up on their findings. There are examples to the contrary, of course, in which medicolegal practitioners have conducted their own research or have planted the seeds of important discoveries by others, but they only point to the potential for gain if these public resources were to be improved.

The press and other media would be among the first to gain from more effective medicolegal work in this country, since the primary function of these programs is to provide public knowledge about medical matters of serious concern to the general population. The relation between forensic medicine and the press is built on necessity, but it should be possible to make it a more positive and less destructive effort on both sides in the future.

COMMENTS

In this column, I took another opportunity to advocate improved medicolegal systems in the United States. This time, I sought the support of the public media in the effort. In the years that followed, the print journalists have often been very helpful in publicizing reform efforts in the field.

In the later 1980s, both newspapers and the television networks have become more sophisticated in the handling of scientific and medical news. However, there are still serious problems with in-depth coverage of complex medicolegal issues. The most obvious problems currently can be found in coverage of human-rights issues and public health requirements related to the epidemic of the acquired immunodeficiency syndrome (AIDS). A recent book explores media coverage of the field. See R. Shilts, *And the Band Played On: Politics, People and the AIDS Epidemic* (New York: St. Martin's Press, 1987).

The Acceptance of Scientific Evidence in the Courts

The Anglo-American common law has traditionally been uncomfortable with scientific evidence. Great reliance has been placed on the lay jury system and partisan advocacy to provide justice. The result, however, is often a rather unstudied lack of reality in the legal system. What is clearly accepted scientifically in the outside world has often been rejected inside the courtroom; and the reverse, brazen charlatanism, has been allowed to sway lay juries with procedures and opinions having little or no credibility in scientific circles.

An effort to provide reform in both these areas has been in progress over a long period of years and is based on the so-called *Frye* rule, which originated in the federal courts.[1] Under this rule, trial-court judges are instructed to allow into evidence the results of scientific tests or procedures only when they have been recognized as reliable and useful by the scientific community as a whole or by the part of the scientific community concerned with the procedure or technique. The trial judges are expected to make affirmative efforts on their own to ascertain the state of acceptance of the procedure in the appropriate scientific community. This can be done by examining the scientific literature and by calling nonpartisan, unbiased experts in the field in question to advise the court concerning the state of the art of the technological procedures whose results are offered in the court.[2] The judges may also have received information (not yet "evidence") from the contending parties regarding the science involved to support or deny admission into formal evidence. In addition, the trial judges must evaluate the competence of the particular witness to have per-

From the *New England Journal of Medicine*
1983; 309:713-714.

formed the test in question and to offer an expert opinion on the meaning and relevance of the results for the case in hand.

The development of the *Frye* rule has been fairly steady over recent years, with most of the appellate litigation being over its particular application, especially in rather obscure and limited fields of expertise, but not in regard to the basic wisdom of the rule itself. When the rule has been criticized at all, most commentary has been concerned with the potential for unnecessary strictness in the efforts to find consensus in the scientific community, thus barring from evidence useful technology that has still not been fully recognized in a wide-ranging scientific community.

This was the situation until the Supreme Court of Georgia, in an appeal from a murder conviction, examined some of the criticism of the *Frye* standard and rejected it outright as an "inappropriate method" for determining admissibility into evidence in courts of law.[3] For a unanimous court Justice Gregory referred scornfully to the *Frye* rule as requiring merely "counting heads" in the scientific community—a phrase used in one other federal decision.[4] Justice Gregory also observed that there were "wide variations in intradisciplinary opinions."

The alternative adopted to replace the *Frye* rule was to leave discretion in the hands of the trial court, requiring a substantially increased burden of proof that the scientific method or procedure offered had reached "verifiable certainty" in its results. This reliance on a personal determination by the trial judge was found preferable to "simply calculating the consensus in the scientific community." The *Frye* rule had never required scientific agreement that a technology had reached certainty in results. The original opinion was concerned with a much different level, the point at which an experimental technique or discovery had "crossed the line" to a "demonstrable stage" where it could be found to have gained "general acceptability" as reasonably reliable and useful in the particular field to which it was applied.[5]

The decision in Georgia, breaking away from over 50 years of structured efforts to conform evidentiary rules of the courts to scientific acceptance and credibility, has received attention from the trial bar. In a special symposium issue examining the subject of science in the courtroom, *Trial,* the newsmagazine of the Association of Trial Lawyers, highlighted the decision and its rejection of the *Frye* rule.[6]

The case had been decided too recently, however, to allow for any in-depth analysis of the opinion in the publication.

As it is contained in the *Harper* case, the Georgia high court's opinion does not seem to be a step forward in improving the condition of science in the judicial system. Cumbersome as it might have been at times and burdensome perhaps to some trial judges not accustomed to searching for scientific acceptability, the new rule in Georgia rejects all this effort and replaces it with the uncontrolled discretion of trial-court judges and a standard of scientific certainty virtually unattainable in practical application.

Under the new rule, the Georgia judges would be instructed in science very heavily by the partisan pleas of the contending parties. Perhaps because such presentations could lead to the acceptance of quack ideas from convincing, self-styled experts allegedly fighting against the entrenched principles of the great majority of the scientific community, the Supreme Court imposed this extreme burden of proof, which it called "verifiable certainty." Neither of these terms was defined in the opinion.

In an effort to find their meaning, we might examine the particular issues in the *Harper* case. The defendant had denied killing the victim, whose decomposed body was found in a field. There were no eyewitnesses to the killing (by gunshot), and the evidence against the defendant was circumstantial. The defendant's lawyer had his client examined by a psychiatrist, who conducted a series of "interviews" with the defendant, aided by injections of Amytal Sodium. At the trial, the psychiatrist testified that on the basis of these interviews he was willing to give his expert opinion that the defendant was telling the truth as he knew it in saying that he did not kill the victim. He was also of the opinion that the defendant had no loss of memory or unconscious blocking out of his memory concerning his participation in any killing.

The trial judge, after hearing the witness, excluded the testimony. As his reason, he stated that the use of "truth serum" was rejected by the majority of American state high-court decisions. There had been no precedent decisions on the admissibility of results obtained with "truth serum" in Georgia, but that state had rejected polygraph evidence of truthfulness unless the parties had previously agreed by formal stipulation not to challenge its admissibility.

The Georgia Supreme Court endorsed this determination by the trial-court judge. Furthermore, it asserted that such a technique would continue to be rejected until it could be found with verifiable certainty that "truth serum compels a person to tell the truth."

Psychiatric testimony has had its detractors in the courts, no matter what the issue at hand. When psychopharmacology has been added, the barriers to admissibility have often been raised to heights not observed with more traditional practices. It is doubtful that the psychiatrist witness made claims that the Amytal Sodium could compel the defendant, or any person, to tell the truth. As indicated, the psychiatrist had probably used the drug to relax the defendant and to help to remove any unconscious psychological blocking concerning past events. The defendant claimed no loss of memory throughout the investigation or on the witness stand, and he consistently denied the killing throughout the psychiatric interviews. The psychiatrist's testimony probably added little to his defense, although it could have hurt his case substantially had he broken down and admitted the killing during or after the interviews with the psychiatrist.

Among the worst aspects of this case as a model for future development was the fact that the Supreme Court of Georgia endorsed the method used by the trial court in rejecting this testimony. The judge may not have counted heads in the scientific community, but he certainly counted courts in the United States on their attitudes toward "truth serum." It is not at all explained why court acceptance should be substituted for scientific evaluation. Furthermore, many of these decisions were decades old and involved different uses of Amytal Sodium and even different drugs not related to psychiatric evaluations of the truthfulness of specific statements.[7]

This particular effort to apply science or behavioral medicine to a courtroom question involved that most sensitive of crimes, first-degree murder. It also concerned what is undoubtedly the most guarded of lay-jury prerogatives, assessing the credibility, the truthfulness, of witnesses. The greatest resistance to scientific intrusion has always been to the mechanization of the search for truth on the witness stand. Georgia's decision to abandon the rule seeking a means of accommodation with acceptable scientific inquiry must be seen in the context of these sensitivities in the judicial system.

REFERENCES

1. Giannelli PC. The admissibility of novel scientific evidence: Frye vs. United States, a half-century later. Columbia Law Rev 1980; 80:1197-230.
2. Davis KD. Judicial notice. Columbia Law Rev 1955; 55:945-83.

3. Harper v. State, 293 S.E.2d 389, Georgia (1982).
4. U.S. v. Williams, 443 F.Supp. 269. Affirmed, 583 F.2d. 1194. *cert. denied,* 439 U.S. 1117 (1979).
5. Frye v. U.S., 293 F.1013 (1923).
6. Georgia rejects *Frye* standard. Trial 1983; 1:10-1.
7. Curran WJ. Expert psychiatric evaluation of personality traits. Univ PA Law Rev 1955; 103:999-1030.

♦

COMMENTS

The American courts have never dealt well with, or even been very comfortable with, scientific evidence, as I have frequently had occasion to point out in *Journal* columns over the years. The *Frye* rule laid down by the federal courts has represented the best of a poor crop of precedents in the field. The Georgia case examined in this essay is the worst attempt at improving on the *Frye* rule—in the wrong direction.

For a survey of decisions in the field, see P.C. Giannelli, "The Admissibility of Novel Scientific Evidence: Frye vs. United States, a Half-Century Later" (*Columbia Law Review* 1980; 80:1197-230). Several alternative plans have been proposed. See A.A. Moenssens, "Admissibility of Scientific Evidence: An Alternative to the Frye Rule" (*William and Mary Law Review* 1984; 25:545-75); E.J. Imwinkelried, "The Standard for Admitting Scientific Evidence: A Critique from the Perspective of Juror Psychology" (*Villanova Law Review* 1983; 28:554-71); and Student Note, "The Frye Doctrine and Relevancy Approach: An Empirical Evaluation" (*Georgia Law Journal* 1986; 74:1469-90).

Forensic Medical Science: The Continued Problems of Judges and Juries

A little noticed but disturbing confrontation between forensic medical scientists and the American judge and jury system occurred in a New York City courtroom in the past year.

The trial was a dramatic situation. The male defendant was charged with the brutal murder of a woman. When he was arrested, blood was found on his jacket. He claimed it was his own, caused by bleeding when he injected himself with heroin. The classic problem of forensic science over the years was again presented: a matter of identification. The prosecution was challenging the defendant's statement by an attempt to show that the blood was female and compatible with that of the victim. The courtroom was unusually quiet and businesslike, since the judge had excused the jury while he heard the scientific evidence hotly contested on both sides. It was a transcontinental confrontation. The prosecution's experts were from Los Angeles; the defendant's were all from New York City. If the judge himself were to determine that the prosecution's scientific contentions were not "competent" and "reliable" under law, the jury members would never even be allowed to hear the evidence or to decide for themselves whether they believed it or not.

What was at issue? The police, using proper investigative techniques, had preserved the evidence, but for some strange reason, the prosecution's experts had not analyzed the blood stains until 22 months later. Dr. Thomas Noguchi, chief medical examiner for Los Angeles, and Dr. Omar Alfi, director of the Cytogenic Laboratory at Children's Hospital in Los Angeles, testified that in their opinion the blood was Type O and female, the same as that of the

From the *New England Journal of Medicine*
1976; 294:1042-1043.

victim. The defendant's blood was also admittedly Type O. Three different tests were conducted that were explained at length in Judge Kapelman's carefully written opinion.[1] They were all examinations of the nuclear sex chromatin material of the cells by the F or Y body test, the drumstick test, and the Barr-body test. Dr. Noguchi testified that all three were accepted in the scientific community, and all had confirmed that the blood was female. However, he admitted that he knew of no other studies of dried blood of this age, or of the interaction of such blood with the chemicals in jacket fiber as in this case. He indicated that a member of his staff in California, a Dr. Ishizu, was currently working on these problems, but had not performed tests on dried blood older than 10 months up to that point.

The defense called three witnesses. The first was an assistant professor of medicine at New York University who was a hematologist specializing in genetic studies. He asserted that he had no experience with one of the tests, the F or Y body test, but was familiar with the other two. He concluded that the cells available were too few in his judgment to allow him to make a reliable identification of the sex of the blood. He said that "where there was an important decision dependent I would require the test be repeated with additional cells provided." The second witness, a full professor at New York University and head of its division of human genetics, testified that extensive controls were needed to identify the sex of aged, dried blood, and, like the previous witness, he found the number of cells available for examination too few to allow him to make a judgment. The last witness was obviously saved to strike the heaviest blow against the prosecution's case. As identified in the judge's opinion, he was "an expert in hematology and in the examination of blood stains and blood smears." His name was Dr. Alexander S. Weiner, and he was described as chief serologist for the City of New York. Actually, this was a judiciously modest description of one of the nation's foremost forensic scientists, a member of the New York City Medical Examiner's Office for nearly 40 years. It seems hardly possible that the trial judge, a New York City jurist, after all, was not very familiar with Dr. Weiner and his experience and reputation.

Dr. Weiner indicated that identification of sex is difficult even from fresh white blood cells and that such identification made only from dried blood is "unrewarding" because the cells are extremely damaged and unrecognizable. In a rather surprising statement, however, he admitted that he had never heretofore even investigated sex analysis from dried blood. His first effort was in this case in cooperation with the second witness when he examined the blood stains in question here. He testified that he could not recognize the cell components in the cells he examined.

On the basis of the evidence presented, Judge Kapelman rejected the prosecution's contentions and threw out the testimony of Drs. Noguchi and Alfi as without acceptance in the scientific community, as incompetent, and as unreliable. The jury was recalled to the courtroom and never heard the evidence.

It should be recalled that under American law, a trial judge's powers to throw out evidence as too weak and unreliable to be heard and weighted by a jury is very limited. He cannot rule it out on the basis of its relative weight in comparison to that of other witnesses. For example, the judge here could not himself rule out Dr. Noguchi's testimony because Dr. Weiner was better known and more highly respected by the courts in New York. These are always issues for the ultimate trier of fact, the jury, to decide.

I do not wish to argue about the weight of the evidence here; I have trouble with it myself. I should also like to have known more about some other questions left unanswered or unraised in this opinion: the reason for the 22-month delay; the need of the prosecutor to go 4800 km for his experts; and other matters. However, I cannot but note that this 9½-page opinion ends with a paragraph that asserts,

> This Court cannot stress too much its fear of undue prejudice to the defendant in the receipt of this questionably accepted scientific testimony. The People's case in chief is bottomed solely upon circumstantial evidence. The admission of this testimony, with a seeming scientific imprimatur, pointing to female blood on the defendant's jacket in contradiction to the defendant's claim that the blood was his blood, would in the Court's view be highly prejudicial to the defendant, far outweighing its probative value.[2]

Here is the real key to the decision, the sensitive nerve end of the jury system exposed in this confrontation. The trial judges are often afraid to allow juries to weight scientific evidence along with the other order of things and existences that they meet in our tightly controlled courtrooms — like so-called eyewitnesses and self-serving statements by interested parties and police and all sorts of other human beings, usually much less reliable, in and out of court, than "circumstantial evidence."

My primary concern here is with the classic barrier, the most difficult legal test, for any forensic science to pass before the trial judge: that of general acceptability in the scientific community. The field is so pitifully small and specialized that it is almost impossible even to apply the concept, let alone to surmount it. This case is an excellent example of what I mean. Medical-school and hospital-based hematologists and geneticists just do not have occasion to deal with dried blood on men's jackets, and do not have to analyze such small samples of blood, fresh or old. They have ample blood available from willing patients along with fully adequate controls, and when in doubt, they nearly always repeat the whole procedure, anyway. (Any patients among my readership will agree with that statement.) Forensic scientists do not have these luxuries. They have to deal with scraps and traces and single chances at analysis. They have to deal with murder and rape and the indifference and callousness of so many people to the growing violence of our times.

Forensic scientists are not asked to deal with old blood stains that often either. Most of the police simply are not trained to collect evidence that well, or to preserve it, in any but the most serious cases in certain of our largest cities. We need to pool the knowledge gained in the few good laboratories and to support effective forensic-science research. A recent national survey of the state of the art in forensic science, the first ever conducted in the United States, concluded that most laboratories "do not have time to engage in research, per se."[3] Most of them cannot get the city and state officials to give them any money or positions for research. Very few of these facilities are associated with universities in America, as they are in continental Europe with the institutes of legal medicine. I have found the attention given to work in forensic blood chemistry to be much greater in Europe than in the United States.

Readers of my writings have heard me sound this call before, most recently for the forensic examination of former President Nixon's physical capacity to give testimony in the Watergate trial of his White House associates. I keep sounding the message, but it does not seem to be heard in very many places. I say it again. We need to improve vastly the quality of legal medicine and forensic science in the United

States, for the safety of all of us and for the sake of effective justice for all, victims and defendants alike, in our courts.

REFERENCES

1. People of the State of New York v. Alston, 362 New York Supplement, 2nd Series 356.
2. Opinion,[1] 365.
3. Field KS, Schroeder O, Curtis IJ, et al. Assessment of the personnel of the forensic science profession: final report of research project. Conducted by the Forensic Sciences Foundation, Inc., 11400 Rockville Pike, Rockville, Md., 1975:V-4. (Department of Justice grant no. 73-NI-99-0052-G.)

♦

COMMENTS

In retrospect, it seems to me that this essay expressed my personal standpoint more effectively than the other columns on medical-examiner systems collected earlier in this chapter, because the case examined here typified the sort of situation in which the medicolegal dilemma most frequently made itself apparent. The judge was reluctant to allow a mere "scientific test" to rebut the defendant's testimony in a murder case. The criminal charge was too grave, the punishment too great, to allow "speculative science" to prevail over the lay jury's common-sense deliberations. The judge feared that the scientifically uneducated jurors would be unduly influenced by the "science" of the prosecution.

This case also illustrated the continued weakness of even the largest of the medicolegal offices, those in New York City and Los Angeles, in conducting forensic scientific research. The service demands on these offices in large metropolitan areas were so unremitting that there was at that time little encouragement or budget for research.

For a general review of the problems of applying forensic scientific evidence in the courts, see the latest edition of my law school textbook, W.J. Curran and E.D. Shapiro, *Law, Medicine and Forensic Science* (3rd ed. Boston: Little, Brown, 1982:138-220). It is also instructive to examine the legal issues as they relate to specific scientific fields. For example, see A.E. James, "The New Medical Imaging Techniques as Evidence" (*Journal of Contemporary Law* 1984;

11:105-31); E. Margolin and S. Coliver, "Forensic Uses of Hypnosis: An Update" (*Trial* 1983; 19(10):44-50, 105-6); R.E. Gaensslen, *Sourcebook in Forensic Serology, Immunology and Biochemistry* (Washington, D.C.: Government Printing Office, 1983); H.C. Lee, "Identification and Grouping of Blood Stains," in R. Saferstein, ed., *Forensic Science Handbook* (Englewood Cliffs, N.J.: Prentice-Hall, 1982); and J.S. Levkov, "A Method for the Determination of MN Antigens in Dried Blood" (*Journal of Forensic Sciences* 1987; 32: 357-63).

Scientific Evidence and the Watts Riots

The court of appeals in California has recently decided a very important case involving the acceptability in court of a new scientific test known as a "voiceprint." The technique consists of a spectrographic, stylus-traced recording of the voice of a person developed from a sound recording on tape. In *The People* v. *King,*[1] the court refused to allow a criminal conviction to stand based on personal identification as a result of a voiceprint. The court held that the technique had not reached a sufficient level of scientific acceptability, particularly since it was still basically the theory and practice of one man.

Essentially, this is the bare-bones, or "black letter" law, of the *King* case. As such, it is a quite significant holding. However, just as there is always a difference between medical science in the laboratory and a living, clinical patient, so there is much more to this courtroom confrontation of the State of California versus one Edward Lee King.

The case arose out of the so-called Watts riots in Los Angeles in 1965. The Columbia Broadcasting System (CBS) did a nationwide documentary television program on the riots on December 7, 1965, and during the show portrayed an unidentified young black man whose voice was heard but who was not shown on camera. The youth made a number of incriminating statements about his own role in the riots and in the starting of fires, particularly that at a Thrifty Drug Store at Central and Washington streets in Watts. After the showing of the film, the Los Angeles police began a vigorous investigation to find the speaker. The CBS people and the announcer, Bill Stout, refused to disclose the name or other identification. On December 25, 1965, the defendant was arrested and booked on a narcotics charge. His property was taken, including a wallet that contained the

From the *New England Journal of Medicine*
1969; 280:771.

business card of the CBS cameraman who had filmed the documentary, a piece of paper with the name of the producer of the film, and a watch and ring later claimed to be identified in the film. The police suspected that King might be connected with the film and the mysterious speaker. They took him to a county jail interrogation room, which was secretly wired to record his voice. They interrogated him on the Watts riots, but got no further evidence from him. However, they took the tape of the interview, which was recorded without his knowledge or consent, and had a "voiceprint" made of it for identification purposes.

At the very long trial of King on an arson charge nearly one year later, the main case against the defendant consisted of the expert-opinion evidence of Mr. Lawrence Kersta, the originator and primary authority on the voiceprint technique. Mr. Kersta testified that the voiceprint was very highly reliable and that no two persons will produce identical voiceprints. He asserted that his technique and his machines have the accuracy of fingerprints in making a personal identification. He testified that he had made voiceprints of the soundtrack of the CBS film and of the defendant's voice taped in the jail interview and that in his opinion the voices were of the same man. The defense brought in a series of experts, all of whom disagreed with Kersta's testimony and challenged the reliability of the voiceprint technique. The trial court admitted the evidence, and the jury convicted King of arson and sentenced him to the state prison.

As indicated earlier, the intermediate appellate court reversed the conviction and threw out the voiceprint as scientifically unreliable. The court denied the defendant's objection to the evidence as violating his constitutional rights against self-incrimination. It held that compelling an accused to repeat words for identification purposes is not incriminating, but "an identification of physical characteristics."

In its finding, the court has agreed with a ruling to the same effect by the superior court in New Jersey earlier in 1968.[2] The only court of record in the United States that has upheld the admission into evidence of a voiceprint is a case in the U.S. Air Force Board of Review.[3] There was a vigorous dissent even in this case.

The courts of this country have generally been cautious about admitting scientific evidence concerning personal identification. There is a long history of the court review of such tests as fingerprints, handwriting, blood grouping, x-ray films, dental charts, and microscopic trace evidence. The battle over the polygraph has been the most hard fought, of course, since this test challenges one of the major issues in all courtrooms, the credibility of the parties and witnesses.

The *King* case brought "science" into the courtroom on the side of the prosecution against defendants in the Watts race riots. There has also been concern about a number of coroner (medical examiner) appearances in Watts riot cases involving police officers charged with killing rioters. The *King* case brought the mass media of television into the courtroom against a single criminal defendant in a mass racial disturbance. We have probably not seen the last of all this.

REFERENCES

1. 72 Ca. Rptr. 478 (1968).
2. State v. Cary, 99 N.J. Super. 323 (1968).
3. U.S. v. Wright, 17 U.S.C.M.A. 183, 37 C.M.R. 447 (1967).

COMMENTS

As indicated in this column, the earlier court decisions generally excluded voiceprint evidence as a means of identifying specific individuals. The turning point came in an important decision passed down in Massachusetts in 1975, which applied the *Frye* rule and found that voiceprint technology was accepted in the scientific community. See *Commonwealth* v. *Lykus,* 367 Mass. 191 (1975). For a reasoned defense of the concept of admitting voiceprint technology into court, see H.F. Greene, "Voiceprint Identification: The Case in Favor of Admissibility" (*American Criminal Law Review* 1975; 13: 171-200). See also the text by the original scientific developer of voiceprint technology, O.I. Tosi, *Voice Identification: Theory and Legal Application* (Baltimore: University Park Press, 1979). See also O.I. Tosi, "Fundamentals of Voice Identification," in W.J. Curran, A.L. McGarry, and C.S. Petty, eds., *Modern Legal Medicine, Psychiatry, and Forensic Science* (Philadelphia: F.A. Davis, 1980). See also H. Hollien, "Forensic Communication: An Emerging Specialty" (*Criminal Defense* 1983; 10:22-9); and H. Hollien, L. Geison, and J.W. Hicks, Jr., "Voice Stress Evaluators and Lie Detection" (*Journal of Forensic Sciences* 1987; 32:405-18).

Medical Patient Management and Confessions to Crime

An important decision from the Supreme Court of California concerning confessions illustrates how poor medical management can substantially affect a criminal case. The case concerns the prolonged attempt in that state to convict the defendant, William Cameron, of the murder of Mrs. Vivian Malone on December 22, 1958.[1]

The defendant has had three jury trials, two resulting in jury disagreements and the third in a conviction of murder in the first degree. Nine years after the crime, the supreme court in a split (four to three) decision threw out the conviction on the grounds that the confessions obtained from Cameron while he was under the influence of alcohol and chlorpromazine were "involuntary."

All the principals in the case lived in a trailer park. On the evening of the crime, Cameron, Mrs. Malone, and another friend were engaged in a drinking bout in Mrs. Malone's trailer. The friend left about 11 p.m. Shortly afterward, Mrs. Malone vainly tried to persuade Cameron to leave. She allegedly began to call him foul names and, in an effort to get him out, may have kicked him in the groin. The defendant's recollection from this point is vague. He remembers being kicked, but not by whom. He remembers standing over Mrs. Malone's body and seeing blood. He went to his friend's trailer and said he thought he had killed Mrs. Malone. The friend called the police.

The police came and found Mrs. Malone's mutilated body in the trailer. Cameron was arrested and taken to the station for interrogation. Liquor was smelled on his breath, and so, before the interview, he was examined by a physician. A blood sample indicated a blood

From the *New England Journal of Medicine*
1969; 280:1008.

alcohol level of 0.18 percent. The physician nevertheless gave it as his opinion that the defendant was mentally competent to be interrogated. Questioning began at about 1 a.m. During the interview, he broke down and cried and asked to be shot. The assistant district attorney, fearing a suicide attempt, stopped the interrogation and ordered him taken to the county hospital for a mental examination.

At the hospital, the physician in charge, not knowing that the defendant had a high blood-alcohol level, ordered him sedated with an injection of 300 mg of chlorpromazine at about 3:30 a.m. Later he justified this very heavy medication on the grounds that the man was being held on a murder charge and that he, the physician, was "quite concerned for the safety of his staff."

The next morning, Cameron was taken to a state mental hospital by the police. The assistant district attorney told the two psychiatrists there that the defendant had been "given sodium amytal" at the hospital the night before. No medical records accompanied the patient, and the psychiatrists did not call the county hospital. At about 11 a.m., an interrogation, with the two psychiatrists as witnesses, took place at the state hospital, and Cameron confessed to the crime and described the mutilations. That afternoon, the defendant was again questioned, this time with the use of a polygraph, and he again confessed. He later gave at least two more confessions.

The majority of the Supreme Court of California found that the three confessions taken after the injection of chlorpromazine were involuntary because of the effect of the alcohol and the drugs in creating a "don't care" attitude in the defendant. Chief Justice Traynor concluded that the defendant's "will to resist was destroyed because he was unable to comprehend the seriousness of his predicament or the significance to him of acceding step by step to 'remembering' the prosecution's reconstruction of his crime."

There was a strong dissent to these findings. However, the majority prevailed, and a new trial was ordered.

Three different physicians were given medical charge over the defendant in less than 24 hours. None knew what the others had done, and none asked. No competent medical history was taken. No delays in the interrogations were requested by the physicians on *medical* grounds to allow examinations and histories to be taken and to allow the effects of the alcohol and the vigorously applied "medication" to wear off. The physicians were greatly influenced by the severity of the criminal charges and allowed the police and the district attorney's office to carry on these interrogations with characteristic haste and inadequate medical advice. Now, 10 years later, the defendant, who was a 22-year-old college student at the time of the murder, and who had had no previous criminal record of any kind, will be returned to the lower court for his *fourth murder trial.* If any case illustrates the need for better medicolegal handling of criminal cases, this is it.

REFERENCE

1. In re Cameron, 67 Cal. Rptr. 529 (1968).

♦

COMMENTS

This column describes the most flagrant example of bungled medicolegal case management that I ever had occasion to describe in any of my writings. The situation appears to have been that an obviously guilty young man wanted to confess and did so repeatedly in a variety of circumstances, but the prosecutors and the medical and psychiatric consultants seemingly made such a mess of the interrogations that the evidence was tainted and therefore inadmissible. The real tragedy was that it took 10 years of litigation to reach even this highly unsatisfactory conclusion.

In more recent years, the handling of defendants in such situations has improved and more voluntary confessions are being accepted by the courts as properly obtained. The reason for this is that under later Supreme Court rulings more sophisticated procedural practices have become routine in law enforcement and prosecution. The polygraph is also used to support or contradict evidence obtained in confessions. See J.A. Matte, *The Art and Science of the Polygraph Technique* (Springfield, Ill.: Charles C Thomas, 1980); D. Lykken, "Psychology and the Lie Detector Industry" (*American Psychologist* 1974; 29:725-39); and I. Nachshon and B. Feldman, "Voice Indices of the Psychological Stress Evaluator" (*Journal of Police Science and*

Administration 1980; 8:40-53). See also G. Ben-Shakhar, M. Bar-Hillel, and I. Lieblich, "Trial by Polygraph: Scientific and Juridical Issues in Lie Detection" (*Behavioral Science and the Law* 1986; 4: 459-79).

Religious Objection to a Medicolegal Autopsy

Maryland was the first state in the United States to adopt an organized, statewide medical-examiner system under a chief medical examiner in its 1939 law.[1] It was also the first of the colonies on the American continent to appoint a coroner. The year was 1637. It took until the Bicentennial Year of 1976, however, and in an opinion printed late in the year, for that state to decide judicially the important constitutional issue of whether religious objections on the part of next of kin could prevent a statutorily required medicolegal autopsy. A Maryland intermediate appellate court has decided that the public interest in having answers to the question of the cause of death in a suspicious or unexplained case covered by the law was paramount to the religious objection of the deceased's father.[2] The highest court of Maryland refused to review the case on a writ of certiorari and so allowed the decision to stand as the law of Maryland and as an important precedent for other states.

The facts of the case are fairly simple. The father picked up his 18-year-old son at school around 1 p.m. The boy and his father were together the rest of the afternoon. They walked about the house. The two were "kidding around" and testing a new electric heater, which gave off a stench. The boy said, "I'm going to get out of here." He went to his room. The father heard a thud. The mother and father went to the boy's room, and when they got there, they found him dead. There was no explanation for the death. The boy was apparently healthy and did not suffer from heart disease or any other chronic condition. He was taken to a hospital, which called the local medical examiner at about 7:15 p.m. The police were also investigating the case. A cursory examination of the body at the hospital revealed nothing as a cause of death. The medical examiner ordered an autopsy.

From the *New England Journal of Medicine*
1977; 297:260-261.

The family of the boy, being Orthodox Jews, opposed the autopsy as against their religious beliefs and practices and filed a suit for an injunction to prevent the autopsy. The agonizingly slow procedures of justice were greatly accelerated in this case, both for the benefit of the family and for the sake of a reasonably fresh postmortem examination. A plenary hearing on the injunction was conducted on the same day. The relief was denied, and an appeal was immediately filed with the Court of Special Appeals and a hearing was ordered and held the next day. The four-judge bench issued an order further denying the injunction, but staying the autopsy itself until the family could appeal to the highest court of Maryland. The court of appeals denied the motion to stay one day later, January 22, and denied petition for a writ of certiorari on February 2, thus ending all appeals.

The opinion of the intermediate appellate court was issued about a month afterward and is the only official opinion in the case. It was printed later in the court reports.

In the opinion by Chief Judge Orth no previous precedent directly in point was cited from Maryland or any other jurisdiction. The court reviewed the statutory grounds for an official medicolegal autopsy and found the case clearly to be covered therein. It was therefore agreed that the autopsy was properly ordered under the classification of a death of a person "suddenly when in apparent health and when unattended by a physician."[3]

The argument of the family was that the autopsy would interfere with their freedom of religion under the first amendment to the U.S. Constitution and Article 36 of the Declaration of Rights in the Maryland Constitution. The court agreed that the family was free to believe as they chose, but not to practice their religion without certain controls in the interest of "the good order, peace or safety of the State." Even though it was granted that the parents were entitled to control of their son's body as next of kin, their property right was held to be a matter of fiduciary trust for the purpose of burial or other disposition of the body. Their property right in the body and their right to practice their religion were held to be subordinate to the state's authority to investigate an unexplained death. In this case it was held that the cause of death could only be determined beyond a reasonable doubt by an autopsy.

The autopsy was performed, and it was clearly revealed that the death was from natural causes, though the delay in the examination left something to be desired in the evidence that could be produced. No criminal or civil charges resulted, and no public health hazard was revealed.

After this decision came down, an effort was made in the legislature of Maryland to limit the powers of the medical examiners in cases of religious objection to an autopsy. Realizing the strongly held beliefs of the proponents of the bill, Chief Medical Examiner Russell Fisher did not stand on previous law or the decision reported on herein. He agreed to an amendment to the law that now requires that in cases of religious objection, any autopsy order by a local (deputy) medical examiner must be reviewed and approved by the chief medical examiner as proper under the law before it can be performed. This compromise did not fully satisfy the religious objectors, but it does ensure consideration of their views in individual cases.

REFERENCES

1. Laws of Maryland, 1939, Chapter 369.
2. Snyder v. Holy Cross Hospital, 30 Md. App. 317 (1976).
3. Maryland Code, Article 22, Section 6 (4).

♦

COMMENTS

It is surprising how few legal challenges there have been to the sweeping powers of medical examiners and coroners to order and conduct mandatory postmortem examinations, including complete autopsies and examination of body tissues and fluids. Today the ruling in the *Snyder* case remains the only high-court decision in which the constitutional issues are analyzed and the exercise of discretionary powers found to be constitutionally valid.

Two other states, New York and Florida, have since enacted statutes that place controls on mandatory postmortem examinations. The Florida law was enacted after a court in that state severely limited the discretionary powers of local medical examiners to order autopsies, even in situations in which there was no religious or other objection by next of kin. The court disallowed autopsies based on mere "suspicion" by the medical examiner and ruled that only "necessary" autopsies could be conducted, in cases in which foul play was quite evident. See *Rupp* v. *Jackson,* 238 So.2d. 86, Fla. (1970). The medical examiner involved in the case published a paper decrying the result of this Florida decision. See J.C. Rupp, "Death of a Medical Examiner System" (*Journal of Forensic Sciences* 1971; 16:420-7).

The Florida statute was designed to counteract the effect of the court decision. The new law authorized local medical examiners to order and conduct autopsies under 12 conditions quite commonly listed in medical examiner–coroner legislation all across the United States (Fla. Ann. Statutes, Section 406.11).

In 1984, after two decisions by courts in that state had, in the face of religious objections by next of kin, limited public investigational autopsies to situations in which the examination was "necessary" to discover illegality or foul play, the New York State Legislature enacted a statute concerning mandatory postmortem examinations. The New York law codifies the requirement of "compelling public necessity" for autopsies to which religious objections are made. The statute defines the required "necessity" as present in any of three situations: (1) when the autopsy procedure is essential to a criminal investigation of homicide in which the deceased was the alleged victim, (2) when the autopsy procedure is necessary to the discovery of a cause of death involving an "immediate and substantial threat to the public health," and (3) when the autopsy procedure is authorized by virtue of the statutory powers of official medical examiners under the state law for medical-examiner systems. (N.Y. Public Health Law, Section 4210-C.)

Damage Suits against Medical Examiners

The increasing vulnerability of physicians to damage suits, usually malpractice actions, has frequently been pointed out in this column. It now seems clear that medical examiners and coroners' physicians carrying out officially authorized or ordered medicolegal autopsies are also subject to these risks. A recent column discussed a suit in Maryland to prevent a medicolegal autopsy on religious grounds.[1] The Maryland court upheld the constitutionality of conducting legally authorized medical-examiner autopsies without consent of the next of kin, even when the objection is religiously based.[2]

I now report on a much more personal attack on a chief medical examiner, this time in the State of Oklahoma. In this case, the autopsy had already been done. Therefore, money damages were sought rather than an injunction. An injunction stops the work of the medicolegal office; a damages action means money—large amounts of money, often beyond any available malpractice insurance. Here, the chief medical examiner for the state was sued both in his official capacity and personally. The total claim was for a half million dollars: \$200,000 in punitive damages; \$150,000 for the mental anguish of the family because of delay in performing the autopsy; and \$150,000 for mental anguish caused by the autopsy itself, especially because it was performed out-of-doors. The chief medical examiner had no malpractice coverage for punitive damages. If he had been found not to have acted with proper authority, the state would not have been liable for his actions.

Some background on this case is necessary. The office of chief medical examiner for the State of Oklahoma has existed for some years, but has not been adequately housed in Oklahoma City. In the summer of 1975, the office was forced to refuse to do autopsies

From the *New England Journal of Medicine*
1977; 297:1220-1221.

because of inadequate facilities and because of fear of contamination of nearby Children's Hospital wards and other hospital and medical school areas. The death in question here was a suspected homicide by violence. The district attorney for Grady County requested a medicolegal autopsy, but the chief medical examiner, A. Jay Chapman, M.D., refused to do the procedure because of the above situation. Two days later, the district attorney obtained a writ of *mandamus* from the Supreme Court of Oklahoma ordering the autopsy.

The chief medical examiner had no choice but to proceed. To avoid the contamination and other dangers in the medical area, Dr. Chapman moved his autopsy table and equipment to an area behind the National Guard armory, screened the area off, assigned guards, and conducted the procedure. The autopsy revealed death by violence from head trauma and a subdural hematoma.

The daughter of the deceased brought the action, alleging that the delay in the autopsy and the manner of its conduct had caused her to suffer mental and physical anguish and personal indignation and humiliation.

A trial court dismissed the suit on the pleadings before trial. On appeal, the Supreme Court of Oklahoma sustained the dismissal of all claims.[3]

The supreme court could find nothing in the facts of the case that could support the plaintiff's allegation of indecent handling of the body, wanton mutilation, and malicious, unlawful, gross negligence. The delay of two days could not itself constitute a "wrongful dissection," and no damages could be seen to have accrued owing to this delay. The autopsy was conducted on order of the court and therefore was not a wanton or reckless action. The court found that conducting an autopsy out-of-doors was not a violation of law or the authority of the medical examiner. The court did not go into the reasons; it concluded, "There may be many legitimate purposes in conducting an autopsy out-of-doors. Accordingly, we hold that conducting an autopsy in such a setting does not constitute a willful wrong."

Because of the above findings, the court decided not to deal with the issues of the chief medical examiner's immunity from suit, even if damages were proved in a case in which the autopsy is ordered by a court, as in the case under discussion, or is conducted within the jurisdictional authority of the chief medical examiner's office. I regret the fact that this issue was not reached. It is a matter that is generally not clear in the medical-examiner laws throughout the country. There is a need to clarify the scope of medicolegal immunity. The general trend of the case law would be to extend immunity for such governmental functions to autopsies conducted in the public interest.

The publicity surrounding this case in Oklahoma did not immediately result in improved quarters. The office has still had to scurry about to obtain facilities and has had to move again and again. I have been told that the state is planning now to build autopsy and laboratory facilities for the medicolegal program. I hope so. Otherwise, the lawsuits may not be over in Oklahoma.

REFERENCES

1. Curran WJ. Religious objection to a medicolegal autopsy: a case and a statute. N Engl J Med 1977; 297:260-1.
2. Snyder v. Holy Cross Hospital, 30 Md. App. 317 (1976).
3. Dean v. Chapman, 556 P.2d 257 (1977).

♦

COMMENTS

Decisions in three other states have found medical examiners and coroners immune from damage suits when the autopsies were performed under statutory authority. *Allinger* v. *Kell,* 309 N.W. 2d 547, Michigan (1981); *State* v. *Williams,* 367 N.E. 2d 1120, Ill. (1977); *Stearns* v. *County of Los Angeles,* 79 Cal. Rptr. 757 (1969). See, however, *Scarpaci* v. *Milwaukee County,* 292 N.W. 2d 816, Wisconsin (1980), in which the court allowed an action for damages for wrongful performance of a medicolegal autopsy. In a confusing opinion, the court found that although the coroner–medical examiner would usually have immunity as a "quasi-judicial officer," such immunity did not apply in this case. The court drew a distinction between actions in excess of jurisdiction and in the complete absence of jurisdiction. It held that immunity applies to the former, but not to the latter.

The latest problem for medicolegal death-investigation systems concerns not so much the original power to order and conduct the postmortem examination, but the "unauthorized release" of information gathered as a result of the procedure. The allegation has been that the privacy of the deceased has been improperly invaded by the publication of details concerning the death. In several cases in point, the information released concerned the alcohol levels in the blood of prominent persons found to have died accidentally, and, very recently, the sensitive point has been the underlying cause of death (again in the case of public figures), particularly when the cause was the acquired immunodeficiency syndrome (AIDS). No court decisions have as yet laid down rules for determining the extent to which the public disclosure of investigative findings in authorized postmortem examinations is allowable. A recent paper examines some of these issues. See S. Asnaes, "The Importance of Medicolegal Autopsies: An Analysis of Complex Problems Regarding Damages" (*Forensic Science International* 1983; 23:123-7). See also C.S. Hirsch, "Forensic Pathology and the Autopsy" (*Archives of Pathology and Laboratory Medicine* 1984; 108:484-9).

Ethical and Legal Problems in Medical Participation in Criminal Investigations

A recent court decision concerning criminal investigational methods has raised, though quite indirectly, serious questions concerning medical participation in such practices. Officers for the California Bureau of Narcotic Enforcement lawfully procured a search warrant authorizing the search of the defendant's home, her automobile, and her person. When they went to apprehend her, she was seen to swallow two balloons and then, in two more quick hand movements, to swallow some other objects, probably also balloons. The investigators thought she had probably swallowed heroin illegally possessed, the criminal activity to which the warrants were primarily addressed. After a struggle, the woman was handcuffed and taken back to her residence, which was searched. After that, she was taken to a hospital emergency service, where the officers showed the physician in charge their warrant and said it authorized search of the defendant's person and requested that her stomach be pumped.

The physician ordered an emetic solution, but the woman refused it. She was forced to lie down on a table, and two nurses tried to strap her down. She struggled strenuously. One of the officers helped to hold her down, and she was strapped across the chest. The nurses forced a tube into her nose in an effort to place the emetic into her stomach. The defendant's continued resistance and thrashing about prevented the nurses from inserting the solution into the tube. The struggle lasted over five minutes when the woman said the tube was "too painful" and consented to drink the solution. She vomited seven

From the *New England Journal of Medicine*
1976; 294:764-765.

balloons containing heroin. She continued vomiting for about 10 minutes and remained nauseated for about 15 minutes more. There were apparently no further ill effects.

The defendant's trial-court conviction of illegal possession of heroin was reversed by the California Supreme Court because of the unconstitutionality of the search and seizure of the drug.[1] It was concluded that the warrant's reference to a search of the "person" did not include the forcible, unpermitted retrieval from the defendant's stomach. The major precedent for the finding was a famous U.S. Supreme Court case in 1952, *Rochin* v. *California,*[2] in which medical personnel had forcibly used an emetic with a person by intubation resulting in the regurgitation of two capsules of narcotics. The Court therein was extremely outraged with this conduct, which it said "shocked the conscience" of the Court and was a violation of due process of law.

The California Supreme Court distinguished the current case from another important U.S. Supreme Court decision in which it was not found unconstitutional for medical personnel to take a blood sample from an unwilling suspect to determine its alcohol content concerning a charge of drunken driving.[3] The court said that this action was justified as an emergency procedure because of the rapid dissipation of alcohol in the blood. In the immediate case, it was concluded that there was a "high probability" that the balloons would pass through the body and could be retrieved from the woman's stool.

In the light of these findings by our American courts, we may question the participation of medical personnel in a practice held, in effect, to be brutal and inhumane. The California court said that the parties had stipulated that, if called as a witness, the attending physician would have testified that he would not have forced the patient to regurgitate over her objections but for the officers' assertion that the warrant authorized the search. In a rather strange footnote to the decision (note 5 at page 533) the court expanded on this observation. It was said that the narcotics officer had expressed to the doctor his concern for the woman's health if the balloons of heroin were to rupture. The court said that the physician "never responded" to the officer's expression of concern. It is then said that it appeared from the stipulation that the doctor thought the woman would probably pass the balloons safely, but he would nevertheless have "recommended regurgitation as a medical precaution." Despite this last remark it seems clear that the court took the doctor's statement to mean that he performed this forced procedure because it was ordered by the narcotics officers on the basis of their warrant.

Questions are currently being raised on the international scene about the ethical justification for participation by medical personnel in penal institutional and police practices that could be considered cruel or inhumane. In October 1975, the World Medical Association adopted the Declaration of Tokyo, which is a set of ethical guidelines for medical doctors in this field. It asserts,

> A doctor must have complete clinical independence in deciding upon the care of a person for whom he or she is medically responsible. The doctor's fundamental role is to alleviate the distress of his or her fellow men, and no motive—whether personal, collective or political—shall prevail against this higher purpose. (Principle 4)

The Declaration specifically prohibits physicians from participating in forced feeding of prisoners who have formed a rational judgment to refuse nourishment.

A United Nations document produced by the World Health Organization for the Fifth United Nations Congress on the Prevention of Crime and the Treatment of Offenders, held in Geneva in September 1975, notes the position taken by the World Medical Association, available then in draft form, but takes pains not to endorse it, saying that medical attitude toward forced feeding of prisoners is by no means unanimous.[4] Nevertheless, it notes that forced feeding by intubation is "disagreeable for all concerned." The forced procedure that it describes is in all essential details the same as that used against the defendant in the *Bracamonte* case earlier described to force the emetic into the suspect's stomach. Furthermore, the same document concludes that this procedure, "especially on resistant patients," can cause fluids to enter the trachea and provoke a pneumonia that could be fatal.

The documents discussed above do not deal with the type of situation described in the California case, and the particular court did not admonish the doctor for his actions. However, one can question whether such forced procedures should be used by medical personnel on any other grounds than medical necessity and perhaps even then, as the Declaration of Tokyo points out, only when the person's resistance is irrational. If medical personnel followed such ethical rules, it seems to me that it would be much more protective of human rights than a higher judicial tribunal's reversal of a conviction months or years after the event and the violation of rights have taken place.

REFERENCES

1. People v. Bracamonte, 124 Cal. Rptr. 528 (1975).
2. 342 U.S. 165 (1952).
3. Schmerber v. California, 284 U.S. 757 (1967).
4. Health aspects of avoidable maltreatment of prisoners and detainees. Paper prepared by the World Health Organization Secretariat. Geneva: United Nations. (Document A/Conf 56/9.)

♦

COMMENTS

Issues of ethical and legal concerns about the participation of physicians in forced interrogations and forced medical examinations, especially those involving invasive and dangerous procedures, have continued to interest me. Most recently my concern was evidenced in my opposition to physicians' participation in the public execution of criminal offenders by lethal injection. See W.J. Curran and W. Casscells, "The Ethics of Medical Participation in Capital Punishment by Intravenous Drug Injection" (*New England Journal of Medicine* 1980; 302:226-30).

For more recent articles examining ethical and legal problems that confront physicians and other forensic scientists participating in criminal investigations, see W.G. Eckert, "Medicolegal Investigation of Problems Involving Criminals and Criminal Activity" (*American Journal of Forensic Medicine and Pathology* 1983; 4:279-86); O. Schroeder, Jr., "Ethical and Moral Dilemmas Confronting Forensic Scientists" (*Journal of Forensic Sciences* 1984; 29:966-86); A.A. Biasotti, "The Role of the Forensic Scientist in the Application of Chemical Tests for Alcohol in Traffic Law Enforcement" (*Journal of Forensic Sciences* 1984; 29:1164-72).

The Law Reform Commission of Canada recently published a thoughtful report recommending that certain limitations be imposed on public prosecutors when they seek to obtain forensic evidence from criminal suspects. Under no circumstances should suspects under arrest be forced or even permitted to allow: the administering of a drug or enema or other substance intended to produce evidence, any surgical procedure (except the taking of blood specimens with the person's consent) intended to produce evidence, any procedure to remove stomach contents, or any procedure to produce an image (e.g., x-ray film of the internal body).

The report also indicated that the possibility had been considered of requiring that licensed physicians aid police and prosecuting attorneys in conducting clinical tests on persons suspected of alcohol- or drug-abuse offenses or of traffic violations. The commission determined not to adopt such recommendations because they would involve "an unconscionable intrusion into the special relationship of doctor and patient." See *Obtaining Forensic Evidence: Report of the Canadian Law Reform Commission.* Report 25, Ottawa, Canada, 1985 (p. 29 [English version]; p. 30 [French version]).

American Personal-Injury Lawyers at Bhopal: Ethics and Public Policy in Mass Disasters

The deaths in Bhopal in December 1984 due to leakage of a highly toxic gas from a Union Carbide chemical plant are estimated at 2500 persons. The injured, in the tens of thousands, are still uncounted in what is well described as the worst industrial accident in world history.[1,2] The aftermath of the disaster has attracted the involvement of many parties, including both lawyers and physicians.

National news magazines and television news programs have shown photographs of American personal-injury lawyers walking through the shantytowns of Bhopal that surround the chemical plant, adding Indian victims and their families to a roster of claimants for a class-action personal-injury suit against Union Carbide in the United States.[1,3] Upwards of 50 suits have already been filed in American courts against the Union Carbide Company and have been consolidated before a single district-court judge.

American medical specialists have also examined Bhopal victims on the scene and made direct reports on their findings to American audiences.

It may be useful to *Journal* readers familiar with personal-injury suits in the United States to review some of the ethical and public policy issues underlying legal involvement in claims resulting from a mass accident. I will try to contrast the legal situation with some aspects of medical practice and ethics in the same type of mass-injury situation.

First of all, how can American lawyers practice their profession on the streets of Bhopal? Ethically, they cannot practice unless licensed

From the *New England Journal of Medicine*
1985; 313:1068-1070.

in the Indian jurisdiction. There are no emergency-practice exceptions for law, as is often the case for medicine. A mass disaster resulting in a medical emergency may warrant considerable relaxation of restrictions on medical support from other countries asked to aid in the situation. I have never seen any such exceptions applied to law practice, no matter how great the demand for personal representation by victims. The ethical claim for the foreign lawyers' presence would seem to be based on the assertion that the Americans were called on by Indian lawyers to advise them on the American rights of their clients. On this basis, the Americans could ethically help in the cases. No independent determination could be made for clients, however, and all actual law practice would be conducted by the Indian attorneys in the area. In the news stories and television scenes of interviews with the American lawyers, this has hardly seemed to be the situation. The American lawyers are described as being in the forefront, organizing activities and answering television interviewers directly on the strategy of their legal efforts. Of course, we see only short excerpts of interviews, which may be very different in context.

The involvement of American physicians in Bhopal, like that of the lawyers, appears to have resulted from requests for consultation by Indian medical sources seeking advice in the assessment of the long-term effects of exposure. The Americans consulted were specialists in lung disease and chronic eye involvement. Their reports indicated that long-term impairment may not be as widespread as expected initially, and little if any blindness has been found. There seems to be little evidence that any foreign physicians were called on to render direct assistance in the care of victims during the height of the emergency. I have seen no reports that any of the medical specialists were asked to assess victims on behalf of the Indian or American lawyers.

Some of the statements of the American lawyers were puzzling. It was asserted frequently that the objective of an American-based lawsuit would be to disclose the gross negligence of Union Carbide and to punish the company for improper standards of plant operation, recovering millions of dollars in damages for individual injuries, thus deterring accidents of this type in the future.

Actually, such assertions would not be necessary were suits filed in the United States. Under American law, in all likelihood, the operation of this plant to manufacture methyl isocyanate would be classified as an ultrahazardous activity, and the company would be strictly liable for direct injury and damage, without the need for proof of fault or negligence. This "ultrahazardous enterprise liability" has been accepted law, especially as it applies to such industries, for several decades at least.[4,5] Ultrahazardous enterprises are described as unusual or unnatural uses of land operations, such as industrial plants or dynamite sites or nuclear energy systems, which necessarily involve, by their character, extreme danger to nearby persons and the surrounding environment and in which no amount of care can entirely eliminate the risk of explosion or leakage.[6] Under English common law, a similar rule in regard to ultrahazardous land use[7] has been recognized since 1868. Indian law, often based on English precedent, may have incorporated this doctrine at that or a later time. These rules of law recognize that the world cannot be made risk-free. The incentive to prevent the loss, or limit the extent of the damage, in an extremely remote but generally predictable explosion, leakage, or other accident does not lie in personal-injury suits. The recovery for personal injury is thus made a cost of operations and is paid from insurance or self-insurance, and disaster coverage is provided by reinsurance with large carriers, such as Lloyds of London. Since negligence need not be proved, the company cannot avoid or defend the suit by showing that it did everything that was technically possible to prevent the accident, or that the accident was caused by the negligence of other contractors or suppliers. The incentive promoted by the no-fault rule is not so much to improve safety, although this is always a thrust of an operational ruling, but to minimize outside damage, should an accident occur. This means encouraging location of plants in remote areas, often offshore, and certainly away from heavily populated areas.[2] That incentive certainly did not operate in India. It is ironic that cities and towns are so often concerned that mental hospitals, drug-addiction centers, and prisons be located in remote areas. These facilities house people who are considered directly dangerous, whereas industrial plants are seen as posing mysterious and only vaguely understood technical hazards. Companies are allowed and often encouraged to locate plants near population centers, providing many more jobs and economic benefits to the community than could ever be achieved with human-services institutions.

In medical malpractice, proof that no negligence has occurred is essentially a complete defense, even in cases involving ultra-hazardous procedures. In fact, the circumstance of inherently high risk provides more, not less, protection for the physician, since it is more difficult for the patient to prove that the poor result was due to preventable negligence by the physician. Lack of negligence is not a complete defense for medical enterprises, such as therapeutic-drug manufacturers or medical-technology companies, in which warranties (or guarantees) of safety and appropriateness for use are made by law. This situation occurred, for example, with the drug thalidomide, which caused relatively large-scale injuries in Europe two decades ago.

An important question in the case of Bhopal is whether any action can or should be brought in an American court. It would be most unusual for such an action to be entertained. The law governing cases like this is the law of India, where the accident occurred and the injuries took place. All the injured were Indians, not Americans. The plant was operated under a joint ownership arrangement in which Union Carbide retained a bare majority of the stock (approximately 51 percent, with 49 percent owned by various Indian parties). The precedent for allowing action in an American court seems to have been established by cases in which the plaintiffs were entirely barred from any action in the original jurisdiction.

It has been observed that American courts should be opened so that American legal expertise can be used to represent the clients and favorable American law can apply, with larger damages recoverable for the Indian claimants. None of these arguments are persuasive. The rule of no-fault recovery leaves little room for any expertise to be applied to the technical aspects of the case. The most feasible defense for the company in individual cases would be to claim that the person involved was not a victim of the accident because he or she was not nearby or that the injury was medically incompatible with the expected patterns of injury. Advocacy of such claims would require the presence of the claimant in court or rather unsatisfactory expense to obtain depositions, medical records, and so forth. These defenses and claims would be extremely difficult to handle in an American court thousands of miles from the scene.

Those who argue for placing the trials in American courts have emphasized the view that larger verdicts or awards may be obtained in American courts. The increases in awards in medical-malpractice and other personal-injury suits in the past five years certainly add credence to this point. However, those awards were based on American standards of living and medical expenses. Such standards are not applicable to wage loss and recoverable expenses and medical benefits in central India. The courts must apply each claim made for compensatory damages to actual losses in India, not imaginary losses in the United States. The American courts could increase awards considerably, however, by applying American standards to general claims for "pain and suffering."

One issue remains clear. If the claims must be filed and prosecuted in India, the attorneys cannot recover a large portion of each award as a contingent fee for professional legal services. Such a system of recovery is not allowed in India on ethical grounds, and the possibility that an exception will be made in this unusual circumstance of mass injury and class action seems legally remote.

Adverse commentary about the efforts of the American lawyers and their Indian colleagues in seeking an American forum for their lawsuit has recently produced a counterreaction.[8] The lawyers are alleging that the Indian courts are too slow and too inefficient to handle the huge volume of claims expected from the Bhopal incident. They predict delays into the 1990s. Problems of delay alone would not seem enough to convince an American court to accept jurisdiction over suits involving only Indian claimants. Delays in personal-injury suits in the United States are also well known; a class action of this type, involving millions of dollars and thousands of plaintiffs, could take years merely for preliminary matters and pretrial motions, many of which might be appealed to higher courts before trial. More serious, however, are allegations that the plaintiffs in India may be required to pay in advance nonrefundable filing fees of 5 percent of the total award sought. Considering the damages contemplated, at least in the cases of death, these extraordinary filing fees could present extreme difficulties for the Bhopal victims. A waiver of the requirement in so notorious a matter, or the posting of a bond for payment, could perhaps be authorized, but it is not clear what the reaction of the Indian courts would be to such a request. Indian lawyers and judges assert that the lack of precedent for issues of this type and for substantive law to support the plaintiffs' claims may further delay progress of the cases in India. Such delays would also occur in the United States, if the courts were bound to apply Indian law, as indicated above, to the substance of the claims. A news story[8] from India reports that Indian public opinion is turning toward support for bringing these lawsuits to the United States.

The expected political reaction in India to the large number of suits brought in American courts has been the enactment of national legislation authorizing the central government to set up a program for exclusive representation of all Indian claimants in any lawsuits brought either in India or in foreign courts.[9] As part of the program, the government will establish a registration system for claimants and will distribute to them all awards made by the courts. This legislation appears to eliminate the requirement that each claimant pay a pretrial filing fee. The program also allows claimants, at their own expense, to have a personal lawyer associated with the trial under the direction of the government's attorneys.

REFERENCES

1. Whitaker M, Mazumdar S, Gibney F Jr, Behr E. It was like breathing fire. . . . Newsweek. December 17, 1984:26-32.
2. Gassed in Bhopal. The Economist. December 15, 1984; 293:12-3.
3. Press A, Gibney F Jr. A lawyers game of chicken. Newsweek. December 24, 1984:23.
4. Morris J. Hazardous enterprises and risk bearing capacity. Yale Law J 1952; 61:1172.
5. Prosser WL. The law of torts. 3rd ed. St. Paul, Minn.: West, 1964.
6. Restatement of Torts. Sections 519 and 520. (Cited in Prosser WL[5]:527, Note 4.)
7. Rylands v. Fletcher, L.R. 3 H.L. 330 (1868).
8. Stewart JB. Why suits for damages such as Bhopal claims are very rare in India. Wall Street Journal. January 23, 1985:1.
9. Riley J. New Bhopal law may affect future role of U.S. lawyers. Natl Law J. March 11, 1985; 26(7):4.

♦

COMMENTS

This essay was one among many commentaries that criticized the conduct of a cadre of American lawyers who rushed to Bhopal to "sign up" the victims and their families for lawsuits in the United States. Among the critics was Chief Justice Warren Burger, who expressed his views in several public speeches made to bar-association groups.

I am glad to be able to report that my legal prediction in this column proved correct. The American suits filed by lawyers engaged in Bhopal by disaster victims were dismissed, and the plaintiffs were directed to seek their legal remedies in India under the procedures indicated in this column. More recently, the Indian courts have approved a settlement including all claims for a grand total of $470 million.

The Medicolegal Lessons of the Airliner Crash at Tenerife

When jumbo-jet passenger aircraft were introduced they meant substantial progress for the air-travel industry and increased comfort for air travelers. The huge aircraft, with seating capacities of over 300, also brought feelings of great uneasiness to experienced medicolegal investigators who had been involved in examinations of the results of previous airliner crashes and multiple-death investigations. The problems of dealing with these crashes and the solving of jurisdictional disputes between investigational authorities had by no means been fully worked out. Now, the jumbo jets would compound the problems by the multiplication of numbers of passengers and crew, massiveness of the aircraft hull, and the great emotional impact for the local community and the world as a whole in being confronted with a sudden, single-site catastrophe involving hundreds of dead and wounded brought to the site from all parts of the world.

There was only limited experience in handling such problems before 1977. The largest was a crash at takeoff in Paris a few years previously involving a DC-10; this crash was blamed on a faulty rear door. Terrorists in the Middle East had destroyed a jumbo jet a year earlier, but passengers were not on board. The first massive test of the world community's ability to cope with a modern air disaster came on March 27, 1977, at Tenerife in the Canary Islands, a not very accessible spot in the world. The crash was at takeoff, a highly predictable risk incident in all aircraft mishaps. But the experts who had thought about such accidents had rarely let their thinking, let alone their active planning and management, reach the proportions of Ten-

From the *New England Journal of Medicine*
1977; 297:986-987.

erife, where not one but two full-capacity jumbo jets hurtled into one another and burst into flame and explosion, killing over 500 on the runway, leaving some 60 or so alive from one of the planes, many of whom died later.

A very interesting report on the lessons learned at Tenerife has recently been published by the International Reference Organization in Forensic Medicine and Sciences (INFORM).[1] One of the two planes was an American-flag carrier, Pan American; the other was a Dutch carrier, KLM. The Spanish government took control of the scene and brought in public health and medicolegal authorities. First efforts were put to clearing the wreckage from the runway, an action that undoubtedly complicated later efforts to reconstruct the patterns of the accident and to separate and classify the victims and physical evidence from both craft. Attempts at identification were made by the local police during the first day. Little could be done. The bodies were severely burned and distorted. Some cursory dental examinations were made, but it is not clear that any dentists were involved in the Spanish group. The authorities decided that the local law requiring embalming and burial within 48 hours of death must be followed. They set about to eviscerate and embalm the bodies and to place each in a casket.

The American legal responsibility at the federal level for investigating commercial-airline accidents now rests with the National Transportation Safety Board (NTSB).[2] The jurisdiction of the Board is limited to U.S. territory.[3] However, the NTSB cooperates in investigations in foreign countries on the invitation of the country when American carriers are involved. Investigations of international air crashes have been conducted according to guidelines of the International Civil Aviation Organization. American investigators, including experts in medicolegal analysis, arrived in Tenerife on the first day after the accident, with a second and larger contingent arriving some 48 hours after the crash. By the time the American pathologists and other experts were on the scene and ready to work, the Spanish authorities had removed the bodies, and the Americans were never given the opportunity of helping in the identification and classification process with the victims. On the other hand, the Dutch investigation team, which arrived sooner, on the morning after the crash, was able to gain permission to examine the bodies designated as coming from the Dutch plane.

The Spanish authorities had taken the living to nearby facilities, including a general hospital. There were no survivors identified with the KLM plane; all the living, some 60 people, were from the Pan American 747. Many died within the next few days. On March 29 the survivors were flown out of Tenerife on Air Force planes to American burn centers.

It was not until the sixth day that the dead were taken out of the Islands. It seems clear that virtually none of the 580 bodies were positively identified at that time. The Dutch buried their dead in a mass grave after recovering as much documentation as possible. The American investigators brought the bodies to an Air Force facility at Dover, Delaware, where a massive interdisciplinary evaluation involving forensic pathologists, forensic dentists, anthropologists, fingerprint experts, and others was conducted. The obstacles to identification were many. The movement of the bodies displaced much useful information and physical materials that could have helped greatly in the task. Fingerprinting was possible in only a few cases. Dental evaluations were useful, but, since many of the passengers were from a group of elderly people on a tour, many of the dead were found to have dental plates that were difficult to trace. Despite these problems, it was reported that almost two thirds of the 331 dead were positively identified.

Investigation of the crash is not over. Lawsuits for damages on behalf of the living and the dead could amount to billions of dollars if "willful misconduct" is proved.

The Tenerife accident underscored the need to reach the scene very quickly if investigation of both the cause of the crash and of medicolegal factors is to proceed effectively. Application of local law again resulted in curtailing widespread international investigation. The problems of international cooperation at the scene were not solved at Tenerife, even though the crash site was an airfield. The field was not equipped for handling jumbo jets in any number on its single runway and limited taxi strips. Yet diversion to such fields can be expected in the future. Worse, what would be the result if a crash were to take place after the craft or crafts were airborne and the remains of planes and victims – over 600 – were to be thrown over a remote region or a crowded urban center? Perhaps the best possible location for proper investigation is, in fact, an airport, the scene of most accidents in takeoffs and landings. Yet the Tenerife incident proves that after the first few hours, both causation evaluation and medicolegal work can be greatly compromised by local law enforcement and local medical and burial regulations.

The INFORM report draws few specific conclusions from the Tenerife disaster: the conclusions noted above are my own. INFORM stresses primarily the development of a voluntary group of regional teams of experts in pathology, dentistry, anthropology, serology, toxicology, criminalistics, and other sciences to aid international air-crash investigation. The suggestion is very worthy of further exploration.

REFERENCES

1. Major air crash investigation: lessons of Tenerife. INFORM Rep 1977; 9(4) 3-5.
2. Transportation Safety Act of 1974, 88 Stat. 2156, 49 U.S.C. 1901.
3. Federal Aviation Act of 1958, 72 Stat. 731, 49 U.S.C. 1301.

♦

COMMENTS

This column was an early expression of a personal interest of mine in the medicolegal aspects of mass-disaster investigations. In the beginning of the jumbo-jet age in the 1970s, I had been consulted on the legal issues presented by airliner accidents of an international character, including the difficulties presented by requests to remove bodies, debris, and other evidence from the scene. The Tenerife crash produced the first international crisis in which all of these issues were raised simultaneously. As indicated in the column, the magnitude of the disaster far exceeded the expectations of those who had been involved in the careful medicolegal planning that had been done in anticipation of such an event. None of the imaginary scenarios that I had heard discussed had involved two jumbo jets from two different nations crashing on a runway, killing so many people, with everything taking place on a remote island in the middle of the Atlantic Ocean.

The circumstances at Tenerife were advantageous to the organizers of a large-scale international investigation in two important respects: the crash occurred on the runway of the airport rather than in midair, and the relatively primitive facilities and resources of the island made it virtually impossible for the local authorities to mount a satisfactory investigation. If an accident of the same proportions had occurred at a large European airport in a metropolitan urban center such as Rome, Athens, or Vienna, or in an Eastern European city such as Warsaw or Moscow, the local authorities might not have been equally cooperative. Most European cities, including all of those mentioned above, have forensic-pathology programs of long standing and high academic prestige that could be quite protective of their own investigative powers. The investigation at Tenerife, difficult as it was to organize, produced impressive results, including the almost complete identification of the American dead. The lawsuits arising out of the deaths were handled expeditiously, and all but 9 of the 664 claims were settled within two years of the accident. For further review of the medicolegal aspects of the Tenerife crash, see J.H. Wolcott and C.A. Hanson, "Summary of Means Used to Positively Identify the American Victims in the Canary Islands Crash" (*Aviation, Space, and Experimental Medicine* 1980; 51:1034-5).

More about Mass Disasters: The Handling of Airliner-Crash Investigations in the 1980s

The interest in my recent column[1] on the ethical and public policy issues surrounding the industrial mass disaster in Bhopal, India, prompts me to offer the *Journal* readership some comments on another form of mass disaster—the airliner crash that results in hundreds of deaths.

Nine years ago, I wrote a column[2] on the worst air-travel disaster in history—the collision of two jumbo jets on the ground at Tenerife in the Canary Islands. I focused on the medicolegal investigation of the cause of the crash and the forensic difficulties involved in identification of the victims.

In this column, however, as in the Bhopal commentary, I will deal mainly with the ethics of the conduct of the personal-injury lawyers and the insurers during medicolegal investigations of disasters, the impact of these incidents on the industries involved, and the aftermath of these events.

The year 1985 was the worst in aviation history in terms of commercial airliner disasters; there were 15 major crashes. Since the advent of superjets that carry more than 300 passengers, the chance that multiple deaths will result from one mishap has greatly increased, and such incidents have begun to occur almost regularly. No country has learned to deal well with the sudden emergencies at the site of the crash. The resources of even the largest airports and metropolitan population centers are taxed by the demand for investigational resources, the identification procedures, the notification of

From the *New England Journal of Medicine*
1986; 314:692-693.

relatives, the need for space for handling bodies and debris from the crash, and many other aspects of post-crash crises.

At the center of a strong controversy this year has been the growing tendency of plaintiffs' lawyers to rush to the scene of airline accidents to sign up the families of the victims in order to pursue millions of dollars in compensation suits. This practice is regarded as a new and more sophisticated form of "ambulance chasing." After the crash of a Delta airliner at Dallas–Fort Worth Airport on August 2, 1985, for example, it was alleged that two attorneys from California set up shop at a Dallas hotel 48 hours after the crash, sought out the victims' families, and filed their first lawsuits within six days of the accident. A complaint against these attorneys of ethically improper solicitation of clients was filed in Texas and later forwarded to a grievance committee of the appropriate bar association in California.

There is a specialty group of personal-injury lawyers in this country who concentrate on investigating airliner crashes and bringing lawsuits in those situations. This group claims that its members are much more skilled and experienced in handling such cases than the local counsel usually retained by victims' families. The movement toward immediately seeking clients at the scene, however, is a new approach by lawyers who, in the past, usually received the cases through referrals from family-retained counsel. Two justifications for the more aggressive style have been cited: the need to be on the scene to ensure effective investigation and preservation of evidence, and the need to counter the efforts of insurance companies and the airlines to get to the families first and talk them out of lawsuits and into quick settlements favorable to the companies.

In the past, there does seem to have been cause for the plaintiffs' attorneys to be concerned about post-crash activity on behalf of the airline companies and other potential defendants. The comprehensive, systematic response of insurers and defense counsel to airline crashes was recently referred to by a leading representative of the defense bar as "a well-oiled machine."[3] In many of these situations, there are more than 80 underwriters of insurance for the various aspects of the airline-company's operation, the airplane, and the parts of the airplane. For each crash, a coordinating team is put together to handle all aspects of the investigation and the early contact with families of victims. Such contact involves none of the sensitive ethical issues surrounding personal solicitation of lawsuits by out-of-state plaintiffs' attorneys, since the companies, because they are insurers with legal liability to pay compensation where it is warranted, have a direct relationship with the families. Early contact is usually justified on the basis of its being necessary to inform the families that the insurance claims–adjustment system exists, that it is available to answer inquiries and, most important, that the insurers may make advance payments to the families for burial costs, personal travel expenses to visit the site of the crash, and matters related to the settling of the deceased's estate. These offers can be most welcome to distressed families.

However, plaintiffs' attorneys have complained bitterly about some practices of the defense teams, such as attempting to discourage families from retaining highly experienced lawyers and cautioning families to avoid "precipitous" lawsuits. Insurance teams have also allegedly advised families to take their time in arranging the settlement of claims and told them that the insurers would arrange a "reasonable extension" of the statute of limitations. Of course, the latter promise is grossly improper and unethical, since only a court, under extremely unusual circumstances, can extend the statutory deadline in individual cases. The leisurely drawing out of settlement negotiations past the deadline for a lawsuit could destroy the claim and leave the family with nothing but what the company wished to pay voluntarily.

These questionable practices by the insurance and legal defense teams seem to have been eliminated, but the "well-oiled machine" is still diligently at work reaching the families and moving them toward settlement.

The insurers vehemently defend their efforts, claiming that they allow the families to receive prompt advice and help, as well as a fair settlement from which they do not have to deduct large sums for legal and investigational fees. The insurers' approach is apparently quite successful; in nearly all airliner crashes in the United States, about 95 percent of all claims are settled out of court. I was particularly interested to read that all but 9 of the 664 death claims from the Tenerife crash (the airlines involved were Pan American and KLM) were settled in only two years.[3]

The very serious business of these lawsuits and settlements is, however, becoming more complex as the circumstances and the parties involved change with each disaster. The planes and the passenger loads are larger; the crashes occur in foreign places, and the equipment and the bodies may not be recovered; and there are bewildering patterns of multiple technical and nontechnical reasons for the disasters. Currently in litigation, for example, are the puzzling and highly sensitive claims that arose when the Soviets shot down Korean Airlines Flight 007 over Soviet territory. What, if any, is the liability of the airline in this situation? Was the pilot negligent in straying into Soviet airspace? Was there a technical failure in navigational equipment? How can the basis of any allegations in this type of case ever be proved?

A recent report[4] in the financial section of the *New York Times* described the experience of Japan Air Lines after the crash of August 12, in which 520 persons died in the worst single-plane, jumbo-jet disaster in history. Even though the management of the airline did not believe it was at fault, the chief executive officer of the company assumed full personal responsibility for the crash and resigned shortly after the event. The airline set out on a vigorous course of aiding the families of the victims, nearly all of whom were Japanese. The company has already paid out more than $17 million in post-crash expenditures, which include funds for two elaborate mass memorial services for the victims and for an unusually broad and generous voluntary program of payments to families for the expenses of identifying bodies, living costs, and scholarships for the children of victims. The compensation payments may eventually exceed $100 million. This response is perhaps a manifestation of the singularly Japanese system of industrial paternalism.

Despite its efforts, however, the airline has suffered grievously in its operations after the crash, mainly because of the reaction of its Japanese customers. Predictions regarding its profits for 1985 were reduced from an estimate of $107.7 million early in that year to an estimate of only $35.5 million at the end of the year.[4] The airline has been severely criticized by the press in Japan and by Japanese government agencies investigating the crash. The investigators have pointed out that this disaster was not the first for the country's largest and most prestigious air carrier. The most cited (and most embarrassing) previous incident was a disaster that occurred in 1982, when a mentally disturbed pilot deliberately crashed his plane into Tokyo Bay.

In comparison with the vast complexities and sensitive qualities of the investigational activities in the international air-travel business, the medicolegal negotiations in Bhopal, India, seem like child's play. Yet many of the same ethical and public policy issues emerge from the two situations. In every mass disaster, hundreds of families are affected by the sudden death of loved ones.

I suggest that when major airline crashes occur in the United States, the involvement of a federal agency—the Federal Aviation Administration (FAA), perhaps—is justified and that such activity would be welcomed, especially by the families of the deceased passengers and crews. This agency could coordinate all aspects of preservation of the evidence pertaining to the causes of the crash and the identification of victims, and it could also monitor the activities of insurance and defense representatives and independent plaintiff's lawyers. The FAA could also produce advisory guidelines for airliner-crash investigations, in cooperation with the American Bar Association, the American Academy of Forensic Sciences, and appropriate insurance and industry groups. We can hope that such activities will lessen the confusion and distress of airline disasters, while preserving the necessary adversary process and preventing the unwarranted exploitation of grieving families.

REFERENCES

1. Curran WJ. American personal-injury lawyers at Bhopal: ethics and public policy in a mass disaster. N Engl J Med 1985; 313:1068-70.
2. *Idem.* The medicolegal lessons of the Tenerife disaster. N Engl J Med 1977; 297:986-7.
3. Tarr A. Lawyers collide over post air crash conduct. Natl Law J. November 4, 1985:1.
4. Chira S. J.A.L.'s post-crash troubles. New York Times. November 8, 1985:D1.

♦

COMMENTS

The handling of mass disasters, particularly those involving airliners, has not noticeably improved since I wrote this column. International medicolegal involvement is still organized on an ad hoc basis as each mass disaster occurs. There is no international office or coordinating body authorized, or generally recognized on an unofficial basis as entitled, to put together a medicolegal investigation team. No international treaties or conventions deal effectively with these aspects of such disasters.

Most of my physician readers were not aware of the extensive efforts of American lawyers and casualty-insurance companies in the "business" of handling personal-injury litigation arising out of deaths in airliner crashes. In fact, plaintiffs' lawyers have had their own national organization with a section devoted to airliner crashes for over 30 years. This section was formerly a part of the National Association of Compensation Claimants Attorneys, organized in Boston in the 1950s, which later became the American Trial Lawyers Association. For a general review of the medicolegal aspects of plane-crash investigations, see L.R. Simson, Jr., "Aircraft Death Investigation: A Comprehensive Review," in W.J. Curran, A.L. McGarry, and C.S. Petty, eds., *Modern Legal Medicine, Psychiatry, and Forensic Science* (Philadelphia: F.A. Davis, 1980).

The Mass Suicides in Guyana: The Medicolegal Investigation

For the second time in only a few years, a huge tragedy has taken place, involving the deaths of hundreds of American citizens in a remote place outside the United States. Once again, the handling of a large-scale disaster by the U.S. government has been evaluated and severely criticized by medicolegal and forensic-science groups in this country.[1]

Previously, the largest disaster involving American citizens occurred in March 1977, when two jumbo-jet airliners collided on the ground at the virtually unknown auxiliary airfield on Tenerife in the Canary Islands. More than 500 people died on the runway.

The second incident, which occurred in November 1978, was even more unbelievable to the entire world, which heard of the place, Jonestown, Guyana, and the dead, more than 900 members of the People's Temple religious cult, with astonishment and shock.

The inadequacies in the handling of these two disasters are disturbingly similar. In fact, it seems that the experience at Tenerife led more to imitation than to correction. In a previous column, I reviewed the problems involved in handling the American dead from Tenerife and the lessons that could have been learned.[2] Now, after this second incident, the same medicolegal authorities are making criticisms similar to those offered after the first disaster.

The two major critical groups are the National Association of Medical Examiners and the International Reference Organization in Forensic Medicine and Sciences. The main points they make are:

Positive identification of bodies was not achieved in nearly two thirds of the cases because of inadequate resources and the failure at

From the *New England Journal of Medicine*
1979; 300:1321.

Jonestown to keep the bodies, including those of the children, in family units and other natural groupings.

The handling of the situation by the U.S. government was marked by conflicting statements and shuffling of responsibility back and forth among federal agencies.

The selection of Dover Air Force Base for the handling of the bodies in the United States unfortunately did not facilitate further investigation of the background of the victims, nor did this location make it easy for relatives to visit and identify and claim bodies. Most of the cult members were from, or related to residents of, the San Francisco–Oakland area. The bodies could have been taken to Oakland, where military facilities are also available. (It is striking that the same difficulty also arose after the disaster at Tenerife when the victims, all from Southern California, were taken to the same Dover, Delaware, facility on the East Coast. Identification of the dead in that situation was much more successful, however.)

There was no prearranged plan for action to handle a mass tragedy of this type outside the United States in a remote location. There was no panel of civilian experts in forensic medicine who could be called on to help in investigation, postmortem examination, positive identification, and proper disposition of the bodies.

Lastly, the medicolegal authorities insisted that, despite the monumental task of handling 911 bodies in a very hot and humid jungle village, where decomposition and putrefaction occur quickly, a medicolegal autopsy should have been performed on every body for the purpose of issuing death certificates (none were ever obtained on any of the persons at Guyana) and accurately determining the manner and cause of death for each person. Future litigation over insurance claims and over the disposition of the remaining funds of the People's Temple — funds perhaps numbering in the millions of dollars — may be hampered by these medicolegal uncertainties.

The primary recommendation of the medicolegal experts resulting from the Jonestown suicides is the same as after Tenerife: The U.S. government, in consultation and collaboration with forensic-medical and scientific groups, should develop a coordinated plan of action for handling disasters involving the deaths of large numbers of Americans in foreign countries.

The criticisms and the recommendations of the medicolegal societies seem well taken and are supported by the events in these two tragedies. A basic plan should help reluctant public officials to take quick action. It may also prove useful to have a list of civilian medicolegal experts willing to fly to God knows where on a moment's notice. Yet, as in the disasters at Tenerife and Jonestown, local authorities will be at the scene and will want to control the situation. Because of their rural nature, developing countries may actually have been more willing to allow outside help than might have been the case in a more industrialized country. Actually, there is no government plan of action for handling disasters involving the deaths of large numbers of Americans in the United States, let alone on foreign soil. There is no federal authority to order autopsies in such situations or to take jurisdiction merely because of the size of the disaster. Where is the medicolegal facility in any state that could handle, preserve, and examine 1000 bodies from one disaster? The main body of experts in this country is the Armed Forces Institute of Pathology, an excellent medicolegal unit that probably should be given more resources and expanded jurisdiction. The possibility that a great disaster could have occurred at the Three Mile Island nuclear power plant should alert us all to the fact that it is folly to continue to expect that "it can't happen here."

REFERENCES

1. The Guyana tragedy: an international forensic problem. INFORM Rep 1979; 11(2):2-8.
2. Curran WJ. The medicolegal lessons of the Tenerife disaster. N Engl J Med 1977; 297:986-7.

COMMENTS

A further report on the results of the investigations by the Armed Forces Institute of Pathology on the bodies recovered from Jonestown has recently been published. The paper was presented at the annual meeting of the Academy of Forensic Sciences in February 1980, but it was not published until March 1987. No explanation for the delay is contained in the article, but it may be related to the sensitive nature of the data and the requirements of the U.S. military for clearance for publication. The article contains no formal summary or conclusion. The most important points made by the authors, all of whom were formerly on the staff of the Armed Forces Institute of Pathology, were as follows: Of the 913 bodies they examined, 666 (73 percent) were identified. Fingerprints matched with immigration records were the most frequent means of identification (in the cases of 441 persons), followed by a combination of fingerprints and dental records (150). Interestingly, one victim, an infant, was positively identified by a footprint. The small number of identifications arrived at solely on the basis of dental records (73) was probably due to the large number of children in the group and the fact that many cult members were drawn from black and other minority communities where dental care was not commonly received and records were not retained, as was the case, for example, among the victims of the airliner crash at Tenerife. The one other positive identification was of a person known to have undergone an amputation.

The paper revealed the reason that no autopsies had been done on victims at Jonestown or shortly after the arrival of the remains at the Dover Air Force Base: attorneys at the U.S. State Department had given the opinion that no autopsies could be authorized in this situation. Therefore, all bodies were embalmed and no plans for later autopsies were made. Nevertheless, the medicolegal investigation team at Dover Air Force Base persisted in urging an investigation into the causes of the deaths. As the authors put it, "Some time later, after much discussion, it was decided to try to get permission from the families to perform autopsies on all bodies with traumatic injuries and on a few with no such injuries" (p. 436).

As a result, on February 15, 1978, seven autopsies were performed. Two of the bodies exhibited traumatic injuries—i.e., gunshot wounds to the head with indications of close contact—which would undoubtedly have caused death. One of the two bodies, but not both, also showed evidence of cyanide intoxication. The other five bodies showed evidence of cyanide intoxication alone. The authors speculated that the two gunshot victims might have been shot because they did not rapidly show signs of having succumbed to the cyanide used to kill the great majority of the cult members. The investigators could not, however, entirely rule out self-inflicted gunshot wounds in these two cases. Because of the limitations of the investigative procedures, the authors asserted, "The manner of death in the cases of the seven bodies that were autopsied was listed as undetermined. It is debatable whether these persons actually took cyanide of their own free will or were coerced" (p. 442). See R.L. Thompson, W.W. Manders, and W.R. Cowan, "Postmortem Findings of the Victims of the Jonestown Tragedy" (*Journal of Forensic Science* 1987; 32:433-43).

4 • Insanity, Psychiatry, and the Armor of the Law

The Armor of the Law

The killing of Lee Harvey Oswald by Jack Ruby deprived the people of the opportunity of prosecuting Oswald under the law for the assassination of President Kennedy. In that trial, they may also have been deprived of a rare moment to make new law on a vexing, still very unsettled medicolegal question: the criminal responsibility of mentally ill persons. There is an indication that Oswald was mentally unstable at various times in his life, and this instability might well have been pleaded in his defense.

The trials of persons accused of assassination or attempted assassination of heads of state have been the occasion for the making of much law in this area. The most important cases in English common law on criminal responsibility have involved assassination attempts. The first was the trial of James Hadfield, in 1800, for an attempt on the life of George III. There were many parallels in this case to the actions of Lee Harvey Oswald. Both were former servicemen. In each case, there was a connection with another public figure who was physically at the side of the head of state. For Oswald, it was Texas governor John Connally, who had been secretary of the Navy and had refused an Oswald request. For Hadfield, it was the Duke of York, under whom he had served. Both Oswald and Hadfield made their attacks by gunfire at public occasions, and both abandoned their weapons at the scene of the crime.

Hadfield had received severe head and brain injuries in battle and was alleged to have suffered psychotic delusions ever since that time. His defense attorney was Thomas Erskine, the foremost barrister in England. In his opening address to the jury at the trial Erskine asserted that the entire manner of the handling of the case was a "perpetual monument to our national justice." Hadfield had fired at the King from a seat in the front of the Drury Lane Theatre. The King had

From the *New England Journal of Medicine*
1964; 270:516-517.

fallen back in his box high above the orchestra seats. "Yet," said Erskine, "not a hair on the head of the supposed assassin was touched." Hadfield threw down his weapon and was taken into custody by bystanders, including an Army officer. He was turned over to the police shortly afterward. Erskine then pointed out that because Hadfield was on trial for his life, accused of the greatest of crimes, treason, he was "covered all over with the armor of the law." He was provided with counsel and was given various other procedural protections.

The trial, according to all reports of historians, was notable for the restraint of all who took part. The plea of not guilty due to insanity was made by Erskine and won. The law at the time was based on an earlier assassination attempt on a high public figure, Lord Ornslow, in 1724. In *Arnold's Case,* the court had held that to establish insanity as a defense, the defendant had to be totally deprived of his reason, so that he did not know what he was doing, any more than an infant or a wild beast would have known. Erskine and the crown prosecutor in *Hadfield's Case* both spoke of this "wild-beast" test. The *Hadfield* decision is notable in adding the significance of insane delusions as a basis for a finding of insanity.

The next great trial of an assassination involved the only successful attempt on the life of an English prime minister, Spencer Percival, in 1812. He was shot by a man named Bellingham, who was very quickly brought to trial, found guilty, and hanged within a week of the crime. Bellingham had pleaded not guilty by reason of insanity. Lord Mansfield, the judge at his trial, asserted that to have such a defense, the prisoner must be incapable of distinguishing right from wrong. The fact that Bellingham considered his act one of justifiable revenge against the government's alleged injustice to him, said the judge, was no defense.

The next case was an attempt on the lives of Queen Victoria and Prince Albert in 1840. The assailant, Edward Oxford, was found not guilty because of insanity on extensive evidence of insanity in his family and on evidence that he had delusions about being a member of a secret society. *Hadfield's Case* was used as precedent for the finding.

The last great case, the most important in all common law on the subject, was the trial of Daniel M'Naughten in 1843. M'Naughten was accused of killing Edward Drummond, secretary to the prime minister, Sir Robert Peel, in the mistaken belief that he was assassinating the prime minister himself.

There are again, as in Hadfield, some strange parallels between Oswald and Daniel M'Naughten. Both were political fanatics. Oswald ran off to Russia but returned to commit his crime against his own country. M'Naughten left his native Scotland in fear of imagined persecution by Jesuit priests. He went to France but returned to England, where he believed he was pursued by spies. He believed that the Tories and the prime minister were after him because he had voted against them in the last election.

M'Naughten's trial and acquittal gave rise to the famous "M'Naughten Rules" pronounced by the House of Lords. Unsettled to that time was the relation between the two types of allegations in insanity defenses: that the defendant did not know right from wrong, and that the defendant acted on an insane delusion. The lords answered by affirming the law on the first type of defense, saying that to be acquitted by reason of insanity the defendant must, owing to disease of the mind, be incapable of knowing the nature and quality of his act, or, if he knows it, unable to understand he is doing wrong. On the second type of defense the lords asserted that only when the delusions, if true, would be a defense as a matter of law could the defendant be excused from criminal punishment.

The M'Naughten Rules are still the law in the great majority of American states. Some reforms have occurred, but as yet no wholesale rejection of them has taken place. Perhaps, if Lee Harvey Oswald had been tried, there would have been a great national reexamination of this law.

There are other lessons in these cases from England. Certainly, Oswald was not "covered all over in the armor of the law." It was a porous law enforcement in Dallas that let the likes of striptease nightclub owner Ruby through. It was an irresponsible press and popular television that broadcast so much about Oswald that led Ruby to kill him and would, in the opinion of many, have made a fair trial for Oswald impossible anywhere in the United States.

There is one further bit of history encountered in the research of these incidents. At the time of the assassination attempt by Hadfield on King George III, a new verse was hastily written and added to the

British national anthem. It might be said by all in President Kennedy's memory and in prayer for President Johnson:

> From every latent foe,
> From the assassin's blow,
> God save the King.
> O'er him Thine arm extend,
> For Britain's sake defend,
> Our Father, Prince and Friend,
> God save the King.

♦

COMMENTS

As noted in the Introduction, this column was the first of my medicolegal essays in the *New England Journal of Medicine*. It was my own personal observation that the law of insanity was most frequently influenced by trials of persons accused of the assassination or attempted assassination of a head of state or prime minister. A review of legal history should make this apparent, but examinations of the law of insanity tend to concentrate on the technical aspects of the subject, rather than political circumstances. See W.J. Winslade and J.W. Ross, *The Insanity Plea* (New York: Charles Scribner's Sons, 1983).

As predicted in the column, the next occasion for a radical reexamination of the insanity plea in the United States was provided by the trial of another defendant accused of an attempted presidential assassination. This was the trial of John Hinckley, Jr., for the wounding and attempted murder by gunshot of President Ronald Reagan. Because the law of the District of Columbia required that the prosecution prove beyond reasonable doubt that the defendant was sane at the time of the crime, both sides produced expert evidence as to Hinckley's mental state at the time of the action. In the end, the defense won its case, and Hinckley is still confined as criminally insane in a District of Columbia mental hospital.

There was considerable public outcry against the verdict at the time, and since the trial, reform legislation has been adopted at the federal level and in at least 20 states. In the federal system, a new definition of criminal insanity has been adopted by statute to apply in all federal courts. Before this new law was passed, there had never been a statutory definition of criminal insanity in the history of the federal system. The federal courts had operated under case law established in each circuit across the country. The statute makes the plea of insanity an affirmative defense that must be proved by the defense on the basis of "clear and convincing evidence." Also, the law eliminates the insanity defense of "diminished responsibility" due to an inability to form mentally the necessary intent to kill. Furthermore, it eliminates the insanity defense of what is commonly called "an irresistible impulse" to kill because of an inability mentally to conform one's conduct to the requirements of the law.

The only basis for a successful plea of insanity remaining under the federal system is thus the traditional, and more strict, standard of the "right and wrong" defense derived from the classic M'Naughten Rules as modified by the Model Penal Code of 1962. This test allows a verdict of not guilty as a result of severe mental disease or defect under which the defendant was unable to understand (or appreciate) that his or her action was morally or legally wrong when committed.

In more recent years, almost every national organization of physicians or lawyers has produced recommendations regarding the insanity defense. The most radical approach was taken by the American Medical Association, which suggested virtual abolition of the defense; see *The Insanity Defense in Criminal Trials and Limitations on Psychiatric Testimony,* Report to the Board of Trustees (Chicago: American Medical Association, 1983). For an analysis of the new laws across the country and a review of the proposals, see S.A. Shah, "Criminal Responsibility," in W.J. Curran, A.L. McGarry, and S.A. Shah, eds., *Forensic Psychiatry and Psychology* (Philadelphia: F.A. Davis, 1986). See also H.J. Steadman and J.P. Morrissey, "The Insanity Defense: Problems and Prospects for Studying the Impact of Legal Reforms" (*Annals of the American Academy of Politics and Social Science* 1986; 484:115-26).

The Supreme Court and Madness: A Middle-Ground Ruling

There has been a great deal of legislative activity in the 50 states of the United States in recent years in the field of commitment for mental illness. Civil-rights organizations have been largely responsible for the changes in the law. Psychiatrists and mental health program planners have recently been concerned that the reforms may have gone too far in many states, where the legal barriers may prevent needed treatment from reaching very sick people.

Much of the focus in the involuntary-commitment procedure has been on the standard of proof that the person is seriously mentally ill or that he or she is a potential danger to self or others if not confined and treated psychiatrically. The strictest requirement, advocated by the most outspoken critics of psychiatric commitment, has been the imposing of the criminal-law standard of proof beyond reasonable doubt. Some 12 or 13 states have adopted such a requirement by statute or by court ruling.[1]

Advocates of this position have been interested in pressing the U.S. Supreme Court to review this issue and to make a ruling that the deprivation of liberty in a civil commitment to a mental health facility is just as great an area of concern as criminal conviction and incarceration in a jail or prison.

The Supreme Court had traditionally been reluctant to review issues in this field. Medical and psychiatric cases involving disputes over adequacy of proof and standards of proof are rarely considered by the nation's highest court. The commitment laws have been rather clearly matters of state concern.

From the *New England Journal of Medicine*
1979; 301:317-318.

To the surprise of many Supreme Court watchers, the justices did consent to review a case this year on issues of proof in civil commitment. Even more surprisingly, they took the case from Texas, where jury trials are required in civil commitments and on issues similar to, or frankly identical to, a case wherein the Supreme Court denied certiorari (declined discretion to review) only two years earlier.[2]

In the current case under discussion, *Addington* v. *Texas,*[3] the Texas Supreme Court had applied the traditional rule of the preponderance of the evidence, a lesser burden of proof than the criminal. Under the traditional rule, the state, in order to commit a person, would merely need to produce more evidence of illness and danger – any degree more – than is produced that the person is not mentally ill or not dangerous. The Texas court had applied this standard of proof because the proceeding is civil, not criminal, and because it questioned whether the state's psychiatrists could be expected to offer expert testimony within the stricter criminal standard on such difficult predictive issues as the person's potential for dangerous conduct in the future.

Faced with arguments concerning these two standards of proof, the civil (preponderance of evidence) and the criminal (beyond a reasonable doubt), the Supreme Court of the United States rejected both views. Instead, the Court chose a middle ground. It applied the test of "clear and convincing evidence" as required under the Fourteenth Amendment to the Constitution. Thus, it reversed the Texas court's decision for applying a lesser test, but refused to require proof beyond a reasonable doubt. On the same basis, Chief Justice Burger, writing for a unanimous bench (Justice Powell not participating in the deliberation or decision), also refused to require that the term "unequivocal" be added as a further modifier of the terms "clear and convincing," because he thought that the latter term could be interpreted to move too close to the criminal-law standard it had rejected.

The importance of this decision to the Supreme Court can be inferred from the fact that the Chief Justice wrote the opinion. The strength of the holding is shown by the unanimity of justices in supporting it.

Most psychiatrists in the country will be pleased with the decision. There was great concern about the movement in so many states toward the criminal standard. First of all, psychiatrists do not generally accept the idea that hospitalization of a mentally ill person, even when formally handled as an involuntary admission, should be equated with conviction of a crime and incarceration in prison. Most hospitalizations across the country, even involuntary, are now of very short duration, perhaps two months on average, often much less. Community facilities are now much more available, and involuntary admissions are being reduced substantially. Most important, however, psychiatrists generally believe that it is much too difficult under the current state of the art in psychiatric practice to be forced to certify patients involuntarily only when they are convinced "beyond a reasonable doubt" that the patient meets the complex legal requirements for the commitment.

Chief Justice Burger seems clearly to have accepted this view. In his opinion, he wrote that the application of the criminal-law standard could result in the denial of needed treatment and hospitalization for "many patients desperately in need of institutionalized psychiatric care."

A strong decision of this type should influence the states considerably. A few already apply the "clear and convincing" test or some version thereof, as a middle-ground standard of proof for involuntary hospitalization. Some commentators may think that all these arguments over the wording of tests of evidence is too much hair-splitting. The Chief Justice admitted that this view could be taken. However, it seems clear that the psychiatrists of the country were very worried and very uncertain about their responsibilities for evaluating mentally ill people. Many were refusing to certify patients when they had any vestige of doubt about their evaluation or prognosis. It is unquestionably difficult to practice medicine on such a standard of certainty, at least if medicine is still to be practiced by sober and thoughtful physicians who must admit that some doubts exist in most areas of clinical judgment. The Supreme Court has now recognized the sometimes inhumane results of placing too high a legal barrier around access to needed treatment for sick people.

REFERENCES

1. Curran WJ. Psychiatric emergency commitments in Hawaii: tests of dangerousness. N Engl J Med 1978; 298:265-6.
2. State v. Turner, 566 S.W.2d 563, *cert. denied,* 435 U.S. 929 (Texas, 1977).
3. Addington v. Texas. US Law Week 1979; 47:4473-7.

COMMENTS

This very well reasoned Supreme Court opinion seems to have had a substantial effect on state legislation in the 1980s. No additional states have enacted laws requiring evidence beyond reasonable doubt in order to hospitalize a mentally ill person involuntarily. The states have, however, shortened the length of involuntary commitments. Most of the states have abolished indefinite periods of compulsory hospitalization and have enacted limitations of from 60 days to one year. The definitions of mental illness for purposes of involuntary commitment have also been amended in most states to limit the application of the law to persons severely mentally ill and dangerous to themselves or to others in the community. Evidence of actual self-destructive conduct, violence, or attempts at violence toward others is usually required for compulsory hospitalization.

See, generally, S.S. Herr, S. Arons, and R.E. Wallace, *Legal Rights and Mental Health Care* (Lexington, Mass.: Lexington Books, 1983); A.A. Stone, *Law, Psychiatry, and Morality* (Washington, D.C.: American Psychiatric Press, 1984). See also D.B. Wexler, "The Structure of Civil Commitment: Patterns, Pressures, and Interactions in Mental Health Legislation" (*Law and Human Behavior* 1983; 7: 1-18); and M. Mills, "Civil Commitment of the Mentally Ill: An Overview" (*Annals of the American Academy of Politics and Social Science* 1986; 484:28-41).

Impartial Expert Witnesses in Child-Custody Cases: The Vulnerability to Countersuits

Among the most hotly contested and emotional courtroom battles are those involving child-custody disputes. These are the cases that could not be settled amicably between the parties in divorce and separation actions. Reforms in divorce law have removed a great deal of the wrangling over grounds and guilt in the marital split itself, but no amount of procedural or substantive reform can eliminate conflict arising from the faith, love, hopes, and dreams wrapped up in the children produced by the relationship. It is estimated that by the end of this decade approximately one third of American children, before reaching the age of 18, will have experienced the divorce of their parents.[1,2] Ten percent of divorce actions lead to court hearings on child-custody disputes.[3]

More and more trial courts are trying to approach these extremely sensitive cases more effectively by encouraging the parties to agree to the appointment by the court of an impartial expert who will examine the matter and make findings and recommendations to the court.[4] Such an expert conducts a thorough review of the dispute and interviews both parties, the child or children, and any other relevant persons, such as grandparents, who have been close to the children. A single report is prepared and shared with the parties and the court, often with recommendations to the court concerning who should receive custody and under what stated conditions. Many times, however, expert consultants will limit their reports to certain findings about the previous care of the child and medical and psychological

From the *New England Journal of Medicine*
1985; 312:1168-1170.

factors of importance, but will not make an actual recommendation about custody. In any event, the report is only advisory, no matter how definitive its conclusions. The judge must make the ultimate decision on the basis of all the evidence received at the hearing.[3,4]

The question that has often worried expert consultants in these emotional disputes has been their own vulnerability to suit by a disgruntled parent still disturbed about losing the custody battle. Can the expert physician who agrees to such a role and recommends that custody be awarded to one parent be sued by the angry loser for malpractice? Does being appointed by the court as an impartial expert afford protection or, better still, immunity from vexatious, nonmeritorious legal action?

A recent decision in a federal court in Colorado offers considerable comfort to court-appointed experts in such cases.[5] The court dismissed all charges of malpractice, negligence, invasion of privacy, and violation of constitutional rights and found that the physician, a psychiatrist, was immune from legal action because of his status as a witness in the court. The court also found the entire case without merit and frivolous. It ordered the husband who brought the case to pay for all the expenses of the defense, including lawyer's fees. The only claim the husband had made was that the psychiatrist had specifically recommended that custody be awarded to the wife. The mere fact of recommendation was found not enough even to require an answer or defense by the expert.

The custody dispute had its bizarre aspects, as long-drawn-out cases of this type often do. Before agreeing to the appointment of the expert to help resolve the matter, the husband had abducted the child from the temporary custody of the wife. After the final hearing wherein the judge awarded permanent custody to the wife, with visitation rights to the husband, the husband again abducted the child during a visit and apparently kept the child from 1980 to 1983. During that time, the husband appeared on a daytime national television talk show, *The Phil Donahue Show,* and according to the court, discussed the case, his abduction of the child, and his refusal to return the child to its mother. The mother sued the producers of the television program and its star, Phil Donahue, and the expert consultant was a witness for the mother in that trial, testifying to his previous evaluation in the custody case and to the effects of the abduction on the child.

Additional lawsuits are often among the expected side effects of such exaggerated confrontations between estranged husbands and wives. This decision in Colorado should encourage experts to help bring about settlement of such disputes without unnecessary fear of vexatious suits directed against themselves, the innocent peace-seekers.

It is to be hoped that other courts will follow the forceful and positive opinion of this Colorado federal judge. Ensuring complete immunity from suit is the only sensible method of discouraging such angry retaliation. There is, however, one remaining problem with the opinion that should be mentioned. The judge granted immunity to the expert only as an ordinary, common-law witness, not as a court-appointed impartial expert. The judge refused to denominate the expert as an "agent of the court" in his actions, despite his appointment as an impartial adviser to the court with judicially determined powers to require attendance of the parties and the child for his evaluations. This refusal was sustained despite the fact that the husband's claim of invasion of privacy was dismissed on the ground that the physician was not in a confidential relationship with the parties but was performing a public duty of evaluation for the court. The fact that the husband paid the expert's fee under order of the court was found insufficient to support a claim that the physician was the husband's witness and could not testify without the husband's permission. If the physician was performing a service for the court and was not the witness of either party, how could he be anything but a nonpartisan agent of the court?

The U.S. Supreme Court, in a very important decision not cited by this federal court, referred to a court-appointed expert examiner of a criminal defendant (in an issue of post-trial sentencing to capital punishment) as "an agent of the court."[6] Apparently, the Colorado judge hesitated to make such a designation because one of the grounds of the suit was a provision of the federal legislation concerning Civil Actions for Deprivation of Rights (42 US Code Section 1983). In order for the action to be brought, the claimed violation of civil rights had to be attributable to governmental (or state) action. The Colorado court admitted that the expert was appointed under federal authority to carry out a court-ordered function, but the judge asserted that the physician was not "a state actor" because his "decision" was not "influenced" by the judge or any other government official. The court cited another, earlier federal decision as having come to a similar conclusion.[7] This may have enabled the court to dismiss another complaint against the doctor without his having to answer it, but the reasoning as applied in this case was quite poor. This physician's role was strictly a court-ordered function, involving a power and authority that could not have existed without a governmental appointment. The expert was "influenced" to make a recommendation within the specified bounds of the court's directive to him. The fact that he arrived at the actual recommendation on the basis of his own professional judgment does not negate his judicially appointed authority to make the recommendation.

My concern here is with the impact of this decision. It could have provided broader protection for this and other types of court-appointed experts and, had it based its finding on the impartiality of the role and its court-appointed authority, could have encouraged the movement toward the use of more impartial consultants in place of partisan "battles of the experts." The court could have admitted that the consultant was an agent of the court, as he certainly was in fact, but ruled that he was still provided full immunity from suit. This would have been a novel approach in keeping with the otherwise forthright and positive character of this excellent ruling. To leave the court-appointed expert protected only as an ordinary witness is to invite further litigation over the obvious difference and greater influence exerted by this type of court-appointed consultant.

REFERENCES

1. Glick PC. Children of divorced parents in demographic perspective. J Social Issues 1979; 35:170-82.
2. Goldstein J, Freud A, Solnit AJ. Before the best interests of the child. New York: Macmillan, 1979.
3. Foster HH, Freed DJ. Joint custody, legislative reform. Trial 1980; 16:22-7.
4. Derdyn AP. A consideration of legal issues in child custody contests. Arch Gen Psychiatry 1976; 33:165-71.
5. Anderson v. Glismann, 577 F.Supp. 1506 (D. Colo., 1984).
6. Estelle v. Smith, 451 U.S. 454 (1981).
7. Watkins v. Roche, 529 F.Supp. 327 (S.D. Ga., 1981).

COMMENTS

Most physicians who talk with me about their courtroom appearances dislike the experience intensely. Most frequently, they favor some sort of reform in the adversarial system of justice in the United States to allow the liberal use of impartial experts appointed by the judge and free of partisan control. The idea always sounds good; its practical implementation is frequently difficult. Such a system would in all likelihood require the appointment of experts—not only in medicine, but in other scientific and technical fields as well—who would be available to the court either full time or on a regular basis for considerable periods of time working on a panel, and whose duties would include making court appearances and preparing legal reports. No such system has ever been installed in a common-law jurisdiction.

The local trial courts do, it is true, make indirect use of what could be called "impartial medical experts" when they call on specialists in forensic pathology and forensic psychiatry employed in public facilities in the local community or nearby state agencies, laboratories, or hospitals. In routine matters, when there is little or no controversy about the medical or psychiatric issues, these publicly employed forensic experts supply the courts with what is essentially impartial testimony, since the expert is not selected or employed by either side in the litigation. If the case is contested, however, the party to whom the forensic specialist's testimony is not favorable may seek out and retain independent expert testimony in rebuttal. At this point, the publicly employed expert's testimony loses its impartial character, and the expert is treated as a witness retained and presented by the party by whom he or she is called. In such situations, it would be legally improper to refer to the public employee as an impartial expert witness.

The particular issue in the *Anderson* case, as reported in this column, concerned vulnerability to countersuits in child-custody cases. Another recent California case indicates that psychotherapists still need to be aware of this vulnerability. In this decision, a California appeals court found a basis for personal damages against a treating psychologist who testified in a case concerned with child custody and visitation rights. The psychologist testified on behalf of the former wife and against the interest of the former husband, his patient, who alleged that the psychologist, testifying voluntarily and without subpoena, had violated confidences by revealing the diagnosis and certain aspects of his patient's illness. The psychologist claimed immunity under a California statute allowing breaches of confidentiality and privacy in judicial proceedings. The psychologist asserted that he had acted in the best interest of the child involved. The trial court dismissed the damage suit on these grounds, but the appeals court reinstated the case, holding that the right to privacy in psychotherapy outweighed the immunity of judicial proceedings when the witness was testifying "voluntarily" on behalf of his patient's adversary. See *Cutter* v. *Brownbridge,* 228 Cal. Rptr. 545 (1986). See also G. Paquin, "Protecting the Interests of Children in Divorce Mediation" (*Journal of Family Law* 1988; 26:279-316).

The Obligation of Confidentiality in Psychiatric Practice

The California Supreme Court continues to make financial awards to patients in suits against physicians with seemingly little regard for the effect of these awards and decisions upon the practice of medicine and the availability of insurance to cover this largesse of the judiciary, and without regard for the social consequences of this "money-for-everything" attitude.

The particular case, *Tarasoff* v. *Regents of the University of California,*[1] has already become infamous among mental health programs in California and among college and university student medical programs all over the country as it has taken its course through the various levels of trial and appeals courts in the Golden State.

The facts of the situation are undisputed. A student at the University of California's Berkeley campus was in psychotherapy with the student health service on an outpatient basis. He told his therapist, a psychologist, that he wanted to kill an unmarried girl who lived in Berkeley but who was then on a summer trip to Brazil. The psychologist, with the concurrence of another therapist and the assistant director of the department of psychiatry, reported the matter orally to the campus police and on their suggestion sent them a letter requesting detention of the student and his commitment for observation to a mental hospital. The campus police picked up the student for questioning but "satisfied" that he was "rational," released him on his "promise to stay away" from Miss Tarasoff. The police reported back to the director of psychiatry, Dr. Powelson. Dr. Powelson asked for the return of the psychologist's letter to the police and directed that all copies of the letter be destroyed. Nothing more was done at the

From the *New England Journal of Medicine*
1975; 293:285-286.

health service about the matter. Two months later, shortly after Miss Tarasoff's return, the student went to her home and killed her.

The parents of Miss Tarasoff brought suit for damages against the university and against the therapists and the campus police, as employees of the university and individually. In suing Dr. Powelson, the plaintiffs sought not only general money damages for negligence in failure to warn the girl and her parents and to confine the student, but exemplary or punitive damages (which could be assessed in huge amounts as multiples of the general damages or in any amount at the determination of the jury) for malicious and oppressive abandonment of a dangerous patient.

The superior court dismissed all these grounds for legal action against the defendants. The supreme court, in a four-to-two decision, reversed the decision and found that on these facts a cause of action was stated for general damages against all the therapists involved in the case and the assistant director and the director of psychiatry and against the university as their employer, for breach of the duty to warn Miss Tarasoff. The court dismissed the claim for exemplary damages against the therapists. It also dismissed the action against the police as protected from a suit by a statutory immunity, as well as the suit against the therapists for failure to confine the student under a commitment order, again because of a statutory immunity. The court implied that without the immunity, both these actions might have been meritorious.

It seems to me most physicians would throw up their hands in dismay over this result and the massive contradictions in the assessment of who was and who was not legally responsible for this death. If I were to describe in detail the reasoning of the court, the confusion of the medical mind would be compounded a thousand times.

The court asserted that the *Principles of Medical Ethics of the American Medical Association,* Section 9, did not bar breaching the confidentiality of this patient "in order to protect the welfare of this individual [the patient] or the community." From this premise the court jumped wholeheartedly to a positive duty to warn Miss Tarasoff. This is not what the *Principles* said. The traditional code of medical ethics allows a physician in his sound discretion to breach the confidentiality, but does not require it. It is almost impossible to draft an ethical principle to force a duty on physicians to breach confidences. Must they always warn of death threats, but have discretion on less dangerous threats? Must they warn if the patient is psychotic, but not if he is less disturbed? Does this case mean that every time a patient makes a threat against an unnamed person, the therapist must take steps to find out who it is and warn him (of anything at all, from vague threats to murder) or suffer money damages in the thousands or tens of thousands if the threat, or an aspect of the threat, is carried out?

This case was greatly confused by the array of immunities from suits created under California law. It can be strongly argued that the thrust of these immunity statutes regarding the duty to warn should also have been applied to the therapists, since the statutes were intended to encourage police and mental health personnel to release patients and not confine them on the basis of unreliable diagnoses of dangerousness. In the past it was thought that too many mental patients were confined for years and years because of their threats to other people, rarely carried out, and because of the conservatism of mental health personnel in exercising any doubt about dangerousness in favor of confinement as the safest way to prevent harm to third parties.

It seems clear that the therapists here thought that they had done all they could to protect their patient and the community by reporting the case to the police. They had exercised their discretion to warn the community and to breach the confidence of the patient, for his own sake, and that of the unknown girl. They could hardly warn her, since she was not even in the country at the time. Also, the threat to Miss Tarasoff might actually have been vaguely directed. The student could well have turned his anger and violence toward another person or toward himself. The only basic recourse was to recommend temporary observational commitment. The practice was to make this recommendation to the campus police. It was the police who acted, and they decided to release the student with a warning and a promise to stay away from the girl. How many thousands of such warnings — and releases — do police departments make every year? How many people then proceed to kill? The immunity statute was established to encourage release in these circumstances. But the statutory armor had a hole in it. The director of psychiatry was found by the court to have a "duty" to warn the girl, irrespective of the police action. The court utilized some precedents, none clearly applicable to this case, to justify its decision. It seems, however, that the real rationale was the aggravated nature of the case — a killing — in which the family was left without someone else to sue. The therapists, particularly Dr. Powelson, could have warned the girl if they had wanted to go against the police action and if they had thought the specific threat to Miss Tarasoff so serious as to warrant that action. The court did not apply any test to ascertain the custom of psychiatrists and mental health programs actually in such situations. The court declared the duty as a matter of law, regardless of the accepted practices of the profession. As in the *Helling* decision[2] discussed in an earlier column,[3] the court made the physician a guarantor against harm to this party, here not even a patient, on the basis of its own concept of monetary justice.

REFERENCES

1. 529 P.2d 553 (1974).
2. Helling v. Carey and Laughlin, 519 P.2d 981 (1974).
3. Curran WJ. Glaucoma and streptococcal pharyngitis: diagnostic practices and malpractice liability. N Engl J Med 1974; 291:508-9.

♦

COMMENTS

There was a storm of protest against the *Tarasoff* decision in psychiatric circles and generally in the public media. A rehearing on the decision was allowed, but the Supreme Court of California reaffirmed the holding. See 131 Cal. Rptr. 14 (1976), generally known as *Tarasoff II.* A well-known forensic psychiatrist severely criticized the decision in the *Harvard Law Review,* but his article failed to dampen the enthusiasm that most legal commentators felt about the ruling. See A.A. Stone, "The *Tarasoff* Decisions: Suing Psychiatrists to Safeguard Society" (*Harvard Law Review* 1976; 90:358-70).

Later case law in California and other states has tended to limit the application of the legal obligation to warn, by confining it to situations in which the identity of the alleged victim is known, or can easily be determined, by the treating psychiatrist. See, for example, *Currie* v. *United States,* 836 F.2d. 209 (4 Cir., 1987). Despite psychiatric criticism of *Tarasoff* and similar decisions in other states, no high court in other jurisdictions has specifically mentioned and rejected the concept of a duty to warn when such situations arise in private psychiatric practice. See J.C. Beck, "Violence and the *Tarasoff* Duty in Private Psychiatric Practice" (*Journal of Psychiatry and Law* 1985; 13:361-76); and W.J. Bowers, D.J. Givelber, and C.L. Blitch, "How Did *Tarasoff* Affect Clinical Practice?" (*Annals of the American Academy of Politics and Social Science* 1986; 484:70-85).

Psychiatric Testimony in Capital-Punishment Cases

The Supreme Court of the United States has instructed the state courts and legislatures that they must not be "arbitrary and capricious" in applying the death penalty in capital cases. This instruction was part of the background when, in 1972, the Court struck down existing statutes permitting the death penalty, as cruel and unusual punishment, in the landmark decision of *Furman* v. *Georgia.*[1]

In response, some states have enacted mandatory death penalties for specified crimes, allowing little or no discretion in the application of the law. The Supreme Court did not agree with this solution. In *Lockett* v. *Ohio,*[2] the Court held that the Constitution required that the sentencers not be precluded from considering "mitigating factors," including individualized aspects of the defendant's personality and character, his criminal record or lack of one, and the special circumstances of the crime. Expert psychiatric evidence could be used to establish mitigating circumstances. Chief Justice Warren Burger wrote the opinion expressing these views in the *Lockett* case.

Then came the important case of *Eddings* v. *Oklahoma,*[3] in which a 16-year-old boy was found guilty of killing a police officer and was sentenced to death under the new mandatory death-sentence law of Oklahoma. Oklahoma was also the first state to install the system of capital punishment by lethal drug injection. Ironically, the new method of execution was introduced in 1977, the same year that this killing occurred.

The action of the Supreme Court in the *Eddings* case does not help much in clarifying the meaning of "mitigation" or the use of psychiatric testimony in such cases. After the conviction, the trial judge was required under the Oklahoma law to hold a presentence hearing. The

From the *New England Journal of Medicine*
1982; 307:1431-1432.

prosecution asked for the death penalty because of the "heinous" nature of the crime. The trial judge agreed with this characterization. In fact, he found the killing to have been heinous, atrocious, and cruel. The judge also found the defendant's youth to be a mitigating factor, but he refused to consider any other aspects of the defendant's background or character, saying that he was bound by law not to consider them. He sentenced the boy to death. The Court of Appeals of Oklahoma upheld the decision.

The circumstances of the crime and the youth's background were described in the Supreme Court's opinions. The probationary report made to the trial court had indicated a troubled boyhood in which the defendant had received little or no care or supervision. His parents had been divorced when he was five years old, and he had lived with his mother until he was 14. His mother had been an alcoholic and "possibly" a prostitute during these years. The mother had claimed that she could not control the child and sent him to live with his father. The father, in an effort to control and discipline him, had beaten him severely.

When he was 16, the boy ran away from home along with several younger companions, taking his brother's car and three guns belonging to his father. Once out on the highway, the group drove off without any set direction or purpose. The inexperienced driver was apparently operating the car erratically and was flagged down on a major interstate road by the Oklahoma Highway Patrol. As the officer approached the car, the Eddings boy reached into the back seat, grabbed a shotgun, and shot the officer before he reached the car.

The murder conviction was a foregone conclusion because of the unprovoked assault on the police officer. In the hearing on sentencing, the defense relied heavily on the juvenile probation report and on psychiatric and psychological testimony indicating the emotional disturbance of the boy at the time he had fled from home and escaped onto the highway with his young friends. The witnesses indicated the boy's panic at being stopped by the police. Evidence was produced that immediately after the shooting the defendant had said, "I'd rather have shot an officer than go back where I live."

On certiorari appeal, the Supreme Court reversed and remanded the Oklahoma decision in a very close vote, five to four, on the basis of the above-mentioned *Lockett* case. The trial judge had refused to consider the emotional status of the defendant, his troubled upbringing, or the circumstances of the crime. The *Lockett* case seemed clearly to require such consideration. Surprisingly, however, the Supreme Court had considerable trouble reaching this conclusion. Only three justices agreed in the primary opinion. Two other justices wrote separate opinions expressing quite disparate views, concurring only in the decision to reverse and remand, but not in the reasoning of the primary opinion.

The four dissenters were led by Chief Justice Burger, who had written the *Lockett* decision on which the primary opinion was supposedly based. The chief justice did not agree to the application of that earlier opinion to this review of a troubled boyhood and the killing of a police officer. This created an odd situation in which more justices agreed on the dissent (four) than on a single opinion (three) favoring reversal. The result was judicial confusion in an important case and little or no guidance for the state courts in future cases involving capital offenses.

The effect of the *Eddings* case in terms of psychiatric evaluation is even more questionable than its usefulness in defining the role of judges and juries in these matters. Much of the strength of the dissenting opinion by the chief justice was drawn from the dissenters' obvious dissatisfaction with some of the psychiatric testimony offered for mitigation. The dissenters were particularly critical of what they considered a very unrepresentative psychiatric evaluation of the defendant's conduct. On the basis of a one-hour interview in the presence of the defendant's attorney, who would not allow questioning about the defendant's mental status on the day of the crime, an imaginative psychiatrist had come up with the opinion that the defendant had acted like a seven-year-old boy and had, in shooting the highway patrolman, been trying to kill his stepfather, a former police officer. This man had been married briefly to his mother and had evidently lived with the child and his mother when the boy was about seven years old. The Court quoted the psychiatrist as asserting that the defendant had been "preordained" to commit the murder since the time of his parents' divorce when he was five. The distaste of the justices for this seeming flight of fancy was obvious. They dismissed this "determinist" view as being rejected by "an overwhelming majority of psychiatrists."

After the *Hinckley* verdict of not guilty by reason of insanity in the assassination attempt on President Reagan, legal reformers have been clamoring to exclude examining psychiatrists from the role of key witnesses on guilt or innocence and to use them only in "the sentencing process." The *Eddings* case involved psychiatric testimony in just such a setting. At least for the purposes of mitigation in capital-punishment cases, the value of psychiatric testimony is still in doubt.

REFERENCES

1. 408 U.S. 238 (1972).
2. 438 U.S. 586 (1978).
3. 102 S. Ct. 869 (1982).

♦

COMMENTS

In recent years there has been an increasing amount of adverse criticism of psychiatric testimony, especially in criminal insanity cases. Most of the adverse comment relates to testimony on ultimate questions of law, such as criminal responsibility and legal competency to stand criminal trial. The American Psychiatric Association has joined in the criticism, even going so far as to make a formal statement advocating limitations on the scope of psychiatric testimony concerning such matters. See "Statement of the Insanity Defense" (*American Journal of Psychiatry* 1983; 140:681-5). See also A. Halpern, "The Fiction of Legal Insanity and the Misuse of Psychiatry" (*Journal of Legal Medicine* 1980; 1:18-74).

For an analysis of the role and contribution of the psychiatrist in the courtroom, see W.J. Curran and A.L. McGarry, "The Psychiatrist as Expert Witness," in W.J. Curran, A.L. McGarry, and S.A. Shah, eds., *Forensic Psychiatry and Psychology* (Philadelphia: F.A. Davis, 1986). See also L.R. Tancredi and D.N. Weisstub, "Law, Psychiatry, and Morality: Unpacking the Muddled Prolegomenon" (*International Journal of Law and Psychiatry,* 1986; 9:1-38). More recently, see "Executive Summary: Final Report of Ad Hoc Forensic Advisory Panel, National Institute of Mental Health" (*Mental and Physical Disability Law Reporter* 1988; 12:78-105).

Excluding Psychiatrists from the Courtroom: The Supreme Court Lays down the Law

The U.S. Supreme Court is heavily involved, to its own discomfort and growing impatience, in reviewing a seemingly endless series of appeals in capital-punishment cases. The defendants wait in death rows while their lawyers process the appeals. At present, most of these appeals are failing.

The latest area in which the Supreme Court has laid down a very firm rule rejecting challenges to state-court impositions of the death sentence is the use of psychiatric testimony to predict future violent conduct by convicted defendants. Under the state law in Texas, one of the grounds for imposing the death penalty is that the defendant constitutes a "continuing danger" to the public safety because of a strong potential for committing future violent crimes. The Texas courts have established a practice in over 50 cases of using psychiatric testimony on this issue from a small group of psychiatrists, usually associated with the prison system, in which the testimony has supported the death penalty.[1,2]

In the most recent review before the Supreme Court, *Barefoot* v. *Estelle,*[3] the issue was presented in stark terms. The defendant was convicted of the murder of a police officer. After the conviction, a special hearing was held before the same jury on the issue of capital punishment. The defendant had a record of five previous offenses, all nonviolent, but two involving possession of a firearm. He had also been arrested and charged previously on several counts of sexual crimes involving children. The defense called no expert witnesses on the issue of the

From the *New England Journal of Medicine*
1984; 310:1651-1652.

defendant's dangerousness. The prosecution, on the other hand, called two psychiatrists, both of whom testified on the basis of a description of the defendant's personal background and criminal record and of the circumstances of this particular killing. Neither physician had examined the defendant personally. One asserted that on the basis of a reasonable degree of medical certainty, he believed the defendant would probably commit violent crimes in the future. The other psychiatrist was even more positive. He asserted that in his opinion the probability of future violence was "one hundred percent and absolute," whether the defendant was in a prison or subsequently released. The jury had no trouble finding that the defendant should be sentenced to death.

The American Psychiatric Association filed an amicus curiae brief in this case, as it did in some others, arguing that the Supreme Court should bar from American courtrooms on Constitutional grounds all testimony by psychiatrists on the likelihood of future violent conduct. The association's brief cited numerous follow-up studies indicating that psychiatric evaluation is unreliable in predicting dangerousness in the long term, especially when the psychiatrist does not conduct a thorough clinical examination of the defendant. (As might be expected, convicted murderers in Texas often refuse such examinations by the prosecution's psychiatrists, and such examinations are not compelled by the courts.) The association relied heavily on the 1981 review by Professor John Monahan of a group of follow-up studies.[4] Monahan concluded that psychiatrists and psychologists were wrong in two out of three predictions over an extended period of time. The association claimed that this two-thirds failure rate should result in the exclusion of all psychiatric prognosis of the potential for violence.

The majority of the Supreme Court (five justices, one concurring, with three justices dissenting) firmly dismissed the arguments of the association and upheld the imposing of the death penalty. The opinion by Justice White treated the position of the association quite abruptly and with a strong flavor of disdain for the cautious statistical approach taken in the brief. Justice White began his commentary by asserting that to accept the argument of the association that all psychiatric testimony about the potential for violence should be totally excluded from evidence was "like asking us to reinvent the wheel." He pointed out that predictions concerning future conduct were made regularly throughout the criminal–penal system in granting bail, imposing sentences, and allowing the release of prisoners on parole. These decisions were generally made by nonprofessionals without the aid of expert evaluations. Justice White observed caustically that it would make "little sense, if any" to argue that psychiatrists, out of the entire universe of persons who might have an opinion on the subject, would "know so little" about the subject that they should be totally excluded from testifying. It should be understood that the Court had no difficulty with a challenge to the relative weight of any particular expert's opinion once admitted into evidence; it was only refusing to agree to a total exclusion of all psychiatric testimony. The Court also observed that not all psychiatrists agreed with the association's position. Furthermore, Justice White demonstrated the depth of the Court's reading of Professor Monahan's 1981 review by pointing out that the author had said that although he had originally believed it was "impossible" for psychiatrists to predict that a given person would probably commit violent acts, by the time he completed his monograph he had come to the conclusion that there may be circumstances in which prediction or prognosis is both empirically possible and ethically appropriate.

As a result of the *Barefoot* decision, defense lawyers have lost one more round in their challenge to the new trend toward reimposing the death penalty in the United States. The prosecution can continue to use psychiatrists who are willing to offer their professional services in finding defendants a continuing menace to society on the basis of their future potential for violence.

Most physicians of ability and ethical sensitivity in any field of clinical medicine are, in my experience, reluctant to be very certain about the long-term prognosis of an illness or the extent of expected recovery in individual patients. Even in terminal illnesses, five years is the usual limit of most clinical prognostic evaluations.

Is the ability to predict violent conduct, directed against the self or others, within the scope of the effective clinical skills of psychiatrists?

The American Psychiatric Association did admit in its brief in the *Barefoot* case that short-term predictions of violence can and should be made in the case of disturbed persons needing emergency psychiatric care and treatment. Is the reluctance of the association related only to the longer-term nature of the legally requested evaluations? Are all such predictions for all types of persons equally unreliable? This seems an extreme position. The Supreme Court observed that the district court, after hearing extensive evidence on the subject, had found that the majority view in psychiatry was that the accuracy of even long-term psychiatric predictions rose dramatically when there was a proved pattern of repetitive assaults and violence in the history of the person being evaluated.

There seems to me to be possibly a deeper meaning in the amicus brief submitted by the psychiatrists that escaped the caustic, rationalistic view of the Court. The American legal adversarial system uses psychiatrists in a particularly shabby way. Cases like the Sirhan Sirhan trial in California and the more recent Hinckley trial in Washington resulted in the heaping of greatly undeserved public scorn on the participating psychiatric witnesses. It often seems that the more ethical, cautious, and professionally skilled the psychiatrist, the less his or her evaluations are welcomed in the courtroom, where certainty and a willingness to play the adversarial game are the attributes most valued not only by the competing lawyers but by the presiding justices, from the lowest to the highest of our courts. The association was perhaps saying that the courts currently seem unable or unwilling to distinguish the good from the bad in psychiatric testimony; the responsible bulk of the profession would like to have this distasteful burden removed from the entire profession by a judicial exclusion from the courtroom, at least until the judicial system is reformed. This underlying dissatisfaction with the legal environment, most glaringly presented in death-sentence cases, may well explain the association's position more fully than most lawyers and judges are willing to admit.

REFERENCES

1. Dix GE. The death penalty, dangerousness, psychiatric testimony and professional ethics. Am J Crim Law 1977; 5:151-214.
2. Estelle v. Smith, 101 S. Ct. 1866 (1981).
3. Barefoot v. Estelle, 103 S. Ct. 3383 (1983).
4. Monahan J. The clinical prediction of violent behavior. Washington, D.C.: Public Health Service, 1981.

COMMENTS

Psychiatrists and psychologists seem determined to limit expert testimony in capital-punishment cases, especially when the expert is called in to predict whether the defendant will be likely to engage in violent conduct in the distant future – i.e., years and decades later – and after a period of high-security imprisonment. See C.P. Ewing, "'Dr. Death' and the Case for an Ethical Ban on Psychiatric and Psychological Predictions of Dangerousness in Capital Sentencing Proceedings" (*American Journal of Law and Medicine* 1983; 8:407-28). See also S.A. Shah, "Dangerousness: A Paradigm for Exploring Some Issues in Law and Psychology" (*American Psychologist* 1978; 33:224-38). One of the psychiatrists who testified in the *Barefoot* case, Dr. James P. Grigson, who is known as "Dr. Death" because of his testimony in such cases, continues in 1988 to be willing to offer expert testimony in capital-punishment cases. See L. Belkin, "Expert Witness is Unfazed by 'Dr. Death' Label" (*New York Times.* June 10, 1988:B9).

The American Bar Association has recently adopted standards for the applicability of expert psychiatric testimony in criminal proceedings. The report was prepared by an interdisciplinary group and includes recommendations for limitations on predictions of future dangerous conduct. *Proposed Criminal Justice Mental Health Standards* (Washington, D.C.: American Bar Association, August 1984). See also R.C. Reinher, H.K. Dudley, Jr., and J.V. White, "Dangerousness Review Boards in Texas" (*Journal of Psychiatry and Law* 1985; 13:449-56); and W. Greene, "Capital Punishment, Psychiatric Experts, and Prediction of Dangerousness" (*Capital University Law Review* 1984; 13:533-53). See also M.W. Jackson, "Psychiatric Decisionmaking for the Courts: Judges, Psychiatrists, Lay People?" (*International Journal of Law and Psychiatry* 1986; 9:507-20).

The Competency of the Mentally Retarded in Criminal Proceedings

One of the continuing fallacies in the law of most American jurisdictions is the assumption that mental retardation and mental illness are the same thing for legal purposes. The fallacy is reinforced by the location in many states of retardation programs in state agencies for mental health operated by psychiatrists.

An impressive and influential blow was struck for a more specific examination of legal issues in mental retardation in a recent decision of the U.S. Supreme Court. In *Jackson* v. *Indiana*[1] a retarded 27-year-old deaf mute was charged with two minor robberies. A question of his mental competency to stand trial was raised. Under the Indiana law, the defendant was examined by two psychiatrists and was given a hearing on his competency. Though the statute did not require it, he was provided counsel. The joint report and testimony of the psychiatrists was to the effect that the defendant had the mental age of a preschool child. He could communicate in only a very limited manner through sign language. They concluded that he was not capable of understanding the charges against him or of aiding his attorney in his defense. They observed that his prognosis was "rather dim" and that it was unlikely he could ever become competent.

On the basis of this evidence, the trial judge found the defendant incompetent and ordered him committed to a state institution until the State Department of Mental Health should certify to the court that the defendant was "sane." The defendant appealed, and the Supreme Court of Indiana affirmed the decision.

From the *New England Journal of Medicine*
1972; 287:1184-1185.

The U.S. Supreme Court on certiorari reviewed this action and unanimously found it an unconstitutional deprivation of the rights of the defendant.

The Supreme Court held that the defendant was entitled to a competency hearing with all procedural and substantive safeguards available to any person civilly committed under Indiana law. Under these statutes, the defendant would be released at any time the superintendent of the institution found that his condition justified it. The Court specifically noted, however, that since the defendant was retarded and not mentally ill, the requirements of regaining "sanity" and, in fact, of becoming mentally competent could not be applied as they are to mentally ill persons who, under psychiatric treatment, may regain normal mental status. To impose this condition on the retarded defendant was to effect his lifelong confinement in an institution. It was admitted that Indiana did not have facilities to help persons like the defendant. Justice Blackmun held that the defendant could only be held for "a reasonable time" during which it could be determined whether or not he could attain competency through available treatment or habilitation "in a foreseeable future." If, as in this case, it was clear that he could not, the defendant must be released, or an independent proceeding must be conducted to commit him civilly.

The Court also discussed the issue of the charges standing against the defendant. In the remand to the Indiana court for a new trial it was suggested that Indiana should consider allowing the counsel for the defendant to raise at least some issues in his defense despite his inability to stand trial. These would include the question of his criminal responsibility owing to his retardation. No Indiana statutes were cited allowing such action, but the Court nevertheless encouraged the Indiana court to examine "these possibilities."

The decision of the Supreme Court adopts with approval the rationale of the *Druken* case[2] in Massachusetts, which had arrived at similar conclusions in an incompetency case. Also, the Court cited with approval statutes in Massachusetts, Maryland, Montana, New York, and Wisconsin that allow the raising of certain defenses on the merits on behalf of incompetent defendants.

Research indicates that mental incompetency to stand trial is a very important issue in any case involving a retarded person—probably much more important than when the defendant is mentally ill. Many, if not most, mentally ill persons are capable of understanding criminal charges and of aiding in their own defense, even where they are psychotic. There has been much confusion in the past between competency and criminal irresponsibility, very different legal concepts often indiscriminately grouped under "insanity." On the other hand, a retarded person below ascertainable levels of intelligence, understanding, and experience, particularly if also handicapped in ability to communicate, may well be incapable of meeting the minimum legal requirements of understanding the charges against him, of understanding what a criminal trial is all about, and of being able to help his lawyers to defend him.

The principles of this case apply to the mentally ill as well as to the mentally retarded and other developmental disabilities. However, it is most encouraging to see the courts make important distinctions between these different kinds of disabilities, which can affect legal rights in greatly different ways.

REFERENCES

1. Jackson v. Indiana, 92 S. Ct. 1845 (1972).
2. Commonwealth v. Druken, 356 Mass. 503, 254 N.E.2d 779 (1969).

COMMENTS

The decision reviewed in this column was the first ruling in the Supreme Court determining rights of the mentally retarded in criminal cases. It was also important in drawing distinctions between the rights of the retarded and of the mentally ill. See, generally, J. Monahan and H.J. Steadman, eds., *Mentally Disordered Offenders: Perspectives from Law and the Social Sciences* (New York: Plenum Press, 1984). See also M. Kindred and B. Sales, "Developmentally Disabled Persons in the Criminal Justice System," in W.J. Curran, A.L. McGarry, and S.A. Shah, eds., *Forensic Psychiatry and Psychology* (Philadelphia: F.A. Davis, 1986).

More recently, however, the Supreme Court has refused to classify the mentally retarded as a protected class and thus impose the requirement that charges of discrimination against them be subjected to "close scrutiny" to ensure that their constitutional rights are not violated. This ruling leaves the retarded outside the cover of specially protected minorities and women. The majority found by six to three that such special protection was not advisable and might lead to the creation of further protected classes encompassing the mentally ill, aged, and disabled. Nevertheless, on a lower scale of scrutiny, in a housing-law action in a case in which a city had denied a permit for group housing to an organization seeking housing for retarded persons, the majority found that the retarded had indeed been improperly discriminated against. See *City of Cleburne* v. *Cleburne Living Center,* 105 U.S. 3249 (1985).

The rights of the retarded are protected under federal law supporting programs that provide services to a range of developmentally disabled persons. See the landmark legislation, Developmentally Disabled Assistance and Bill of Rights Act, Public Law 95-602. The Supreme Court, however, has recently restricted the jurisdiction of federal courts in applying this act and has allowed state agencies to follow their own state laws in determining the rights of the retarded.

The Management of Psychiatric Patients: The Legal Right to Refuse Treatment

A serious loss of judicial confidence in the efficacy of psychiatric treatment is clearly reflected in two decisions reached in the federal courts in recent months. The cases were hard fought on both sides, and the opinions are laboriously well thought out and soberly written.

At the district-court trial level in the federal system, the judges heard evidence of inadequate treatment of patients in public mental hospitals in Massachusetts and New Jersey. The Massachusetts case, *Rogers* v. *Okin,*[1] decided by Judge Tauro, consumed 72 trial days, 8000 pages of transcript testimony and exhibits, and more than 2300 pages of argument in post-trial briefs by the lawyers for each side. The New Jersey case, *Rennie* v. *Klein,*[2] decided by Judge Brotman, was equally long and drawn out. Both decisions are now on appeal.

Neither the evidence nor the opinions can be summarized adequately in these pages in a manner that does justice to the impact of these cases on the law in the field of psychiatric treatment. I can only try to call attention to the major results of the rulings.

Both judges found that involuntary as well as voluntary psychiatric patients in state institutions have the constitutional right to refuse treatment that psychiatrists or other hospital personnel offer or attempt to force on them. The right to refuse treatment was firmly associated with the constitutional right of personal privacy, which has now been related to many areas of medical treatment and personal integrity.

From the *New England Journal of Medicine*
1980; 302:1297-1299.

There is no doubt that the judges were disturbed at what they saw and heard about dirty and drab facilities, inadequate staffing and care of patients, overuse of psychotropic drugs with serious side effects (particularly drugs resulting in tardive dyskinesia), and forced seclusion as a means of general discipline of patients. In addition to affirmation of their clients' rights, the patients' attorneys in the Massachusetts case sought a sizable financial award in damages. Judge Tauro refused to find either professional negligence on the part of individual practitioners or any wholesale violation of personal rights resulting in damages action against individual defendants. One suspects in reading the opinion that the judge had little sympathy with the poor quality of the overall management of the hospital. Nevertheless, he did not see fit to justify a damages award for what he found to be a sincere effort by the staff to do the best that they could under the standards of psychiatric care and the low budgets that prevailed in state institutions in the years covered by the lawsuit, 1973 to 1975.

Judge Tauro did authorize a very limited use of forced medication of psychotic patients in acute stages of illness. He found the defendants' definition of "psychiatric emergencies" too broad, subjective, and prone to abuse. He limited temporary forced medication and restraint or seclusion to unequivocally serious cases with substantial likelihood of physical harm (not property damage or anxiety or bizarre behavior) to the patient or to other patients or staff at the hospital.

It should be understood that both Judge Tauro and Judge Brotman rejected the traditional assertion that an involuntary-commitment order contains within it an inherent legal authority to treat the unwilling patient, for his or her own good, as a mentally incompetent person. Commitment alone was found not to render the person incompetent, even regarding decisions about treatment.

It seems clear that the courts found a common lack of individualized attention to many patients' complaints and a disregard for the patients' refusals to accept certain treatments. The only way that the judges could see to break what they believed was inhumane inattention to the patients' conditions was to erect a new legal barrier that the hospitals would have to respect, no matter how inconvenient and rigid the new standard might seem, at least in its general application.

Along with the appeal of the case in Massachusetts, attempts are being made to explore with the probate courts methods of appointing guardians for those psychiatric patients who clearly are mentally incompetent. These guardians would make general decisions concerning the treatment of their wards. It is not at all clear how many psychotic patients might be covered by such a guardianship arrangement.

The New Jersey decision, actually passed down shortly before the Massachusetts case finally moved out of the system, is, in my judgment, the more imaginative in suggesting administrative methods for allowing greater scope to patients' refusals of treatment and yet allowing medication under controlled conditions for patients clearly in need of such treatment. It also seems that the New Jersey court was more willing to allow (or to prod) the professional system to readjust itself and to meet the new demands placed on it. The order of Judge Brotman contains a series of steps to safeguard patients, but it also allows necessary medication in controlled situations without the need to obtain courtroom or judicial review of each case or to seek general guardianships that could, for indefinite periods, deprive patients of the right to refuse.

The first requirement under the New Jersey order is that the state hospitals must seek and obtain the written informed consent of both voluntary and involuntary patients before administering a specific psychotropic drug. The written document must describe the specific medication, its intended benefits, possible risks and discomforts, and short-term and long-term side effects, if any. One form may seek permission for administration of up to three different medications, concurrently or alternatively in a treatment plan. Even after a form is signed, however, the patient may refuse orally to accept any specific administration by a physician or nurse, and the oral refusal must be respected. The written consent document must explain in plain language all rights of the patient under the new system.

Next, the state of New Jersey must set up a system of patients' advocates or representatives who are to be made available to patients to assist them concerning their rights and to facilitate communication concerning medications. These advocates or representatives are not to be responsible to the individual hospital to which they are assigned but are to be recruited, trained, and employed by the Department of Human Services. The representatives may be drawn from different backgrounds and must receive special instruction on the effects of psychotropic drugs and the principles of legal advocacy. They are to be supervised by a psychiatrist and an attorney in the central office of the Department of Human Services.

In the event of a patient's refusal of treatment that the psychiatric staff believes that he or she should receive, and if the staff believes that the patient is at that time "functionally incompetent" in refusing the medication, a new procedure for independent psychiatric review may be called into play. Outside psychiatrists who are not on the hospital staff will be engaged to conduct these independent reviews with an informal hearing attended by a representative on behalf of the patient. The patient may also have legal counsel at the hearing at the patient's expense or supplied by outside agencies. The independent psychiatrist must render a written opinion in such cases. He or she can negotiate with the patient to accept medication or with the staff to modify its treatment plan, or the psychiatrist can prohibit the use of psychotropic drugs altogether. The psychiatrist can also authorize specific forced medication, following the court's standards, for a period not exceeding 60 days.

Judge Brotman also dealt with emergency situations and general guardianships. He would allow forced medication for committed patients for no longer than 72 hours during a sudden, serious change in the patient's condition that creates a clear danger (physical) to the patient or to others in the hospital. Certification by the hospital director of continued acute danger to life or limb of the patient may allow extension of forced medication for another 72-hour period. Concerning patients under guardianship as mentally incompetent, consent would have to be sought and obtained from the guardian under strict application of New Jersey law. In addition, the patient's advocate or representative at the hospital must be consulted on the patient's behalf. The representative is expected to review the case and the patient's feelings about the drug and possible side effects in the case. The representative may contact and consult with the guardian and is also authorized, under his or her own judgment, to institute examination and hearing on the case under the independent psychiatric review procedure described.

There is no doubt that these courts have (with perhaps overreactive zeal) suggested a solution that itself may create havoc on the wards as it seeks to redress serious patient problems. I am not sure of the wisdom of this judicial confrontation.

REFERENCES

1. Rogers v. Okin, US Law Week, 478 F.Supp. 1342 (1979).
2. Rennie v. Klein, 462 F.Supp. 1131, 1978; Preliminary injunction, September 1979. Action to stay enforcement declined, December 1979.

♦

COMMENTS

Despite subsequent developments that have somewhat changed the picture, I still believe that the lower court opinion in *Rennie* v. *Klein* is the best approach to a reasonable application of a "right to refuse treatment" that any American court has come up with. Unfortunately, the U.S. Supreme Court remanded the *Rennie* case to the Federal Circuit Court with orders to reexamine the role of professional psychiatric decision making in view of the Supreme Court's previous rulings on right to treatment. The circuit court largely reaffirmed the approach that Judge Brotman had originally taken to the case and ordered that those directives that had been reinstated be implemented in accordance with rather complex administrative procedures that had subsequently been adopted in New Jersey. See *Rennie* v. *Klein,* 720 F.2d 266, Third Circuit (1983).

The *Rogers* case has had just as checkered a career in its course through the courts, finally reaching the U.S. Supreme Court, which remanded it as it had *Rennie,* finding that the state law of Massachusetts was controlling on the issues. The implication of the Supreme Court's opinion was, however, that the lower federal courts had not given enough weight to psychiatric professional opinion as to whether a disturbed mental patient should be forcibly treated when such treatment appeared to be in his or her own best interest. The Supreme Court remanded the *Rogers* case to the Massachusetts Supreme Judicial Court, directing it to provide rules for the implementation of the decision that mental patients have a right to refuse psychiatric treatment in that state's public mental hospitals. The high court of Massachusetts subsequently produced a set of guidelines that provide wide latitude for competent patients to refuse treatment in state institutions. See *Rogers* v. *Commissioner of Mental Health,* 390 Mass. 489 (1983). The decision also provides for the appointment of guardians to exercise "substituted judgment" on behalf of incompetent mental patients in regard to needed psychiatric treatment.

At present, nearly all American states have provided mental patients with at least a qualified right to refuse psychiatric treatment that could be harmful to them. See L.A. Callahan and D.R. Longmire, "Psychiatric Patients' Right to Refuse Psychotropic Medication: A National Survey" (*Mental Health Disability Law Reporter* 1983; 7:494-9). For a general review of decisions in the field, see D.J. Kemma, "Current Status of Institutionalized Mental Patients' Right to Refuse Psychotropic Drugs" (*Journal of Legal Medicine* 1985; 6:107-38). For a provocative critique of the right to refuse treatment from the point of view of treating psychiatrists, see P.S. Appelbaum and T.G. Gutheil, "'Rotting with Your Rights on': Constitutional Theory and Clinical Reality in Drug Refusal by Psychiatric Patients" (*Bulletin of the American Academy of Psychiatry and Law* 1979; 7:306-15).

The Right to Psychiatric Treatment: A "Simple Decision" in the Supreme Court

> A finding of "mental illness" alone cannot justify a State's locking up a person against his will and keeping him indefinitely in simple custodial confinement.
>
> Justice Stewart

The idea of a constitutional right to psychiatric treatment has been around now for some 15 years, having been articulated by Morton Birnbaum in an article in the *American Bar Association Journal* in 1960.[1] It received statutory recognition in the District of Columbia in 1965 and was supported in an opinion by Judge David Bazelon in 1966.[2] In this first case, the specific basis of the opinion was the 1965 statute, which required treatment of committed patients. In later cases, however, it was often held or implied that the right to treatment was constitutionally guaranteed. These later cases extended the doctrine to sexual psychopaths, alcoholics, defective delinquents, and juvenile offenders. Some of the later cases were much more sophisticated than the earlier ones in applying the doctrine to general conditions at the Patuxent Institution in Maryland[3] and in Bridgewater Hospital in Massachusetts.[4] Its broadest application, however, came in 1971 and 1972, when a federal district court in Alabama imposed very detailed conditions for treatment of mentally ill persons and for habilitation of the mentally retarded.[5] Implications of this decision were examined in an earlier *Journal* column.[6]

During all these years, no decision of the Supreme Court of the United States supported this widespread judicial activism in the field

From the *New England Journal of Medicine*
1975; 293:487-488.

of clinical psychiatry. It seemed to be assumed by all commentators that the principle would be supported without doubt or controversy. As pointed out in the earlier column,[6] the Alabama judge did not even bother to cite any authority whatsoever for his pronouncement of the constitutional basis for the right.

Then things changed. The Supreme Court decided to review a Florida case in which the Federal Court of Appeals had recognized the constitutional right of a committed patient to adequate treatment while confined to a Florida state hospital. Nearly every constitutional lawyer and psychiatric law specialist expected the Supreme Court to deal with the full implications of the doctrine for the guidance of courts and legislatures all over the country.

In the decision, *O'Connor* v. *Donaldson,*[7] the Supreme Court, in a unanimous opinion, treated the subject much more cautiously than expected. The Court held only that when a patient is not dangerous to himself or others and, if he is mentally ill, is not currently receiving any treatment, he must be released from custody at his own request.

The Court refused to deal with the full scope of the questions that it could have examined. It was observed, "We have concluded that the difficult issues of constitutional law dealt with by the Court of Appeals are not presented by this case in its present posture."

In a rather ingenious way, Justice Stewart asserted that the case was really very simple. He concluded, "As we view it, this case raises a single, relatively simple, but nonetheless important question concerning every man's constitutional right to liberty."

Thus, the Supreme Court completely avoided the crucial question: If a patient is mentally ill and is dangerous to himself or others, can he be held involuntarily in a mental hospital without treatment?

Newspapers throughout the country have treated the case as a major landmark in American law. The *New York Times'* headline on page 1 read: "High Court Curbs Power to Confine Mentally Ill."[8] The *Washington Post* went much farther and devoted much more space to the subject. One story was headlined: "'Right to Liberty' Proclaimed for Thousands of Mentally Ill."[9] After a few days had passed and time for reflection had occurred, the *Post,* in an editorial, took back some of its enthusiasm for the implications of the decision. In a much soberer fashion, the editorial started out with the key observation, "The decision by the Supreme Court last week on the constitutional rights of the mentally ill will undoubtedly spawn more litigation."[10] The *Post* now admitted that the principle laid down in the case was so simple and fundamental that it could not understand why it had not been stated long before!

With this observation of the *Post* editorial writer we are in full agreement. It is an unfortunate commentary on the mental hospital system and on psychiatry in this country that in 1975 the Supreme Court had to order the State of Florida to release a person who had been confined against his will and who was admittedly not dangerous and who was receiving no treatment. This person, Mr. Kenneth Donaldson, was confined for nearly 15 years. He made repeated attempts to gain his release, both informally and through the courts. He continuously asserted that he was not mentally ill. He had had a job before he was hospitalized by his parents, and he obtained a position again shortly after his release. At various times during the 15 years he was able to show that, if necessary, other responsible adults were willing to help him upon his release. The superintendent during nearly all these years, Dr. J.B. O'Connor, refused all these efforts. Upon Dr. O'Connor's retirement after this litigation had begun, the hospital staff changed this decision and released Mr. Donaldson.

Dr. O'Connor himself was a key defendant in this case. The trial-court jury returned a verdict against Dr. O'Connor and a co-defendant of $38,500 for compensatory damage and $10,000 punitive damages. The court of appeals had confirmed this finding. The Supreme Court returned the case for trial against Dr. O'Connor on instruction that he would not be personally liable for damages unless he knew or reasonably should have known that his action in continuing to confine Donaldson against his will and without treatment would violate the patient's constitutional rights, or if he took such action with malicious intent to deprive the patient of his constitutional rights or otherwise to injure him.

Chief Justice Burger wrote a concurring opinion in which he agreed with the result reached, but in which he went into much greater detail about the implications of the decision and the simplistic approach taken by the Court. It seems clear that the chief justice, and perhaps other justices, will have trouble in agreeing to extend the principle of the Donaldson case into the more troublesome aspects of the asserted constitutional right to psychiatric treatment.

REFERENCES

1. Birnbaum M. The right to treatment. Am Bar Assoc J 1960; 46:499-505.
2. Rouse v. Cameron, 125 U.S. app. 366, 373 F.2d 451 (1966).
3. Director of Patuxent Institution v. Daniels, 243 Md. 16, 221 A.2d 397 (1966).
4. Nason v. Superintendent of Bridgewater Hospital, 353 Mass. 604, 233 N.E.2d 908 (1968).
5. Wyatt v. Stickney, 325 F.Supp. 781, 1971; 334 F.Supp. 1341 (1972).
6. Curran WJ. The "class action" approach to protecting health-care consumers – the right to psychiatric treatment. N Engl J Med 1972; 289:26.
7. US Law Week 1975; 43:4929-37.
8. New York Times. June 27, 1975:1.
9. Washington Post. June 27, 1975:1.
10. Washington Post. July 2, 1975:19.

♦

COMMENTS

This opinion is still the only decision of the Supreme Court that deals with a right to psychiatric treatment for committed mental patients. A later decision extended a limited right of "habilitation" to retarded persons in state institutions. These rights include the basic necessities of life in the form of food, clothing, and shelter, reasonably safe environmental conditions, adequate training or education within the limits of the resident's capacities, and protection from physical abuse and unnecessary restraint. See *Youngberg* v. *Romeo,* 102 S. Ct. 2452 (1982). A more recent decision in a lower federal court applied the ruling of *Youngberg* to a failure to afford these "fundamental rights" of habilitation to a retarded resident who died after an allegedly excessive drug treatment administered for purposes of restraint. See *Sabo* v. *O'Bannon,* 586 F.Supp. 1132, East. Dist. of Pa. (1984).

Since the *Donaldson* decision, the movement in both the mental health and the retardation fields has been toward deinstitutionalization. This trend was greatly encouraged by case law and state statutes mandating that mental patients and mentally retarded persons receive treatment or habilitation only in the "least restrictive" environment applicable to the person concerned. The movement was not, however, accorded support by the Supreme Court. In *Pennhurst State School and Hospital* v. *Halderman,* 451 U.S. 1 (1981), the Court refused to find a mandate in the federal Developmental Disabilities Assistance and Bill of Rights Act (Public Law 95-602) for requiring that all state governments provide treatment or habilitation in the "least restrictive" environment or lose federal aid under the act.

In a second review of the same case, *Pennhurst State School and Hospital* v. *Halderman,* 104 S. Ct. 900 (1984), the Supreme Court issued an even more restrictive ruling on the authority of the federal government to order compliance by institutions with their own state's legal requirements. A sharply divided court (five to four) decided that the 11th Amendment to the Constitution prohibited a federal court from ordering a state agency to comply with state law. These decisions and others on the right to treatment provoked a psychiatrist to describe the Supreme Court as hostile to mental health reform, despite the fact that several decisions have displayed a willingness on the part of a majority of the Supreme Court to defer to professional psychiatric judgment rather than impose strict legal rules. See D.H. Brandt, "The Hostility of the Burger Court to Mental Health Law Reform" (*Bulletin of the American Academy of Psychiatry and Law* 1983; 11:77-82). For a more recent study, see J.P. Morrissey and H.H. Goldman, "Case and Treatment of the Mentally Ill in the United States: Historical Developments and Reforms" (*Annals of the American Academy of Politics and Social Science* 1986; 484:12-27). For a collection of papers on different aspects of the subject, see "Symposium on the Right to Refuse Treatment" (*Behavioral Science and the Law* 1986; 4:247-345).

5 • Ethics in Medical Practice

Breaking off the Physician–Patient Relationship: Another Legal Hazard

The practice of medicine in the United States is still a matter of free determination. There are no compulsory duties on the part of physicians – or of patients, for that matter. One of the unclear aspects of this freedom, however, is the proper method of breaking off an existing professional relationship with a patient. As it is usually stated, the attending doctor should continue to treat a patient under care for a particular disease or condition until the patient no longer needs care or dismisses the doctor. Termination of a continuing relationship is clearly allowed, but the physician must take precautions to give the patient adequate time and opportunity to find another appropriate physician. In an area well served by medical facilities and practitioners, this time need not be very long. In remote areas, however, the physician should allow a considerable period before ending the professional service. The problem is most difficult when the patient's condition is chronic and requires regular medical attendance. Failure to follow the proper method for ending a relationship with such a patient may result in ethical charges against the doctor and, if harm comes to the patient, a legal action for "abandonment" of the patient. When the method of ending the relationship is proper, it has always been held that the physician need not state reasons for the termination.

A recent decision of the Supreme Court of North Dakota places this last statement in some doubt. In this case, *Moritz* v. *Medical Arts Clinic,*[1] the plaintiff sued the group-practice clinic, its administrator,

From the *New England Journal of Medicine*
1982; 307:1058-1060.

and all 23 of the physicians associated with the clinic for libel in sending her a letter of notice terminating her care at the clinic. The plaintiff had previously brought a claim for malpractice against the clinic, which was settled out of court at a compromise evaluation. It was after this event that the clinic attempted to break off the professional relationship with the plaintiff and members of her family who were enrolled as regular patients of the group practice.

A letter was sent to the plaintiff through the regular mails, stating that the clinic and its physicians wished to "withdraw from further treatment." The letter went on to assert, "The reason for this withdrawal should be obvious to you. The physicians are extremely uncomfortable treating you and do not find that they can do so in the physician–patient relationship that they would want to offer." It was indicated that the "past actions" of the patient had made it "difficult" for the doctors to continue to treat her as a patient. The clinic and its doctors "respectfully ask you to place yourself and other members of your family in the care of some other physician in this community." The letter indicated that the clinic would continue care until another arrangement was made, but not to exceed 10 days from the date of the letter. Since the community was well served by physicians, the letter stated, this period should be "ample" for making such arrangements. The letter concluded that, with the patient's approval, the clinic would send her medical records, case history, and other necessary information regarding diagnosis and treatment to her new doctor or doctors.

The clinic administrator had signed the letter, and it had been typed by his secretary. The clinic had apparently acted in this matter with legal advice. In fact, the letter of notice of withdrawal from service was modeled on a form letter for such purposes contained in a well-known legal textbook.[2] Imagine the surprise of the clinic when the patient protested this action by bringing a suit for – of all things – libel. The letter admittedly did not contain disparaging or defamatory statements about the patient. Furthermore, the letter was sent only to the patient. For any libel action, the alleged defaming statement must be received by, or published to, a third party. To collect any appreciable award, the plaintiff must also suffer damage, usually monetary, as a result of the alleged libelous statement. There was no indication that the plaintiff was inconvenienced or harmed in seeking other medical services.

After allowing discovery proceedings, the trial judge dismissed the lawsuit against all the defendants. Finding the action "frivolous" and entirely without merit, the trial court took the added step of requiring the plaintiff to pay all the attorneys' fees of the defendants, amounting at that time to $7,611.

The supreme court upheld the dismissal of the case on the grounds that it lacked merit but reversed the decision of the trial court to award attorneys' fees, which the higher court deemed an abuse of discretion. Higher courts rarely find trial judges to have "abused their discretion" in cases of this type. Wide latitude is usually given to the judge hearing the case and observing the parties in court. The result of the supreme court's decision in this case is that the plaintiff has succeeded in much of the underlying purpose of the lawsuit to the extent of forcing the clinic to expend a large sum of money in defending the action. If we include the costs of the appeal, the loss of the clinic probably exceeds $10,000. It is doubtful that any ordinary liability insurance policy would cover this type of action for libel, which is generally not considered part of professional malpractice coverage.

The supreme court reached its decision to disallow attorney-fee costs because the judges were divided on dismissal of the case. The majority of the court found that the letter could not be taken to have any defamatory meaning. It did not accuse the plaintiff of any wrongful acts or any immoral or antisocial behavior. The chief justice concurred in the result, but found that he would add the fact that an affidavit was received from the secretary who typed the letter. She swore that she did not take it in a defamatory sense. She was aware that the reason for the letter was the malpractice claim of the plaintiff.

Only Justice Sand dissented. In a very puzzling opinion the justice concluded that the letter was susceptible of a defamatory meaning but did not indicate what this defamatory meaning could be. The justice observed only that "extrinsic evidence" was necessary to arrive at any evaluation of whether the letter was or was not libelous. Justice Sand would have allowed the plaintiff to examine the secretary and other witnesses at a trial to seek to reveal some hidden defamatory substance in the letter. Justice Sand also noted that the letter closely followed the suggested legal form, but that the clinic did not include one paragraph from that form and did not give any specific reason for the termination notice. The justice concluded, "If the letter had given the reason for the termination, the innuendoes would not be left and the reader would not be in the position to speculate."

As indicated earlier, the clinic and its physicians were indisputably within their rights not to give reasons for the termination. The North Dakota court did not dispute this right. No allegation was made that the notice failed to give the plaintiff adequate time to find another doctor or that the patient had trouble finding one. No allegation was made that the letter was seen by a third party outside of the clinic. How, then, could it defame the plaintiff? Both the plaintiff and the secretary knew the reason for the termination. As the letter made clear, the clinic doctors were "uncomfortable" in continuing to treat her. In fact, the opinion of Justice Sand, not the majority opinion, disclosed that the termination was "most likely" to have been prompted by the malpractice claim.

The dissenting Justice Sand would seem to have reached two conclusions: that failure to give reasons for termination of a professional relationship leaves the notice susceptible of a defamatory meaning and requires that a jury examine extrinsic evidence to determine the actual meaning, and that the recipient of a medical termination letter can claim libelous publication merely because an employed medical secretary typed the letter. There was no discussion of the fact that secretaries to physicians are frequently privy to private information about patients and are required to maintain strict confidentiality concerning that information.

Justice Sand went on to observe, "I am not implying that the clinic or any association of doctors may not terminate its services to any person except under the possibility of penalty. Nor am I implying that the letter can only be viewed as being libelous." Justice Sand gave no further explanation. It is evident that, to this justice at least, not giving a reason does carry a penalty. The penalty is having to meet and defend a charge of libel.

The other judges did not agree with this sobering idea, but because of one justice's dissent, the majority denied the imposition of attorney-fee costs on the plaintiff. The majority made it clear that this dissent was the only reason for their reversal of the trial judge's decision on this matter.

It is regrettable that the effort of this clinic and its professional staff to avoid stating specific reasons for its action resulted in a penalty of $10,000 or more in attorney fees. Generally speaking, when a free agent can end a relationship without substantive grounds, it is advisable (and good manners) not to state the grounds. An enumeration of the reasons for termination merely tends to encourage arguments over justification. It is usually wise to provide a polite notice, state no reason, and let it go at that.

In this case, however, when the doctors said that they were made uncomfortable by the plaintiff's "past actions" but did not indicate what those actions were, there was speculation over the provocations. It is apparent from the North Dakota case – one of the very few state appellate court decisions concerned directly with correspondence to break off a physician–patient relationship – that some judges may be willing to read a possibly false and defamatory implication into such wording.

Health maintenance organizations and professional groups that enroll patients for care on an indefinite basis must give some type of notice for termination of service. These types of medical practice may be most vulnerable in the future to the problems of stating or not stating reasons for breaking off patient relationships. Providing reasons for termination might be the legally prudent way to avoid the type of issue that Justice Sand raised in North Dakota. This judge's view was clearly a minority position, however, and the adoption of such a precautionary practice would seem destined to provoke more problems with former patients than it would avoid. Statements of reasons for termination would tend to cause disputes and lawsuits over the adequacy and truth of the reasons given. The complexities and vulnerabilities of medical care delivery will continue, and the cost of providing such care could be increased even more by the kinds of problems in patient relationships that this North Dakota case suggests.

REFERENCES

1. 315 N.W.2d 458 (N. Dakota, 1982).
2. American Jurisprudence, Physicians and Surgeons, Section 10:1515, 1981.

♦

COMMENTS

This column was selected to lead off this chapter because it involves issues concerning the ethical principle that physicians are free to choose their circumstances of medical practice (salaried practice, fee-for-service practice, family medicine, obstetrics, etc.) and are generally free to choose their patients and to break off a physician–patient relationship as long as proper notice is given in adequate time for the patient to seek other services. This standard is contained in the latest version of the American Medical Association's *Revised Principles of Medical Ethics,* adopted in 1980. It is asserted, "A physician shall, in the provision of appropriate patient care, except in emergencies, be free to choose whom to serve, with whom to associate, and the environment in which to provide medical services" (Principle VI).

The common law is even less demanding than the AMA's ethical standard. Privately practicing physicians are not legally bound to render aid in emergency situations, in the sense that they are not liable for financial damages if they fail to do so. The various Good Samaritan laws adopted in 49 of the 50 states provide an immunity from damage suits for malpractice in order to encourage doctors to render voluntary, nonpaid services in emergencies, but they do not make such services a legal requirement. Only one state, Vermont, does impose a legal duty to render emergency care under its Good Samaritan law, except in cases in which to do so would endanger the physician or in which such action would interfere with "important duties" to other patients (Vermont Statutes Ann., title 12, section 519). See also M.A. Franklin, "Vermont Requires Rescue: A Comment" (*Stanford Law Review* 1972; 25:51-61). A few additional states have included the requirement that physicians render emergency services among their duties under state licensure. These provisions are regulations, not statutes, and are difficult to discover or interpret. It is doubtful that these provisions would make the giving of emergency care an affirmative duty entailing financial damages in the event of breach. The reason for this is that the American common law has been very reluctant to impose affirmative duties of rescue on private parties.

On the other hand, breaking off a clinical patient care relationship without adequate notice can result in a damage suit for "abandonment." Nevertheless, there have been few suits reported for outright abandonment of patient care in recent decades. Patients are apparently more apt to file ethical complaints with local medical societies or state medical licensing and disciplinary boards. Failure to respond to patients' requests for services or premature discharges of patients from hospitals or emergency services can, however, result in malpractice claims that are quite close in conceptual terms to "abandonment." These cases involve significant delays in treatment resulting in severe injury or death. See A.R. Holder, *Medical Malpractice Law* (2nd ed. New York: John Wiley and Sons, 1978:372-88). See also L.L. McIntyre, "The Action of Abandonment in Medical Malpractice Litigation" (*Tulane Law Review* 1962; 36:834-55).

The most extraordinary feature of the case reviewed in this column was the cause of action chosen by the plaintiff—that of libel. It was probably selected in frustration when the plaintiff was advised of the weakness of an "abandonment" case since she had no serious damages to claim and had been given adequate notice to seek other medical services.

The North Dakota court did not, however, examine any special obligations of health maintenance organizations and similar forms of medical practice, since the plaintiff's suit did not relate to such groups in any way, nor have any later cases against such medical care organizations dealt with the issues of their specific responsibilities. However, it is conceivable that a broadened obligation will be imposed on such groups, requiring them to continue their services, especially in rural areas, at least for the length of a contractual period and perhaps beyond that time. The medical advertising of health maintenance organizations as "total services to maintain health" may also encourage courts to limit the right of such organizations to cut off services or to refuse renewal of contracts for services to patients found not to be profitable enough for purposes of the fiscal aims of the group. The courts may impose affirmative duties of care on the corporation (health maintenance organization, preferred-provider organization, etc.) that would not be imposed on the individual medical practitioner.

The Freedom of Medical Practice: Sterilization of the Poor

The pages of the *Journal* have been open to controversial positions on the freedom of physicians to practice medicine as they see fit,[1] particularly in the face of economic changes in medical practice and the strident claims of our day concerning a legal right to treatment by patients. In a recent column, I described a California decision that found invalid a hospital's attempt to make admission conditional upon an alleged "agreement" to arbitrate any malpractice claim.[2] An earlier California case had also found that a "charitable research hospital" could not make admission conditional on the patient's signing of a release of legal liability for any injury incurred during hospitalization.[3] It has also been said that a hospital, at least a public institution, cannot make admission dependent upon the patient's willingness to engage in research studies. These cases were dealing essentially with improper coercion of patients regarding their medical care.

Earlier in the 1970s there was considerable national publicity and Congressional inquiry about family-planning programs and coerced sterilization of poor black women in the South. In 1977 one of the cases arising out of these incidents was decided by a higher federal court with what many observers consider a very surprising result—i.e., affirmation of the right of a physician to practice medicine freely, even when he places conditions on his patients concerning the care that he will give.

In *Walker* v. *Pierce*[4] it was alleged that an obstetrician in South Carolina required certain patients to agree to a sterilization after their third child; otherwise, he would not accept them as patients for

From the *New England Journal of Medicine*
1978; 298:32-33.

prenatal care and delivery. However, he did not impose this condition on his private, paying patients but only on the poor, the charity cases, and Medicaid patients. The court quoted his position as follows:

> My policy was with people who were unable to financially support themselves, whether they be on Medicaid or just unable to pay their own bills, if they were having a third child, to request they voluntarily submit to sterilization following the delivery of the third child. If they did not wish this as a condition for my care, then I requested that they seek another physician.

Two Medicaid patients sued the doctor for violating their civil rights, among them being the right of privacy, due process of law, and equal protection of the law. The lower federal court dismissed one of the cases because the woman was not actually sterilized. The other case was more serious. Mrs. Walker was expecting her fourth child. She was black, had a seventh-grade education, and was separated from her husband. She was on Medicaid. During prenatal care, Dr. Pierce discussed family planning and advised a tubal ligation after the birth. The patient refused. In a subsequent visit, the issue was again discussed, and she again refused. Mrs. Walker alleged that the doctor threatened to have her state assistance cut off if she did not agree—an allegation that the doctor denied. However, he did send a social worker to talk with Mrs. Walker about the sterilization. She alleged that the social worker said he could do nothing about the doctor's position, but would try to get her another doctor. Mrs. Walker tried another physician, but he was taking on no new patients at the time. She went back to Dr. Pierce and signed a consent to a tubal ligation after delivery. When the child was delivered, Dr. Pierce was not present. She was attended by another physician. After her baby was born, she signed two more consent forms, and Dr. Pierce performed a sterilization procedure. Mrs. Walker said at the trial that she had given in to the procedure because she believed any further protest was futile.

The jury found Dr. Pierce guilty of violating Mrs. Walker's civil rights and awarded nominal damages of $5.

The Court of Appeals for the Fourth Circuit reversed the jury verdict and dismissed the action, finding that Dr. Pierce, as an independent, fee-for-service physician, could lay down terms for rendering his medical services. It concluded that there was no legal basis on which to prevent a physician from pursuing his own "personal economic philosophy." It was found that he had not forced his views on his patients. The court was impressed that Mrs. Walker had signed three consent forms.

One of the judges filed a vigorous dissent. Judge Butzner would have found the doctor guilty of discrimination because he based his policy upon "economic factors." He admitted that the Medicaid law barred interference in a physician's medical judgment as well as interference with physician–patient relations. However, he asserted that Dr. Pierce's actions were under the color of state law (since he was acting as an agent of the state) and thus constituted discrimination under the Fourteenth Amendment. He asserted: "Had Dr. Pierce's decision to sterilize his patients been based upon their medical needs, he would not have acted under the color of state law. . . ."

Judge Butzner's concerns about Dr. Pierce's policy may be understandable, but his reasoning is difficult to follow. He admits the doctor is legally free to make medical judgments and is not an agent of the state, even though he is paid for his services under Medicaid. Yet his conduct can be controlled, and he is an agent of the state if his reason for refusing care, or his reason for a sterilization, is based on "economic factors." But if the physician's decision can be prohibited, why not also the patient's? What if the patient wishes a sterilization for social or economic reasons? On the basis of Judge Butzner's reasoning, the patient could be controlled also because it would not be a medical need. Currently, the debate is not over sterilization, but abortion. Next year it may again be "economic" – i.e., the high cost of psychiatric care or a kidney transplant. The scope of the benefits in a universal governmental medical care plan should not depend upon a judge's determination of what are proper medical, social, or economic reasons for either a physician's or a patient's decisions about medical care.

To this extent, I agree with the majority opinion in the *Pierce* case. Nevertheless, I would not apply its findings too broadly, and I find its decision on the facts of the case disturbing. I would say that the Medicaid program should be able to prevent a physician from using coercive measures against his patients and making his obstetric services conditional upon "agreement to" a tubal ligation after the delivery. The patient's free choice, especially in a Medicaid program, is compromised too much by this action on his part. I would hold to this position even if the physician imposed the same condition on his private patients. The issue to me is not discrimination. It is also not the fact that Dr. Pierce's policy was based on his economic philosophy or his ideas about family planning that concerns me. It is the fact that it was inherently coercive of the free choice of his patients.

REFERENCES

1. Sade RM. Medical care as a right: a refutation. N Engl J Med 1971; 285:1288-92.
2. Curran WJ. Malpractice arbitration and conditional medical treatment. N Engl J Med 1977; 296:1045-6.
3. Tunkl v. Regents of the University of California, 60 Cal.2d 92, 383 P.2d 441 (1963).
4. Walker v. Pierce, 560 F.2d 609 (1977).

♦

COMMENTS

This column now strikes me as rather too subtle and too complex for a brief essay. I did not receive much comment on it from medical readers. Nevertheless, it is one of the essays I cite quite frequently in teaching medical students about the freedoms and duties of medical practice in America. The majority of the court in this case took a firmly libertarian view of the freedom of the physician to practice medicine as he saw fit and to attach whatever conditions to his services that his moral or economic philosophy led him to require.

As I saw it, there was a fine line between the doctor's freedom to practice, which I accepted, and his alleged freedom to impose his views on his patients, especially poor patients, by coercing them to undergo unwanted medical procedures. The women's rights movement has been particularly critical of what its adherents have considered coercive practices engaged in by male obstetricians and gynecologists in previous decades.

In some states there are statutes and regulations that limit the freedom of private medical practitioners to deny services to patients on grounds of race, religion, or Medicare or Medicaid status. Where this is the case, the penalty is usually exclusion from participation in the Medicare–Medicaid programs. In Massachusetts, for example, physicians are prohibited by regulation from "acting differently toward a recipient of public assistance in any medical way." See 243

Code of Mass. Reg. 2.07 (9). On other aspects of physicians' battles with medical care programs for recipients of public assistance and with the antitrust laws, see M.D. Raup, "Medicaid Boycotts by Health Care Providers" (*Iowa Law Review* 1984; 69:1393-415). See also the discussions of other aspects of the impact of the antitrust laws on the freedom of medical practice in Chapter 2 of this collection.

Dumping the Poor: Economic Considerations in Emergency Medical Services

The Arizona Supreme Court recently reviewed a case in order to clarify the law regarding the obligations of physicians and hospitals in rendering emergency care to indigent patients. The opinion could have far-reaching implications, not only for clinical obligations to patients but also for the importance of economic factors in emergency care medicine.

In *Thompson* v. *Sun City Community Hospital,*[1] a minor, age 13, was injured in an accident (not otherwise described) and was rushed by ambulance to a nearby private hospital. The patient suffered, among other injuries, a full or partial transection of the femoral artery high in the left thigh. The emergency room physician consulted an orthopedic surgeon on the staff, and a vascular surgeon was also consulted by telephone. It was agreed that the patient required immediate emergency surgery. After his condition was described as stabilized, however, the decision was made to transfer him to the county hospital. It was never made clear at the trial who made that decision. The evidence indicated that the emergency care physician, Dr. Lipsky, determined that the patient was "medically transferable," but he described the actual decision to transfer him as having been made "for economic reasons."

At the trial, an administrator of the hospital testified that it was the policy of the institution (and common practice at other hospitals in the area, according to other witnesses) to transfer indigent patients to the county public hospital whenever, in the judgment of a physician, the transfer "could occur." An hour after he was stabilized, the patient was taken by ambulance to the county hospital. The patient's

From the *New England Journal of Medicine*
1985; 312:374-375.

condition was described as worsening after the transfer. A few hours later, he underwent abdominal surgery and repair of the femoral artery. He was left with a permanent impairment of the left leg, seriously limiting his growth and development. The patient's mother brought suit against the emergency room physician and the consultant physicians at the private hospital and against the hospital itself, charging that the transfer was inappropriate and led to the patient's permanent injury.

The trial lasted for three weeks and was described by the high court as hard fought and often acrimonious. However, the hospital never denied that the patient was transferred solely for financial reasons. In fact, attorneys for the defense stipulated (made binding agreement with the court) that this was the case. The Arizona Supreme Court concluded that the transfer was made solely on financial grounds and "not because surgery at County Hospital could be performed more quickly or by a more skilled surgeon."

The private hospital based its defense on the point that the financial considerations, commonly a factor in such decisions by area hospitals, did not affect the clinical determination that the patient was stabilized and could be transported without further clinical danger. It was alleged by witnesses for the hospital that the chances were great that the patient would suffer permanent impairment because of the original injury, no matter where the surgery was done.

The Supreme Court of Arizona wrote a detailed and thoughtful opinion on all the aspects of this complex case.

The court declared that the obligations of the physicians involved in the matter were considerably different from those of the hospital. The physicians were found to have no liability, and the cases against all of them were dismissed. It was found that they had met their obligations fully in treating and evaluating the patient. The emergency care physician had done all he could for the patient within the limits of his own competence and the resources of the emergency room. He could not require that the hospital admit the patient, and he could not prevent the transfer. In this regard, one matter of evidence was observed by the high court, and it undoubtedly influenced the trial and upper courts. It was indicated that Dr. Lipsky had said to the patient's mother, "I have the shitty detail of telling you that Mike [the patient] will be transferred to County. . . ."

The suit against the consultants was dismissed on the grounds that their evaluation was not questioned and that they had been quite willing to provide treatment at the private hospital. They also could not have prevented the "economic transfer" to the county institution.

The bulk of the opinion dealt with the hospital's liability. The Arizona court confirmed an earlier and well-known decision, *Guerrero* v. *Copper Queen Hospital,*[2] which held that a private institution has the same legal obligation as a public hospital to render all needed care to emergency patients.

In regard to the transfer of such patients, the court cited the standards of the Joint Commission on Accreditation of Hospitals concerning emergency services: "No patient should arbitrarily be transferred if the hospital where he was initially seen has means for adequate care of his problem."[3] The court pointed out that among the "arbitrary" grounds found inappropriate by the Joint Commission (in its standards concerning patients' rights) was the consideration of the source of payment for the patient's care.

Furthermore, the court seemed to find no obstacle in the county's medical-benefit system to the retention of the indigent patient in the private hospital for the needed emergency surgery. The court quoted the local regulation (Section 11-297.01), which provides for payment to local private hospitals delivering emergency care

> for the reasonable costs of all medical services rendered to such indigent by the facility *until such patient is transferred* by the county to the county hospital, or to some other facility designated by the county [emphasis supplied].[4]

The court interpreted this requirement to apply only when transfer was actually completed. If this patient had not been transferred, the county would have been responsible for the reasonable costs of the emergency surgery determined (without question) to be needed and available at the private hospital. The claimed "common practice" of transferring patients earlier to avoid surgical costs was not provided for in the regulation and was found to be "arbitrary" when resorted to solely for economic and not clinical reasons.

The last issue reviewed by the court was the hospital's contention that the plaintiff must prove that the injury was itself caused entirely by the delay in treatment. The court took this issue very seriously and ruled that where the actions of the hospital increased the risk of permanent harm to the patient, it would be up to the fact finder (the jury) to determine whether that increased risk had led (in probable cause) to the result of a permanent impairment of the child's left leg.

This does not mean that the hospital would lose its case; it means only that a jury could find enough evidence to hold the hospital liable if the case presented in court warranted such a determination.

This decision, by finding that a strong case could be made against the hospital but not the physicians, accelerates the trend, noted in an earlier Law–Medicine Notes column,[5] toward hospital corporate liability. By dismissing as arbitrary and improper a transfer made solely for economic reasons, the Arizona court disagreed with the few earlier precedents in the field in which economic transfers were not found legally improper.[6,7] It should be noted, however, that the court did not make this ruling solely on its own but relied on an expressed standard of the hospitals and the professional groups themselves, in the form of the Joint Commission on Accreditation of Hospitals.

Cost controls and reimbursement standards will continue to place pressure on physicians and hospitals to limit their own financial output for patient care. This decision is a clear indication that the courts will not allow such considerations to absolve the hospitals of responsibility for the risk of permanent harm to the patient when that harm could be avoided by proper clinical determinations uninfluenced by arbitrary financial demands.

REFERENCES

1. 141 Ariz. 597 (1984).
2. 112 Ariz. 104 (1975).
3. Joint Commission on Accreditation of Hospitals. Manual for hospitals. Section 36-405. 1976.
4. Quoted in the Court's opinion (slip opinion) p. 5, note 1, supra.
5. Curran WJ. A further solution to the malpractice problem: corporate liability and risk management in hospitals. N Engl J Med 1984; 310:704-5.
6. Harper v. Baptist Medical Center, 341 So.2d 131 (Ala., 1976).
7. Birmingham Baptist Hospital v. Crews, 157 So. 224 (Ala., 1934).

♦

COMMENTS

This column illustrates one of the most terrible dangers that can arise when economic constraints are allowed to affect the availability of medical services. The vulnerability of the population in general, and the poor in particular, stands forth starkly when emergency services are denied or patients are "dumped" inappropriately from one hospital to another on economic grounds. This column was published in the *Journal* along with a highly supportive editorial and a short paper by a medical resident in training in which the personal frustrations he endured in an institution engaging in such practices are vividly described. See K. Wrenn, "No Insurance, No Admission" (*New England Journal of Medicine* 1985; 312:1522-4).

Medical readers may find it surprising that such practices have not provoked a larger number of malpractice complaints, but, as pointed out in the column, the Arizona case was the first of its kind in which the courts have found malpractice liability. In the previous decisions, the plaintiff failed to prove that "dumping" to a public hospital had caused or substantially aggravated the alleged injury. Earlier courts did not seriously examine the legal justification for the dominant role played by "economic considerations" in decisions to transfer patients.

Since the Arizona decision, a few other jurisdictions, notably Florida and Texas, have enacted statutes to prevent inappropriate transfers of patients to public hospitals. In 1986, the federal government adopted standards under the Medicare system to require hospitals to follow strict procedures in transfers of patients to other medical facilities. The statutes require prior contact with the other hospitals to ensure acceptance of the patients. No patient may be transferred unless the emergency situation is stabilized and the "medical benefits" of the transfer "outweigh the increased risk to the individual's medical condition from effecting the transfer." The statutes do not mention "economic reasons" for such transfers, but they also do not prevent hospitals from applying economic criteria as long as the medical standards for the transfer are followed. See 42 U.S.C. Section 9121, entitled "Responsibilities of Medicare Hospitals in Emergency Cases."

On the broad legal issues of health care services for the poor, see F.H. Marsh, "Health Care Cost Containment and the Duty to Treat" (*Journal of Legal Medicine* 1985; 6:157-90); S. Dallek, "Health Care for America's Poor: Separate and Unequal" (*Clearing House Review* 1986; 20:361-71). For a provocative recent book by a leading medical ethicist on limitations on the treatment of the elderly, at least if they are poor, see D. Callahan, *Setting Limits: Medical Goals in an Aging Society* (New York: Simon and Schuster, 1987).

Medical Ethics and the Conscience of the Practitioner

An aftermath of the recent changes in abortion laws in various states has been the fear of some medical practitioners that any refusal on their part to perform an abortion or to take part in an abortion procedure might subject them to legal action, or to harassment, or to discharge from the staff of a hospital. The serious discussion of a constitutional, legal right to an abortion on the part of a woman has provoked the argument that the pregnant patient can require her physician to perform an abortion at her request.

In New York, after the decision of *Stewart* v. *Long Island Hospital,*[1] these fears were not without some basis. In this case a lower court in New York upheld a malpractice claim against the hospital for failure either to perform an abortion on the plaintiff or to provide her with information about other hospitals that would perform the procedure in the state, even though, at the time, the procedure was still illegal in New York. (No danger was alleged to the mother in the case, the problem being the likelihood of congenital defects in the fetus; the child was born deformed.)

During this year, a bill was filed in the New York legislature to amend the Civil Rights Law to provide: "When the performing of a medical procedure on a human being or assisting thereat is contrary to the conscience or religious beliefs of any person, he may refuse to perform or assist in such medical procedure by filing a written refusal with the appropriate and responsible hospital, person, firm, corporation, or association, and no such [institution or person] shall discriminate against the person for refusing to so

From the *New England Journal of Medicine*
1971; 285:1306-1307.

act."[2] The next section asserted, "No civil action for negligence or malpractice shall be maintained against a person so refusing to act. . . ."

This broadly worded legislation was not passed, however. The law as actually adopted limits the scope of the protection to performing or assisting at an abortion and requires the filing of "a prior written refusal setting forth the reasons therefor with the appropriate and responsible hospital. . . ."[3]

Apparently, there was some fear that the more broadly worded provision would cover refusals to grant blood transfusions and refusals to perform general medical procedures. The rather strict and formalistic nature of the law, requiring as it does the filing of a "prior written refusal" to perform an abortion, may limit its actual implementation. Doctors and nurses may not wish to file such statements, or they may inquire about the need to do so only after refusal. Also, it is not clear whether one blanket refusal to engage in all abortions would be sufficient, or whether specific refusals would be required in every case. Also, the statute seems to require that the refusal notice be sent to the "appropriate and responsible" hospital, etc., but not directly to the patient.

Malpractice actions are a great source of anguish and danger to physicians and medical people today. It was perhaps inevitable that a clash between the requirements of conscience and the requirements of law would give rise to the need for further law such as this New York statute. Yet it does seem a rather formalistic approach to a delicate human dilemma.

REFERENCES

1. 966 N.Y.S.2d 41 (1969).
2. Assembly Bill no. 1781-B; Senate Bill no. 1764.
3. Laws of New York, 1971, ch. 1098.

♦

COMMENTS

This was probably the first column in which I commented on a purely ethical issue, a question of a highly sensitive nature that arose just at the time when the "abortion problem" was heating up as a major medicolegal controversy in American law.

It is fortunate that I was able to obtain the original wording of the New York statute before its application was restricted to abortion. As filed, the bill was much more sweeping in its philosophical thrust and more of a "conscience statement" than it would be when it emerged in its final form, after the legal technicians had gotten their hands on it.

As pointed out in the first two columns in this chapter, the original bill also adhered much more closely to common-law principles pertaining to freedom of medical practice than its medical supporters realized. Its objective, however, was to avoid malpractice suits and to prevent what it vaguely described as "discrimination" against physicians who refused to participate in abortions (and later against other medical personnel, such as obstetrical nurses, who took the same stand).

This column provoked many letters from medical readers and gave further publicity to the New York statute. Despite its weakness as a legal instrument, the statute did become a model for "conscience laws" across the country after the Supreme Court's decisions on abortion in 1973. By 1987, over half of the American states had adopted such "antidiscrimination" legislation.

The federal Congress also acted quickly in adopting a "conscience law" after the *Roe* v. *Wade* decision. For the current law, see Health Services Extension Act, 1983, title IV, section 401. As early as 1973 a federal court broadened the concept of the conscience laws to make them apply to an entire hospital's philosophy. The court ruled that a Roman Catholic hospital operated by an order of nuns could refuse to allow a non-Catholic doctor on its medical staff to perform legal abortions within the hospital; *Watkins* v. *Mercy Hospital Medical Center,* 364 F.Supp. 799, Idaho (1973).

For analyses of the ethical issues of refusal to participate in, or to refer patients to, abortion services, see H.J. McCloskey, "Abortion and the Right to Privacy" (*Philosophy* 1980; 55:17-38); D. Callahan, "Abortion and Medical Ethics" (*Annals of the Academy of Politics and Social Science* 1978; 437:116-27); and W.A. Regan, "Constitutional Rights of Catholic Hospitals" (*Hospital Progress* 1973; 54: 66-9).

Compulsory Drug Testing: The Legal Barriers

If I were to identify one current medicolegal public policy issue as paramount in serious constitutional debate at the close of 1986, it would be compulsory urine testing for drug abuse. A year ago at this time, the most controversial medicolegal policy issues were compulsory diagnostic testing for the human immunodeficiency virus (HIV) as indicative of the acquired immunodeficiency syndrome (AIDS), and compulsory quarantine of all persons with AIDS.

At this writing, no American jurisdiction, state or federal, has enacted a compulsory screening program for HIV for any group in the general population, and no jurisdiction has adopted a program of compulsory isolation or quarantine of persons with AIDS or HIV infection. The proposals concerning the AIDS epidemic have not been totally abandoned, but support for them has quieted considerably because of the recent report of the Institute of Medicine[1] and the institution of educational programs and anonymous voluntary diagnostic services.

The movement for compulsory drug testing seems currently to be considerably stronger and more strident than the AIDS proposals of last year. It had its greatest impetus in 1986 with the sudden death of college basketball star Len Bias. A task force at the University of Maryland recommended a widespread program of drug testing among the college's students, staff, and faculty.[2]

Support for compulsory drug testing is vigorous and steadfast among political figures, particularly in preelection speeches. It is seen as a "no-lose" proposition; the general public is clearly opposed to drug abuse, and since Bias' death, the issue has escalated to become one of life-or-death importance.

From the *New England Journal of Medicine*
1987; 316:318-321.

President Reagan issued an executive order on September 15, 1986, ordering all federal agencies to introduce programs to achieve a "drug-free workplace" throughout the federal government.[3] The program includes authorization to establish compulsory testing for illegal drug use of all new job applicants and also of current employees when there is reasonable suspicion of drug use. The order also declares a policy that "persons who use illegal drugs are not suitable for federal employment."[4] In late November, further guidelines were released to implement the President's program, despite what were described as serious reservations about the constitutionality of the program among high government officials and advisors.[5]

The doubts about the constitutionality of compulsory testing to detect drug abuse or, in the President's order, the "use of illegal drugs," arise particularly as the result of three recent cases decided by federal district courts in New Jersey, Tennessee, and Louisiana. These cases, in firm and outspoken language, ruled programs of drug testing among public employees invalid under various constitutional provisions. An analysis of these cases may shed some light on the legal barriers to the enforcement of at least some aspects of the new federal program.

The first case to be reported was *Capua* v. *City of Plainfield,*[6] which concerned a drug-testing program for municipal firefighters. The plan was implemented without notice to the employees; one workday, all the fire stations in the city were suddenly closed and locked and all employees in the building were ordered to submit to a surprise urine test under the direct surveillance of "bonded testing agents," who watched each firefighter (all were men) while he produced the sample for analysis. A few weeks later, several firefighters were informed that their urine had tested positive for "controlled substances," although they were not told what the substance was or its concentration in the urine. All were immediately fired. In an action seeking reinstatement, the firefighters claimed violation of their constitutional rights. The district court found for the plaintiffs.

The first or threshold issue, of fundamental importance in the case, was whether or not the compulsory testing of urine constituted a "search and seizure" under the Fourth Amendment. It seemed clearly a "search," because of the analysis for drugs, but was it a "seizure"? The landmark precedent cited by the plaintiffs' attorneys was *Schmerber* v. *California,*[7] a famous case decided in the U.S.

Supreme Court in the mid-1960s, in which the compulsory taking of a blood sample was assumed to be a "seizure" because it was an invasion of the body. However, the Court in *Schmerber* held, by a narrow majority, that the taking of blood involuntarily under the circumstances of that case—arrest for drunk driving—although it was a "seizure," was not "unreasonable" and therefore not illegal, as long as the blood was drawn under antiseptic conditions in a hospital or under medical supervision. The Court also held in the same case that the involuntary taking of blood was not a violation of the Fifth Amendment protection against self-incrimination, since the amendment covers testimony, not the use of bodily substances.

The argument against identifying urinalysis as a "seizure" is that, unlike a blood test, it does not involve the use of an invasive technique; the person merely excretes the waste product from the body. He or she is not touched in the procedure. In my medicolegal casebook, I examined a similar distinction made in connection with the use of a Breathalyzer test.[8] In refusing to find the forced use of the Breathalyzer improper, even when the person was strapped to a chair, an Arizona court[9] asserted that the person was not forced to exhale, but that after he had done so, into an instrument held to his mouth, he could not "control" his breath and it merely became part of the "surrounding atmosphere."

In the *Plainfield* case, the court refused to accept these distinctions. It found the involuntary taking of urine under direct observation to be both a search and a seizure. The court concluded, "The city's mass testing program subjected firefighters to a relatively high degree of bodily intrusion." It was observed that the discharge of body-waste products was usually done in private. The city's requirement of surveillance forced the men to expose parts of the anatomy "in a manner akin to a strip search."

Having found the collection of urine and its testing a search and seizure, the court went on to find it "unreasonable" as a matter of law in these circumstances. The city argued that firefighters have no expectation of privacy in such a matter and that the large-scale drug use in all segments of the population in New Jersey warranted a logical and reasonable implication that such persons may have been employed as firefighters. The court dismissed these arguments completely. It held that firefighters had not waived their privacy rights in so intimate an area as urination and had not surrendered their protections under the Fourth Amendment. The court concluded that the plan in operation "sweeps the innocent with the guilty" and sacrifices the individual's rights for a presumed public good. The court admitted that the city could have a legitimate interest in the ability of public-safety officers to perform their duties properly, but found the program in question to be an inappropriate and unreasonable way to accomplish that goal.

In the second case, *Lovvorn* v. *City of Chattanooga,*[10] the group involved was again firefighters. The city had introduced mandatory testing of all firefighters in both 1985 and 1986. All employees who tested positive on a confirmatory test were suspended from duty and presumably discharged. The firefighters brought action for an injunction finding the program in violation of the Fourth Amendment.

The Tennessee court found that the city, when it reactivated the plan in 1986, did so without any objective evidence that the performance of any member of the department or of the department as a whole had been affected by the use of drugs.

The city tried to distinguish its case from the *Plainfield* case on the basis of the fact that the firefighters in Chattanooga regularly undressed in each other's presence and used a common toilet facility. The court was not impressed with the argument. It found that the firefighters still had the expectation of some privacy in the act of urinating, which was clearly invaded during a personal observation by testing agents.

In the most important part of the case, going beyond the conclusions in the New Jersey case, the Tennessee court examined the issue of the reasonableness of the search and seizure. It found that firefighters, like police officers, may not have as much right as "the general citizenry" to resist efforts to determine whether their job efficiency is affected by illegal drug abuse. On this basis, "probable cause" for believing a particular firefighter was a user of illegal drugs and was affected in his work may not have been required. A lesser standard of "reasonable suspicion" would be enough. This standard was defined as "some articulated basis" for suspecting the use of illegal drugs. The court pointed out that the city had no such grounds for their mass testing program and no objective grounds for concern about job performance. It asserted that evidence of deficient performance by individuals should be detectable to a considerable degree by the examination of such factors as job absenteeism, aberrant behavior, and personal financial difficulties.

The third and most recent case is perhaps the most relevant for its application to the President's order, since it involved federal employees. An injunction was sought in the federal district court for eastern Louisiana to stop the compulsory drug-testing program of the U.S. Customs Service. Like the other courts, this one granted the injunction. In *National Treasury Employees Union* v. *Von Rabb,*[11] the court applied both the Fourth and Fifth amendments to the case at hand.

The Customs Service plan applied to employees seeking promotion to certain "covered positions." It required compulsory urine testing under "close observation" by testing agents. In addition, however, the applicants were required to fill out a pretest questionnaire containing questions about their history of medication and illegal drug use and the circumstances under which they may have been in contact with illegal substances in the previous 30 days. Employees with positive tests for illegal drugs were subject to loss of consideration for career advancement and discharge from government service.

Citing the *Plainfield* case, the court found the taking of urine under surveillance an unreasonable search and seizure. Most important, it refused to agree with the government contention that application for promotion implied a waiver of the right of privacy and the right to refuse the urine test. The court concluded, "It is unconstitutional for the government to condition public employment on 'consent' to an unreasonable search."

The Louisiana court, unlike the others, went on to find the drug testing for illegal substances and the questionnaire about the use of illegal substances to be violations of the Fifth Amendment protection against self-incrimination. In regard to the drug testing, the court stressed the lack of a reasonable suspicion of drug use by the employees. It found that the *Schmerber* case, cited in both earlier cases, was different on three grounds: First, the *Schmerber* court had found that there was "plainly probable cause" to arrest and charge the defendant with driving under the influence of alcohol. Second, the *Schmerber* case did not involve what the Tennessee judge described as a procedure that "detracts from human dignity and self-respect." The court described the compulsory urine taking under personal observation as a gross invasion of privacy and a degrading procedure that offended the court's sense of justice. Third, the *Schmerber* case did not involve either an involuntary test or a questionnaire requiring disclosure of illegal conduct.

The question at issue now is whether these decisions represent major barriers to the President's sweeping plan to introduce compulsory urine testing into all federal agencies. Newspaper accounts, as previously noted,[5] have reported that "court decisions" have made the President's program unworkable. I am not at all sure that this is correct.

The executive order does attempt to meet several of the objections raised in these decisions. The testing of existing employees is left to the discretion of agency heads but must be based on the nature of the agency's mission and the danger to the public health, safety, or national security that could result from the failure of employees to discharge their duties adequately. This standard seems to require a program based on job-related physical or mental impairment, not merely the illegality of the drug use. Nevertheless, the order does establish the policy that illegal drug use itself is incompatible with federal employment. There are mixed messages here that may need clarification.

A later part of the order establishes an employee-assistance program for assessment, counseling, and referral for treatment. It indicates that no employees may be discharged or disciplined for illegal drug use if they voluntarily seek counseling or treatment and thereafter refrain from illegal drug use. However, employees in "sensitive positions" can be suspended from duty while undergoing drug treatment. Furthermore, the executive order concludes by asserting that the program shall not be conducted for the purpose of gathering evidence for criminal prosecution.

Regarding the methods used to collect urine samples, the order directs that the procedure "must allow individual privacy" unless the agency has reason to believe that a particular individual may alter or replace the specimen to be provided.

These specific provisions could go a long way toward encouraging a court concerned with individual liberties to find that the program was a reasonable effort to combat drug abuse and drug dependence in current federal employees. The courts would still be opposed, however, to widespread general testing of new applicants for federal positions or of present employees in "sensitive positions" (however defined) if there is no reasonable basis for suspicion that the person has used illegal drugs.

Perhaps the most disturbing aspect of the program, when these specific problems have been faced and solved, is the breadth of discretion afforded agency heads in the executive order. (This broad discretion is, in fact, cited as one of the most important parts of the program.) Agency heads are told that "illegal drug use" will not be tolerated in the federal government. They are told that the President's goal is a "drug-free federal workplace." The emphasis in these ringing phrases is not on rehabilitation and treatment of the ravages of drug dependence. They can be read as encouraging zealotry against the wickedness of illegal behavior. Some agency heads may heed that message and enforce its objectives without due respect for individual rights. The courts will still be needed to guard against potential excesses in the enforcement of the executive order.

REFERENCES

1. Confronting AIDS: directions for public health, health and research. Washington, D.C.: National Academy Press, 1986.
2. Vesey T. U-Maryland Drug Task Force backs expulsion, testing. Washington Post. October 23, 1986:81.
3. Executive order no. 12564. US Law Week 1986; 55:2177-8.
4. Executive order no. 12564. US Law Week 1986; 55:2177-8. section 1(c).
5. Williams L. Reagan drug testing plan to start despite court rulings opposing it. New York Times. November 29, 1986.
6. Capua v. City of Plainfield. US Law Week 1986; 55:2170-2.
7. Schmerber v. California, 384 U.S. 757 (1966).
8. Curran WJ, Shapiro ED. Law, medicine, and forensic science. 3rd ed. Boston: Little, Brown, 1982:138-44.
9. State v. Berg, 76 Arizona 96 (1953).
10. Lovvorn v. City of Chattanooga. US Law Week 1986; 55:2277-8.
11. National Treasury Employees Union v. Von Rabb. US Law Week 1986; 55:2284-5.

♦

COMMENTS

Later court decisions have arrived at similar conclusions to those reached in the cases examined in this column. The Reagan administration has gone forward with its program of random drug testing of federal employees, despite these court decisions. For a defense of the administration's position, see R.K. Willard, "Toward a Drug-Free Work Place" (*Federal Bar News & Journal* 1987; 34:74-6). See also a collection of articles on drug testing in the workplace, "Testing for Drug Use in the American Work Place: A Symposium" (*Nova Law Review* 1987; 11:291-893).

The withdrawal of Judge Douglas H. Ginsburg from consideration for appointment to the Supreme Court because of his admission of casual use of illegal drugs while an adult and during the time he was a faculty member at the Harvard Law School raised issues about federal policy on asking prospective employees about illegal drug use during the period before their applications for federal employment. A story in the *Washington Post* reported on a survey of agencies in the Washington area. The story indicated a wide variety of practices in federal agencies at that time, shortly after Judge Ginsburg's withdrawal. It was reported that the Office of Personnel Management was expected to adopt a new program based on a new questionnaire required to be answered by applicants for presidential appointments and for persons seeking security clearances. The new program would inquire about alcohol abuse and the use of illegal drugs in the previous five years. Decisions on employment would be left to the hiring agency.

In the survey, it was found that most agencies had not previously sought information on prior drug use by job applicants. Questioning about drugs was more common in law-enforcement agencies. At the Central Intelligence Agency, it was reported, questions were asked about drug use, including details concerning types of drug, quantities, and over what period of time the drug abuse had taken place. Applicants were asked "to be honest" about prior drug abuse. However, applicants were also double-checked about drug abuse on the standard polygraph test, also required of all applicants for employment at the agency. At the Justice Department it was reported that prior drug use was not an automatic disqualification for most employees. However, any applicant for appointment as assistant district attorney who admitted the use of illegal drugs after becoming a member of the bar as an attorney in any state or in the federal courts would be barred from appointment to that position. Admission of use of illegal drugs prior to becoming an attorney would not bar appointment but would require case-by-case analysis. See M. Thornton, "Questions on Drug Use Vary Widely by Agency" (*Washington Post,* November 17, 1987:A25).

The most controversial new area of compulsory testing for employment is testing for the acquired immunodeficiency syndrome (AIDS) and human immunodeficiency virus. The federal government initiated compulsory testing for new recruits to the Armed Services in 1985. In January 1987, the State Department became the first federal agency to establish a policy of mandatory testing for civilian employees and new applicants for employment. At the end of the year, it was still the only federal agency with such a program. The described objectives of the program are to avoid sending employees with AIDS or with the potential to have AIDS (persons infected with human immunodeficiency virus) to locations overseas where medical treatment would be inadequate, to reduce the costs of medical treatment abroad, to avoid disruptions in employment service abroad, and to reduce the potential for anti-American responses in countries where the disease is rare or nonexistent. See a detailed story concerning operations of the program by E. Sciolino, "Fear of AIDS Prompts State Department to Act" (*New York Times,* November 29, 1987:26).

Confidentiality in Epidemiologic Investigations

The Centers for Disease Control (CDC) in Atlanta, Georgia, a part of the U.S. Public Health Service, is one of the nation's primary resources for epidemiologic investigations. Much of the work of the CDC is conducted in cooperation with state health departments; together, these agencies collect a large amount of information from a variety of sources. Within the limits of the freedom of information laws, the CDC makes a substantial effort to maintain the confidentiality of personal records and personal identities in its investigational work.

The protection of personal confidentiality and privacy in CDC records has rarely been challenged in the courts. The issue was raised in *Farnsworth* v. *Procter & Gamble Company,*[1] and this case is therefore of considerable importance in this country for setting public policy in this area. The Procter & Gamble Company was sued by a number of plaintiffs in several states across the country for injuries due to the use of tampons that were alleged to have caused toxic shock syndrome. The plaintiffs' suits were alleged to be relying heavily on studies done by the CDC that according to the plaintiffs supported a relation between the use of the defendant's product and toxic shock syndrome.

Before the trial, Procter & Gamble indicated its intent to criticize the CDC's epidemiologic investigations concerning the experiences of particular women who used the tampons during the time period of the studies. Therefore, the company, through pretrial subpoenas and other discovery procedures, sought to obtain from the CDC all the evidence it possibly could on how the studies were conducted and

From the *New England Journal of Medicine*
1986; 314:1027-1028.

how their results were supported by the data collected. Procter & Gamble also sought the names and addresses of all women in the study so that they could go to these women and ask them directly about their use of tampons and about circumstances of the studies that might cast doubt on the validity of the results claimed by the CDC and the plaintiffs.

The lower court granted a protective order to the CDC that prevented Procter & Gamble from gaining access to the names and addresses of the women in the studies. The case was appealed to the Court of Appeals for the Eleventh Circuit.

It is obvious from the opinion given that the public policy issues in the case were very troubling to the higher court. At the outset, the court admitted that the American legal system and the specific rules of the federal courts "strongly favor full discovery whenever possible." The court observed that it was a time-honored tradition that "the law's basic presumption is that the public is entitled to every person's evidence."

Despite these factors in favor of granting access to this evidence, which the court admitted was important to the company's defense, the higher court upheld the district court's protective order. The appeals court stated that the case required a balancing of Procter & Gamble's interest against the interest of the CDC in keeping information confidential. The court found the CDC's interest to prevail. The opinion pointed out specifically that the national mission of the CDC was the "protection of the public's health," and that central to this goal was the ability of the CDC to conduct probing "scientific and social research supported by a population willing to submit to in-depth questioning." It was the view of the court that the breaches of confidentiality that would result from disclosure of the names and addresses of the study subjects could seriously damage this voluntary cooperation. The opinion also pointed out the highly personal, sensitive nature of the information sought from these women, which included details about their habits, their experiences in using tampons, their medical histories, their contraceptive practices, and their menstrual histories.

The opinion did not examine what assurances of confidentiality were given by the CDC to the subjects; consent forms and written promises of nondisclosure were not reviewed. In addition, in reaching its decision, the court did not cite any precedents for its conclusion (either cases involving the CDC or those involving any other epidemiologic research group). The court, in fact, asserted at the end of its opinion that its decision did "not depend upon any *legal privilege*" (emphasis added). The reference to legal privilege is important. It means that the court was not relying on any other legal–ethical privilege of professional confidentiality to protect the names and addresses of the subjects of the study. These women were not patients to whom an obligation of confidentiality is traditionally owed by physicians. They were revealing information about their personal lives and experiences to an investigator for a federal agency. The court was well aware that it was establishing new ground in supporting a confidentiality posture in this situation.

It is also evident that the court of appeals was influenced by the cooperative attitude of the CDC in providing Procter & Gamble with a great deal of information about the studies, including personal data about the subjects (short of names and addresses). The CDC had also agreed to release the names and addresses of women who agreed to be interviewed by representatives of the company. (Although some women consented to be interviewed by the company, a larger number refused; several others could not be reached at the addresses available.) The court apparently thought that the company had already achieved a great deal of its purpose in seeking discovery and that it would not be materially damaged by not having a complete list of the subjects.

It is important to note that the court did not find that the CDC was bound by freedom of information laws to make full disclosure. The court did not, in fact, review any obligations of the CDC beyond the procedural discovery covered under the Federal Rules of Civil Procedure. In a conversation with attorneys at the CDC, I was told that in all of its negotiations with Procter & Gamble, the CDC had followed its own policies of disclosure, which are based on the freedom of information laws. At this time, there is no indication that the company intends to appeal this case to the Supreme Court. In one important aspect, the CDC has achieved an important victory for all researchers who ensure the confidentiality of personal identity in voluntary epidemiologic studies that are conducted in the interest of the public's health.

REFERENCE

1. Farnsworth v. Procter & Gamble Co., 758 F.2d 1545 (1985).

COMMENTS

The *Farnsworth* case was not appealed to a higher court by the Procter & Gamble Company. The Centers for Disease Control later commissioned a research study of the legal and social issues related to requirements for confidentiality in epidemiologic work. See G.R. Smith, "Health Care Information: Confidentiality and Privacy" (*Epidemiological Investigation,* Atlanta: Emory University School of Law, 1987).

AIDS Research and the "Window of Opportunity"

The urgent effort in the science community to develop a test and a national screening program to detect antibody to the viral agent for the acquired immunodeficiency syndrome (AIDS) is nearing completion. The federal government has selected four companies to conduct the complex investigations. Until a reliable test that can screen donor blood for the existence of the antibody is available, the entire supply of blood products used in therapeutic procedures throughout the country will continue to carry the risk of producing disease in blood-product recipients. A recently published study indicates that an initial screening test based on an enzyme-linked immunosorbent assay will have a relatively high degree of sensitivity (82 percent positive in a group of patients with previously diagnosed AIDS).[1] The study also offers evidence that a general screening for AIDS antibody in national blood supplies for transfusion may not cause major disruption in blood-bank programs by unnecessary exclusion of large quantities of donated blood.

Another interest is currently occupying the federal authorities. During the period before the development and widespread use of a reliable screening test, there is an opportunity to learn more about the natural transmission of this highly puzzling and devastating disease.[2,3] To what degree has the disease progressed through the American population? How many recipients of contaminated blood will contract full-blown AIDS? These and other issues strongly merit investigation. The National Cancer Institute sees this period as a one-time-only "window of opportunity" (in the language of the space program) to obtain the answers to these questions.

A large-scale research project is being developed that will enlist in a first phase some 200,000 healthy volunteer blood donors. They will

From the *New England Journal of Medicine*
1985; 312:903-904.

be asked to allow the researchers to retain a sample of the donated blood for storage at the blood bank and for analysis after an AIDS screening program has been initiated in this country.

A news article in *Science* indicates that the federal government has serious concerns about the ethical aspects of this proposed study.[4] The article examines two major issues: First, should the donors be told later whether their blood has been found to be positive or negative for AIDS? Second, should recipients of positive blood products be traced and told that the blood they received was contaminated?

The *Science* article treats the two issues as ethical, not legal, problems. Both are described as "creating terrible dilemmas." The key point of the dilemma in both issues seems to be the fact that there is currently no cure or effective treatment for AIDS. The author of the article believes that the subjects could do nothing with the information in the absence of available treatment, so that disclosure could only cause needless concern and anxiety. The author indicates, however, that after considering ethical and public-relations implications, the National Cancer Institute decided to require full disclosure. It seems to me that this was a wise decision. It is supported on both ethical and legal grounds. Ethically, full disclosure should be made unless there are compelling reasons not to do so. In this situation there are strong legal reasons to disclose information to both donors and recipients of blood.

I will first explore the issue of whether the donor of a stored blood sample should later be told that he or she has AIDS antibody, according to a screening test. The legal aspect of this question was largely settled when the federal authorities decided to gather their information in the context of a formal research project wherein the blood donor would become a subject entitled to the protections afforded to research subjects in federally supported studies under federal law and regulations. Another approach might have been taken. The data might have been gathered by mutual agreement with the blood banks to set aside suitable blood samples without the knowledge or consent of the donors. Such an approach has been used in the past for certain screening or research purposes. It is commendable that the federal government did not choose this alternative—a choice that might have been attractive under less ethically sensitive circumstances.

Because of the decision to undertake a formal research study, the legal requirements for fully informed consent will apply. The only way an investigator could avoid these requirements would be to have no contact with the donor and not to retain the name of the donor or information leading to his or her identity. This will not be feasible under the study design, since considerable data about the donors are apparently needed and desirable. The federal authorities, according to the *Science* article, have decided to seek fully informed consent from the donors and to retain their names and other information about them. Under current regulations that are highly detailed, disclosure of the purposes of the study and its inherent risks and benefits is legally required. In explaining the purposes, the investigators must reveal that the blood will be retained and tested later for AIDS antibodies. Such disclosure obviously raises the issue of what is to be done with subsequent information. Full disclosure of later findings would be legally required unless later disclosure were waived by the subject. Currently, it is the practice of most institutional review boards at the local level to require disclosure of test results either to the subject or to his or her personal physician unless the subject specifically waives that right on a consent form.

Are there important reasons for the donors to want this information? I would say there are several ways in which the test results are valuable to the donors even if no current treatment is available. Treatment may be available at a later time, and with this knowledge, donors will be able to obtain treatment promptly, once it becomes available. Other personal precautions may also be taken by the donors for their own protection before that time. Most compelling at present are the precautions such persons should take for the protection of others with whom they are in intimate contact and in the donation of blood on subsequent occasions. Subjects with positive tests should be advised not to give blood in the future.

A remaining issue not raised in the *Science* article is the problem of false positive results in the screening program. The study noted above did not produce evidence of large numbers of false positive results in the healthy population tested.[2] However, the researchers did suggest that the blood banks should develop and use a second, confirmatory assay for use in all seropositive donors, in order to minimize "the psychic trauma to donors" who may have an erroneous diagnosis.

Next, I should comment on the issue of whether the recipients of blood later determined to be contaminated should be told that the blood contained AIDS antibody. The law that applies to this situation primarily concerns the legal duties of the blood bank as distributor of the blood product and the health care provider, usually a hospital, that performs the transfusion. The obligation of the research investigator would be secondary to the obligations of these other parties.

The law would require that the recipient of a blood product subsequently found to be contaminated be given this information, if it is feasible to find the patient and make the disclosure. In states where the transfusion of blood is deemed a sale, the recipient could bring an action for any harm due to the contamination, because the law of sales would attach a warranty of purity and fitness to the supplied blood product. In states where the transfusion of blood is deemed a clinical service, no warranty would be attached. In the latter situation, since the blood bank and hospital did not know of the contamination and could not test for it at the time of the transfusion, no liability for negligence in supplying impure blood would be imposed. Nevertheless, the law in both types of situations would require disclosure to the recipient of the subsequently discovered information, so that even patients without symptoms of AIDS would be made aware of the fact that they carried AIDS antibodies from the transfusion. Considering the social stigma involved, this information is of more than incidental value to the recipient, even if he or she cannot sue the blood bank or hospital for the transfusion itself.

It can reasonably be hoped that this "window of opportunity" will be used, and valuable results obtained for the benefit of science and humanity. No matter what the outcome, however, personally relevant information should be shared with the donors and with the recipients of the blood products under observation in the investigation.

REFERENCES

1. Weiss SH, Goedert JJ, Sarngadharan MG, et al. Screening test for HTLV-III (AIDS agent) antibodies: specificity, sensitivity, and applications. JAMA 1985; 253:221-5.
2. Hardy AM, Allen JR, Morgan WM, Curran JW. The incidence rate of acquired immunodeficiency syndrome in selected populations. JAMA 1985; 253:215-20.
3. Selik RM, Haverkos HW, Curran JW. Acquired immune deficiency syndrome (AIDS) trends in the United States, 1978-1982. Am J Med 1984; 76:493-500.
4. Culliton BJ. Crash development of AIDS test nears goal. Science 1984; 225: 1128-31.

COMMENTS

Almost seven years after cases of the acquired immunodeficiency syndrome (AIDS) were first recognized and reported by physicians in the United States, AIDS remains at the center of an intersection of complex legal and ethical issues. Unable to agree on a comprehensive prevention strategy, policy makers at the state and federal levels continue to debate the appropriateness of traditional disease-control measures in preventing the spread of the epidemic. Measures such as quarantine and mandatory testing of populations, such as applicants for marriage licenses or prisoners, have been proposed in a number of states. Civil libertarians voice serious objections to such measures, focusing attention on the delicate balance between individual rights and social interests. The literature examining legal issues relating to AIDS is extensive. For an overview of traditional disease-control measures and the implications of their use in the AIDS epidemic, see W.J. Curran, L. Gostin, and M. Clark, "Acquired Immunodeficiency Syndrome: Legal and Regulatory Policy" (Washington, D.C.: Department of Health and Human Services, 1986). For a comprehensive treatment of the area, see the papers collected and published in a two-part symposium on AIDS in the journal *Law, Medicine and Health Care* (1986; 15 (1 and 2)), guest eds. L. Gostin and W.J. Curran; see also H. Dalton and S. Burris, eds., *AIDS and the Law: A Guide for the Public* (New Haven, Conn.: Yale University Press, 1987).

A question of fundamental legal and ethical importance for physicians is whether medical personnel may, in nonemergency situations, choose not to treat patients with AIDS. A recent survey of residents training in New York City hospitals reported that 25 percent of those responding indicated that they would prefer not to treat patients with AIDS and that they believed that it was not unethical to refuse to care for patients with the disease. One third of those responding indicated that house officers should be given a choice as to whether they should have to care for persons with AIDS. See J.A. Kelly, "Medical Students' Attitudes towards AIDS and Homosexual Patients" (*Journal of Medical Education* 1987; 62:549-56); and J.P. Whalen, "Participation of Medical Students in the Care of Patients with AIDS" (*Journal of Medical Education* 1987; 62:53-4).

Recently, the American Medical Association released a policy paper affirming the position that physicians have an ethical obligation to provide care for persons with AIDS; see Council on Ethical and Judicial Affairs, "Ethical Issues Involved in the Growing AIDS Crisis" (*Journal of the American Medical Association* 1988; 259: 1360-1). For a cogent discussion of physicians' obligation to their patients, see A. Zuger, "Professional Responsibilities in the AIDS Generation" (*Hastings Center Report* 1987; 17:16-20). For a review of lawyers' activities in the courts concerning AIDS, see D. Weisenhaus, "The Shaping of AIDS Law" (*National Law Journal* 1988; 10(47):1, 30-32).

The Proper and Improper Concerns of Mankind and Medical Ethics

On my return from a sabbatical year in the proper and orderly Swiss canton of Geneva, I find American physicians as beleaguered as ever with problems in law and ethics. The malpractice crisis seems unabated. Physicians whom I have met express to me their resentment at the continuing and deepening incursions of ethical and legal decision making into traditional areas of clinical medicine.

The Karen Ann Quinlan case occurred during my sabbatical. A major part of the decision of the highest court of New Jersey, unexpected by ethicists with whom I talked, would allow some medical decisions to end efforts clinically to prolong life in some patients if an "ethics committee" were involved in helping to determine the condition of the patient, the prognosis, and the scope of continuing use of life-prolonging measures.

Some writers have greeted the court's opinion as an effort to keep these difficult and delicate matters within the realm of professional medical determination. Others assert that a traditional, though largely hidden and private, medical responsibility has now become too open and has been improperly labeled an "ethical" decision.

Another area of unease has been the controversy over certain forms of genetic research, with the opponents charging that the efforts are "unethical" because of their uncertainty and their potential danger to mankind.

In each case, one can understand the source of the unease. The facts and opinions to be considered by an "ethics committee" modeled after that suggested in the Quinlan case would be related to

From the *New England Journal of Medicine*
1976; 295:1057-1058.

clinical patient management. For genetic research, it is also said that there is no ethical dimension in examining the vastness of the possible risks and benefits from highly technical, very specialized genetic studies. If mankind should study man, as Alexander Pope admonished, rather than waste time searching for answers to the mysteries of God, so also should man learn to leave mankind's and the earth's most delicate and uncertain studies to those who spend a lifetime in developing the skill, the knowledge, and the maturity to understand them.

These are persuasive arguments. Most of the time, they prevail, if only for the practical reason that most decisions in these fields are made in private by the knowledgeable few, perhaps with little realization of their ethical, social, legal, or political impact. What is ethical and legal in these issues? Are men discovering in 1976 a truth unknown to philosophers and scientists, lawyers and ethicists, in previous centuries?

In the Quinlan type of ethical review, it seems to me that the ethical dimension arises out of the traditional ethical obligation of every physician to do all that he or she can for every patient, regardless of clinical condition. The high court of New Jersey in the Quinlan case recognized an exception to this general rule under which the attending doctor acts ethically in ceasing to apply life-prolonging measures to certain patients. Some physicians and some ethicists deny this exception, or quarrel about an added qualification that the only measures that can be stopped ethically are "extraordinary," or merely say that they do not think the court should have applied any such exception to Ms. Quinlan. All this seems enough ethical controversy for me. What are the review committees expected to do? Is their power limited to advising on the medical management of the patient, or, in the sense their titles as "ethics" committees imply, can they also interpret the meaning and application of the exception to the general ethical rule? I submit that they will inevitably do the latter, owing to the uncertainty of the meaning of the exception and the lack of broad experience anywhere with its application to individual cases.

In genetics research, the basic ethical demand of the scientists is to do no harm. (This is also the quintessence of the promise of every Hippocratic physician to his patient.) No one argues with the general rule, but it is said that some risk can be taken if it is balanced by great potential for benefit to mankind. It is in measuring these risks and benefits, and in determining the justification for observable, potential risk, that nonscientific judgment seems involved. There is enough experience with disaster in the world to be wary of strident voices on either side of these arguments. Anti-intellectual and reactionary fears would stop much research that should be allowed. On the other hand, there is a great uneasiness with the scientist who cannot or will not adjust his research design to alleviate reasonable fears about potential danger in his actions and who defends his position with vague reference to potential benefits, wholly unmeasurable, to what he calls "mankind."

As may be drawn from the above rather tortuous explanation, I can see ethical considerations in both these issues. I am not sure, however, how much is gained by this jurisdictional position, or by identifying the ethical content. If broadly representative ethics committees consider such matters as a right to die, the removal of measures to prolong life, experimentation on human subjects, or specific studies of genetic manipulation, does this action remove the case from court review? If courts do review, will they consider the matter afresh, applying their own sense of justice and ethics, as if the matter had never undergone such a deliberative ethical process?

Very few cases have gone to the courts challenging ethics-committee decisions. However, in one case that has been greeted with quite universal legal approval, *Kaimowitz* v. *Dept. of Mental Health,*[1] a lower court in Michigan arrived at its own decision that a research project would be legally improper in attempting to conduct psychosurgery of uncertain benefit on a subject who was in compulsory confinement. This decision was made despite the fact that two different prestigious committees, one called a "Scientific Review Committee," and the other a "Human Rights Committee," had approved the project and its informed-consent procedure for application to such a patient subject. I am not here arguing the merits of this case. I am pointing out that the court did not give binding weight, or even very great consideration, to the decisions of these bodies. The court took its own evidence from a range of sources (not heard at all by the committees, which merely reviewed the protocol and the researchers' plans) when the court found itself confronted with a case involving the rights of human subjects and the protection of their safety and welfare. Would the court have had any greater hesitation in reviewing other "ethical decisions" applied to individuals to their possible detriment, or involving potentially serious harm to populations of people, the community as a whole, or the earth's ecologic balance?

The proper boundaries of medicine and ethics, science and law, are no closer to being airtight compartments of jurisdictional certainty now after the Quinlan case and a year's passage of time than before I left for Geneva.

REFERENCE

1. Civil Action no. 73-19434-AW, 42 US Law Week 2064, Wayne County, Michigan, 1973.

♦

COMMENTS

This column, too, was rather subtle in its approach to issues of ethics and moral reasoning. Its thesis was that most physicians and clinical scientific investigators were uncomfortable with the idea that ethics committees should be given regulatory power over medical decision making and the design of clinical investigations. As Alexander Pope admonished mankind to concern itself with its own problems rather than God's, so physicians and scientists thought that the technical aspects of their fields ought to be left to scientifically trained people.

After the *Quinlan* decision in New Jersey, the attorney general's office adopted regulations that required hospitals to set up review committees in accordance with the court's ruling. However, as my column predicted, the attorney general and his medical and hospital advisers avoided calling these panels ethics committees and also avoided naming any nonphysician members to the panels. The title chosen for the review groups was "prognosis committees," a good parochial term that justified appointing a committee composed exclusively of members of the hospital's medical staff. For a review of committee functioning in New Jersey, see R.L. McIntyre and D.N. Buchalter, "Institutional Committees: The New Jersey Experience," in R.E. Cranford and A.E. Doudera, eds., *Institutional Ethics Committees and Health Care Decision Making* (Ann Arbor, Mich.: Health Administration Press, 1984).

The avoidance of the term "ethics committees" has persisted into the Reagan administration; the federal regulations relating to life-sustaining measures for handicapped infants are a good example. These directives include a suggestion that hospital review committees be set up to deal with such matters, but the federal authorities specifically rejected the expression "biomedical ethics committees" and instead adopted the term "institutional child-care review committees." In similar fashion, federal regulations on the protection of research subjects refer to the committees in that field as "institutional review boards."

On the other hand, there is not much resistance to the concept of ethics committees in the American Hospital Association. See a report by a group of lawyers in the field of hospital law gathered by the American Hospital Association to advise it on the establishment of such review bodies in hospitals. See *Legal Issues and Guidance for Hospital Biomedical Ethics Committees: Report of the Adjunct Legal Task Force on Biomedical Ethics* (Chicago: American Hospital Association, January 1985). See also A.L. Merritt, "The Tort Liability of Hospital Ethics Committees" (*Southern California Law Review* 1987; 60:1239-97).

Quality-of-Life and Treatment Decisions: The Canadian Law Reform Report

The recent "Baby Doe" decision in New York, concerning clinical choices regarding treatment for a child with severe birth defects, and the murder indictment and trial in California of a group of physicians who discontinued treatment and feeding of a brain-damaged patient have provoked reexamination all across the country of the legal and ethical rules concerning the medical obligation to continue vigorous treatment in terminally ill patients or patients whose "quality of life" has deteriorated to unacceptable levels, as in patients in constant, intractable pain or irreversible coma.

These issues have received attention in other parts of the world as well as in the United States. One of the most important recent examinations of the subject has been conducted in Canada by the Law Reform Commission, an official national body charged with periodically recommending the substantive reform of federal law applicable all across Canada. In 1976 the commission established a special study group called the Protection of Life Project. The issues examined in a series of working papers and reports have included abortion, sterilization, criteria for determining death, and consent to medical treatment.

The latest study combines recommendations on the law concerning euthanasia, aiding suicide, and cessation of medical treatment.[1] The final report was prepared after very wide circulation of a preliminary working document prepared by the project staff.[2] After comments were received and considered, the commissioners prepared the final report with their commentary and conclusions.

From the *New England Journal of Medicine*
1984; 310:297-298.

The report is refreshingly brief and concise (35 pages in the English-language version), particularly as compared with the very lengthy document (545 pages) published earlier in 1983 on much the same subject by the American study group known as the President's Commission for the Study of Ethical Problems in Medicine and Biomedical and Behavioral Research.[3]

The first two issues were dealt with quickly and without elaborate discussion. The commissioners recommended that euthanasia – the intentional killing of a person for compassionate motives – remain covered by the criminal code as culpable homicide. Specifically mentioned was the intentional killing of a patient by medical personnel, even when requested by a patient who was terminally ill or in great pain. The commissioners also recommended retaining as a crime an action that would help a patient to commit suicide, such as furnishing a gun, a poison, or a lethal medication that the patient would then self-administer. It was admitted, of course, that prosecutions were rare for helping a suffering patient to commit suicide and that convictions were virtually nonexistent. Nevertheless, it was thought that aiding suicide should not be condoned and that the circumstances of such alleged actions should be investigated, since they could be motivated by improper purposes in some cases.

Most of the report, however, dealt with the third area – decisions to end medical treatment, thus leading to death. First of all, it was recognized that competent patients could refuse treatment, even if the refusal would inevitably lead to death. The physician's duty in such situations was described as the obligation to inform the patient fully of the options open to the patient and of their consequences. It was asserted that physicians could not treat patients against their wills and that to do so would be an assault under both criminal and civil law in Canada. The commissioners refused, however, to recommend the establishment of a new, specific penalty for such medical actions, as had been recommended to the commission by various commentators. Although the commissioners were very strong in their support for patient autonomy, they did not seem to want to single out the physician who treated patients against their will for criminal prosecution (and stronger penalties) any more than any other person in Canada who committed assault and battery.

The commission went on to find that medical treatment of the incompetent patient should be discontinued only for very serious reasons. It was firmly asserted that "in the medical context" the legal presumption in favor of life should always be recognized. However, the commissioners said that this principle was not absolute but applied only when the treatment was "reasonable and useful." The burden was placed on those who would stop treatment, or not initiate life-supporting treatment, to justify a decision resulting in a patient's death.

In an important discussion the commissioners went on to assert that under the federal law, the value of human life should be considered not only from a "quantitative" perspective but also from a "qualitative" viewpoint. It was aptly observed that when the law upheld the patient's freedom to choose to refuse treatment, it was recognizing that the patient's choice was often based on quality-of-life considerations. On the same basis, it should be legally justified to consider quality of life when making "substituted consent" for incompetent, seriously ill patients. The commissioners stressed that they wanted to prevent the possibility that the patient's inability to give or refuse consent because of mental incompetency should impose on the physician a legal duty to provide aggressive treatment under all circumstances. On the contrary, it was found that incompetent patients should be considered within the same context as competent patients. Therapeutically useless treatment should not be begun "to prolong unnecessarily the patient's agony." It was concluded that incompetent patients should also have the right to die in peace and dignity, assisted by whatever palliative care is needed at the time.

The report examined three alternative mechanisms or models for ensuring consent and protection for patients in such situations. These were the judicial model, the family or guardian consent model, and the medical model. Under the first, the decision to treat or to stop treatment would be made by a judge or a quasi-judicial body such as a hospital ethics or administrative committee. It was indicated that the large majority of comments received by the commission was against this alternative as unwieldy, complex, and inappropriate. Specifically, the commissioners rejected this model because of its potential for becoming "confrontational" and "adversarial." They found no advantages to be gained in requiring "every decision concerning treatment of an incompetent person to be automatically subject to the formal and initial order" of a court or quasi-judicial body.

The second alternative was also rejected, although it was found to be supported by a number of Canadian organizations and individuals in their commentaries. The commissioners saw serious disadvantages in this proposal, which would delegate consent and decision making solely to the family, next of kin, or a guardian for the incompetent patient. It was observed that to do so would place an extremely heavy psychological burden on the family, often on persons not equipped emotionally or intellectually to bear it. Also, the family members could have conscious or unconscious conflicts of interest with the incompetent person.

Having dismissed the other alternatives, the Law Reform Commission, composed of leading Canadian lawyers, embraced the third alternative of placing primary responsibility on the physician treating the patient. Since the matter involved was found to be primarily medical in nature, physician responsibility was considered the most satisfactory solution. However, it was indicated that the medical decision to treat or not to treat should be made "after discussion, explanation and consultation with those close to the patient." These persons would not, however, have veto power over the physician's decision. The commission recommended that there be no criminal liability on physicians for decisions in these situations, including decisions not to treat or to discontinue treatment previously instituted, as long as the decision was valid medically – that is, made on reasonable medical grounds under the circumstances, in the best interest of the incompetent patient and in conformity with other standards set by criminal law. It was also indicated that the commissioners would expect, but not require, that serious medical decisions such as these would involve the treating doctor's seeking an independent second medical consultation supportive of the physician's judgment or the advice of "an interdisciplinary hospital committee."

The rejection of criminal liability (a murder charge if the patient died) by the commission in cases in which the treating physician determined that further treatment would be medically useless and in which the quality of life of the patient was unacceptably compromised was the most forthright of any of the ethical–legal pronouncements on the subject that have been published to date. Most of the court cases in the United States have hesitated to accept a broadly worded "quality-of-life" test for removal of life-support systems, except for the universally adopted concept of "brain death" — a form of irreversible coma, which is a quality-of-life standard.

States in our country that have not yet established ethical–legal standards in this field would do well to study and consider the wisdom applied to these difficult issues by the Law Reform Commission of Canada.

REFERENCES

1. Law Reform Commission of Canada. Report 20. Euthanasia, aiding suicide, and cessation of treatment. Ottawa, Canada: Law Reform Commission of Canada, November 1983.
2. Law Reform Commission of Canada. Working paper 28. Euthanasia, aiding suicide, and cessation of treatment. Ottawa, Canada: Law Reform Commission of Canada, 1982.
3. President's Commission for the Study of Ethical Problems in Medicine and Biomedical and Behavioral Research. Deciding to forego life-sustaining treatment: a report on the ethical, medical, and legal issues in treatment decisions. Washington, D.C.: Government Printing Office, March 1983.

COMMENTS

Even now that many other useful commentaries have been published, this Canadian report remains one of the best reasoned of the official documents in the field. It is perhaps most noteworthy for its advocacy of leaving medical decision making in the hands of the treating doctors and its rejection of the most popular of the American solutions suggested up to that time. The report rejected both prior court review of all cases of removal of life-supports, at least in the case of incompetent patients, and the establishment of hospital-based bioethics committees to review all such cases. These approaches were rejected as too formalistic, confrontational, and adversarial.

The report and the working paper that preceded the report were well received in Canada. A symposium on the working paper, consisting of four written discussions of it — two by lawyers, one by a physician, and one by a nurse — was published in a Canadian journal on health law. For a general review, see J.L. Bandouin, "Cessation of Treatment and Suicide: Proposal for Reform" (*Health Law in Canada* 1982; 3:72-3).

Issues concerning euthanasia and assisting in suicides were also dealt with in the Canadian report. These aspects of the subject received very little attention in reports and commentaries in the early 1980s. The Canadian report dealt with these matters because the Canadian Law Reform Commission was focusing on the national criminal code, which is applicable in all Canadian provinces. In the face of the epidemic of the acquired immunodeficiency syndrome (AIDS) in the later 1980s, these aspects of the law may begin to receive more attention. It has been indicated that suicides, the aiding of suicides, and euthanasia are phenomena commonly associated with AIDS in some parts of the world. In the Netherlands, where active euthanasia by physicians is not illegal, it is reported that as many as one in eight deaths due to AIDS has been hastened by medical action. A physician representing the main treating hospital in Amsterdam indicated that the lives of at least 10 patients had been ended in their homes by family doctors at their own requests. See "Netherlands AIDS Euthanasia Rises" (*International Herald Tribune,* April 7, 1987; United Press International Report).

A decision of the high court of the Netherlands (the *Alkmaar* case) has interpreted the National Criminal Code in such a way as to exclude physicians from criminal liability for active euthanasia when the patient is in constant suffering and can no longer die with dignity. Efforts to adopt a legislative standard have failed as a result of conflict between the major political parties in the Netherlands. See H.J. Scholten, "Justification for Active Euthanasia" (*Medicine and Law* 1986; 5:169-72). See also J.K.M. Gevens, "Legal Developments Concerning Active Euthanasia on Request in the Netherlands" (*Bioethics* 1987; 1:156-74).

Care for the Dying Patient: Legal Standards for Denying Nutrients and Hydration

The New Jersey Supreme Court first attained national prominence in medicolegal issues of obligations to critically ill patients in the Karen Ann Quinlan case. The high court in New Jersey issued an eminently sensible opinion in that case, allowing the patient's guardian, her father, to use his discretion in removal of life support from his daughter, who was then irreversibly comatose.[1] The court directed that in future cases, the attending physician and the family be advised in such matters by a hospital-based ethics or prognosis committee, which could avoid a case-by-case judicial review. It was expected that the patient would die soon after removal of the respirator, but she did not. Although the hospital physicians, still opposed to the court's decision that she be allowed to die, removed the respirator, Ms. Quinlan remained alive for nine years in a New Jersey nursing home.

The same high court has rendered a new decision in an even more troubling area: the obligation to provide nutrition and water to elderly patients in nursing homes who are greatly impaired and dying. The difficulties in these cases are manifold. The patients have often lost all control of bodily functions, cannot communicate, are experiencing varying degrees of pain and discomfort, and must be fed intravenously or by a nasogastric tube in order to survive in an extremely feeble condition. The patients are maintained by nursing staff and are rarely seen by physicians except in the event of radical changes in their condition. When, if ever, are the staff and the supervising physician

From the *New England Journal of Medicine*
1985; 313:940-942.

justified in withdrawing (or withholding) nutrition and hydration, allowing the patient to die quietly rather than linger on in such a condition?

There has been a concern that the failure to provide food and water is, in some deeply symbolic way, different from the cessation of medical treatment, whether described as "ordinary" or "extraordinary." Food and water seem to be a key part of the care given in medical and nursing services. In the latest version of the federal government's efforts to prevent "child abuse" in the case of severely impaired infants (the Baby Doe law and regulations), the law does not allow removal of nutritional and hydration care under any circumstances.[2,3]

In a case named *In the Matter of Claire Conroy,*[4] the New Jersey court has determined that removal of the nasogastric tube should be viewed in the same way as other medical and nursing treatment provided to elderly patients in nursing homes. Removal of the tube was found to be legally proper under detailed judicial guidelines. A comprehensive review of the decision is not possible in this limited space, but the highlights can be outlined.

The patient was an 85-year-old woman with irreversible physical and mental impairments, including arteriosclerotic heart disease, hypertension, and diabetes. She could not speak or move on her own and responded only by moaning or smiling in response to certain stimuli. She was essentially unaware of her surroundings. She had no control of her excretory functions and required nasogastric feeding. She was not brain-dead or in a coma. Her guardian since 1979 had been a nephew who visited her each week. She had no other living relatives. The nephew had earlier opposed any efforts to end life support, and he had nothing to gain financially by her death. He petitioned the court to allow removal of the nasogastric tube. The physician in charge opposed removal, since he considered it "unacceptable medical practice." During the litigation, the patient died with the nasogastric tube in place.

The trial court ruled in favor of the petitioner, but an intermediate appellate court reversed that ruling. The supreme court, although the patient had died, retained jurisdiction in order to make its own decision. The case by this time had received considerable publicity. In the appeal to the high court, national attention was enhanced through amicus curiae briefs filed by several groups, including the New Jersey Hospital Association, a group of former members and professional staff of the President's Commission for the Study of Ethical Problems in Medicine and Biomedical and Behavioral Research, the National Citizen's Coalition for Nursing Home Reform, Concern for the Dying, and the New Jersey Concerned Taxpayers.

In their latest ruling, the New Jersey Court established three separate tests or standards under which patients like Ms. Conroy (those in nursing homes who are suffering from "serious and permanent mental and physical impairment," will "probably die within approximately one year" even with treatment, are incompetent to make decisions about life support, and are unlikely ever to regain competence) need not be given nasogastric feeding and other forms of life support.

The first test was described as a "subjective standard" under which the wish of the patient not to receive further treatment or feeding would be followed. The evidence of this refusal could be found, said the court, in specific communications, such as a "living will" stating the person's wish not to be treated or sustained under certain circumstances; in an "oral directive" to a family member, friend, or health care provider; or in a durable power of attorney or appointment of a proxy or representative to make such decisions on the person's behalf.

The second and third tests would be used if it was not clear that the patient had expressed a specific desire not to be treated or fed under the circumstances. These tests would apply the *parens patriae* power of the state to act in the best interests of an incompetent person. The second test was described as a "limited objective standard" to be applied if there was only "some trustworthy evidence" that the patient would have refused treatment and feeding. This evidence could include casual comments to family and friends, the life style of the person, attitudes and actions of independence, and the person's concern for dignity and the ability to sustain his or her own capacity. According to the majority opinion, however, the patient would have to be suffering from unavoidable pain, thus making continued life too heavy a burden to bear.

In the absence of any reliable evidence of the patient's wishes, the court indicated that a third test could be applied, a "pure objective standard" under which feeding and life-support systems could be removed. In such a situation, a stricter standard of the patient's unbearable life would need to be indicated. The net burdens of continued life should "clearly and markedly" outweigh any benefits. This would be the case if the patient met all the conditions stated above and suffered from recurring, unavoidable pain that was so severe that administering life-sustaining treatment or feeding would be "inhumane." The court expressly denied authority under this third test to remove life support from any patient on a "quality-of-life" basis other than extreme pain or on the ground that the patient's "value to society" was negligible.

One might have expected that the high court would end its opinion at this point, except to indicate that guardians could exercise these new standards under the guidance of ethics or prognosis committees set up in New Jersey hospitals and in some nursing homes as well, under the *Quinlan* decision and a procedure formulated by the New Jersey attorney general's office.[5,6] In a move that came as a surprise to most observers of the decision in the lower courts, the supreme court took no notice at all of the ethics–prognosis committee approach so strongly supported in the *Quinlan* opinion. Instead, the majority of the court recognized another administrative system, set up in New Jersey in recent years, as seemingly more acceptable for nursing home oversight. This is the state ombudsman program established to investigate physical and mental abuse of patients in nursing homes. The court determined that this program should be called on to examine all identified cases in nursing homes in which life support, including feeding and hydration, would be withheld or withdrawn under any of the three tests described above and in which the request to investigate was instituted by a guardian, family, friends, or the attending physician or nursing home. (An independent person could also make a complaint to the ombudsman concerning a case in which these guidelines were not followed and abuse of the patient was suspected.)

The ombudsman would be required to conduct an immediate review of the matter and report within 24 hours to the commissioner of human services and other appropriate authorities. The ombudsman would seek appointment of two physicians not associated with the facility to examine the patient and provide an opinion on his or her condition and prognosis. In order to authorize that life support, feeding, and hydration be withheld or withdrawn, the ombudsman would have to agree that the applicable standard was met and obtain the concurrence of the two examining physicians, the attending doctor, the guardian, if any, and the patient's family or next of kin. It was pointed out in a footnote that in the *Quinlan* case the court had allowed the guardian to replace a reluctant or unwilling attending physician with another physician of his choice who was willing to support the guardian's wishes to remove life support. If all these steps were taken and recorded, the authorization of the ombudsman would, in the absence of bad faith, immunize all participants from civil and criminal liability for actions taken.

The importance of this decision in the growing court literature on medical obligation to the dying cannot be overstated. It is the most far-reaching of the judicial opinions in laying down general guidelines for the care of patients in nursing homes. The court's position in allowing removal of nutrition and hydration as well as other forms of life support is without precedent in the American courts. Equally impressive is the willingness of the court to articulate three separate legal standards that can support and justify such removal. Other courts have tended to rely only on the first type of standard, the subjective test, or "substituted judgment," in which a guardian may act only when there is clear evidence of a previously indicated desire on the part of the patient that life support be removed or treatment withheld, under the circumstances prevailing at the time. There has been less support recently for a "best interests" test, no matter how expressed, despite a long history of use of the *parens patriae* doctrine in English and American common law. The *Conroy* case reinforces the legitimacy of this traditional doctrine and supports the actions of guardians who, in good faith and without a conflict of interest, determine that the patient's best interests will not be served by prolonging a painful, hopeless existence.

The *Conroy* opinion is thoughtful and well constructed, not only in the breadth and clarity of its guidelines but in the accomplishment of the court in bringing six of seven judges to full concurrence in the opinion. Only one justice dissented in part. This justice would, in fact, have gone further than the majority by allowing removal or withholding of life support, including nutrition and hydration, on the basis of a "best interests" determination, without the stricter qualifications in regard to pain and suffering. The result, therefore, is a strong position and a firm consensus of the court on the basic philosophy to allow termination of life support in stated circumstances.

The wisdom of the *Conroy* decision in actual operation, however, has yet to be measured. The involvement of a state ombudsman may prove to be a useful and welcome alternative to the continuous involvement of courts and may be more suited to the environment of nursing homes than the ethics–prognosis committees in hospitals. On the other hand, the legislature, in its parsimony, may never provide adequate funds to allow the program to operate effectively. Even if the ombudsman program is broadly successful, New Jersey will have two different systems functioning to deal with similar clinical situations in nursing homes and hospitals, since the *Conroy* guidelines are specifically applicable only to nursing homes. Legislative action to clarify problems of interpretation across the systems is advisable; otherwise, further high-level judicial involvement, no matter how much the New Jersey Supreme Court would like to avoid it, seems inevitable.

REFERENCES

1. In re Karen Ann Quinlan, 70 N.J. 10 (1976).
2. Child Abuse Amendments Act of 1984, Public Law 98-457.
3. Proposed Rule and Interim Guidelines, 45 CFR Part 1340. December 10, 1985.
4. In the matter of Claire Conroy, 98 N.J. 321 (1985).
5. New Jersey Guidelines for Health Care Facilities to Implement Procedures Concerning the Care of Comatose Non-Cognitive Patients. January 27, 1977.
6. McIntyre RL, Buchalter DN. Institutional committees: the New Jersey experience. In: Cranford RE, Doudera AE, eds. Institutional ethics committees and health care decision making. Ann Arbor, Mich.: Health Administration Press, 1984:106-17.

COMMENTS

The complexity of the New Jersey decision in the *Conroy* case obliged me to make this the longest column that I have ever written for the *Journal*. The opinion read more like a legislative bill than a common-law court opinion in that it set forth a series of alternative standards for the care of dying patients. Usually, a high court avoids such detailed standard setting, assuming that later cases will provide opportunities for embroidering the text of the original opinion. But this leisurely approach could not be adopted in this case. In order to persuade a majority of the judges on the bench to accept the ruling terminating food and water for Ms. Conroy, the judge writing the opinion had to spell out the implications of the decision in full. The judge even took the extraordinary additional precaution of bringing in a state regulatory agency, the ombudsman for the investigation of abuse of the elderly in nursing homes, to oversee the implementation of the standards set forth in the opinion.

In a bitterly divided opinion (four to three), the Massachusetts Supreme Judicial Court arrived at a similar finding in that it authorized the removal of a gastrostomy tube from a patient in a persistent vegetative state. In this case, however, the patient was otherwise in good physical condition and not close to death. The majority based its decision on the concept of "substituted judgment," evidence that the patient, before his surgery, had frequently indicated orally his preference not to be continued on artificial life support. The majority asserted that it was recognizing the patient's right "to avoid circumstances in which the individual himself would feel that efforts to sustain life demean or degrade his humanity"; *Brophy* v. *New England Sinai Hospital,* 398 Mass. 417 (1986).

The Massachusetts court in the *Brophy* case did not, however, order the hospital involved and the treating physicians to act against their own philosophy of care by removing the feeding tube from the patient. The majority asserted that in such circumstances, the patient's guardian was authorized to remove the patient from the hospital to another institution or to bring the patient to his or her home.

In a California case that received a great deal of media coverage over a period of years, the court authorized the removal of a feeding tube attached to a quadriplegic woman who did not wish to continue to live under such conditions; *Bouvia* v. *Superior Court,* 225 Cal. Rptr. 297 (1986).

For a comprehensive review of the subject by an interdisciplinary group of extraordinary background in the field, see President's Commission for the Study of Ethical Problems in Medicine and Biomedical and Behavioral Research, *Deciding to Forego Life-Sustaining Treatment: Report on Ethical, Medical, and Legal Issues in Treatment Decisions* (Washington, D.C.: Government Printing Office, March 1983). For another, later report by an interdisciplinary group convened by the American Hospital Association, see *Values in Conflict: Ethical Issues in Hospital Care: Report of the Special Committee on Biomedical Ethics* (Chicago: American Hospital Association, January 1985). See also E.R. Grant and C.D. Forsythe, "The Plight of the Last Friend: Legal Issues for Physicians and Nurses in Providing Nutrition and Hydration" (*Issues in Law and Medicine* 1987; 2:277-99).

Laetrile for the Terminally Ill: The Supreme Court Stops the Nonsense

Over the past five years there has been a growing wave of loudly expressed and widely distributed protest against what has been called "improper interference" by hospitals, physicians, and government regulatory agencies in the "free choice" of patients with cancer to obtain Laetrile, a compound of seeds and kernels of various fruits, as a cure for the disease. The stridency of much of the public media in supporting this movement has been especially painful to us in Massachusetts, the home state of the tragic case of Chad Green. Chad Green died of leukemia in Mexico after being taken there by his parents for Laetrile therapy in defiance of a court order.

A number of badly decided court cases have failed to stop much of the nonsense, the utter cruelty to dying patients – and ones who are not dying – that has resulted from this strange movement. The decisions in these cases have largely agreed with a policy of increased availability of Laetrile, a substance that the Food and Drug Administration (FDA) has consistently barred from interstate commerce as an unlicensed, untested drug whose safety and efficacy have not been proved. One of the few exceptions in court decisions has in fact been the intelligence shown by the Massachusetts Supreme Judicial Court in handling the case of Chad Green, but the effort of that court to ensure proper treatment for a sick child was frustrated in large measure by this ill-conceived national effort in favor of Laetrile availability.

One of the sorriest spectacles was the case in New Jersey in 1977, in which a 78-year-old woman was alleged to be dying of cancer and in

From the *New England Journal of Medicine*
1980; 302:619-621.

a condition described by the court as "steadily deteriorating."[1] The hospital had refused to allow a doctor to administer Laetrile to the patient because doing so would violate FDA regulations and would be an unacceptable method of treatment in the hospital. The court nevertheless ordered the hospital to violate its own standards of practice and to allow the doctor to follow the patient's (and family's) wishes, irrespective of the essentially fraudulent nature of the intended medication. The court blatantly forced the hospital to allow an action that it considered grossly unethical to be committed within its walls. The judge would not even allow the patient to be transferred to another institution whose scruples might be different. In an ironic twist of judicial moral reasoning, the judge said that he could not "in good conscience" allow referral of the patient to another hospital, with consequent "disorienting effects," as a condition of being able "to enjoy whatever benefits may be derived" from Laetrile. Yet this same judge obviously had no confidence in the therapeutic effects of the drug he was forcing the hospital to make available to its patient. The court said, "The efficacy of Laetrile does not enter into this case." Perhaps the most telling observation of the court was to call the substance "a mildly toxic placebo."

The most influential case, however, which was relied on heavily in the New Jersey decision cited above, has been *Rutherford* v. *United States*.[2] It has been making its way, agonizingly slowly, through the federal court system, back and forth from district court to court of appeals, since 1975. I am pleased to report that the substance of this case has finally been addressed in a superb opinion by Justice Thurgood Marshall writing for a unanimous bench.[3]

In this litigation, a federal judge in Oklahoma had allowed a group of patients who were alleged to be terminally ill with cancer, some of whom have since died, to join a so-called class-action suit to enjoin the FDA to permit them to purchase and use Laetrile. The district court granted the order. The court of appeals, in its first review, did not disturb the order but instructed the district court to seek an FDA determination of whether Laetrile was a "new drug" and, if so, whether it was exempt from licensing regulations.

The FDA conducted its investigation and found that Laetrile was a new drug and was not exempt from premarket regulation. The result of this finding should have been that Laetrile could not be sold in the interstate market in the United States, since it had never been offered for testing and no manufacturer had ever sought a license for it as a new drug. But the district-court judge was not to be deterred in his efforts to get Laetrile to patients with cancer. He refused to accept the FDA's finding that the drug was not sold commercially and used as a cancer cure and was not recognized by experts in the field as safe before October 9, 1962, when the Drug Amendments of that year went into effect. Alternatively, the judge held that even if Laetrile was not exempt from premarket regulation, denying patients use of the drug would be an improper infringement on their constitutionally protected rights to privacy.

The federal court of appeals then had another opportunity to review the matter. It did no better the second time. As Justice Marshall said in his review of the lower-court opinion, the court of appeals "addressed neither the statutory nor the constitutional rulings of the District Court." Instead, it went off on its own tack: It determined that the standards of safety and efficacy required under the law by the FDA could not have any reasonable application to terminally ill persons. The court of appeals therefore ordered the FDA to promulgate regulations "as if" the alleged therapeutic drug, Laetrile, had been found safe and effective for terminally ill patients.

In the only concession to therapeutic caution that one can find in the order, the court of appeals, apparently concerned that the FDA had found some evidence that Laetrile was toxic when taken orally, issued its order to the district court to authorize the drug's use only by means of intravenous injection under a physician's "supervision."

When the case reached the Supreme Court, Justice Marshall found no merit in the reasoning of the court of appeals. He quickly disposed of the notion that the FDA had no legal authority to protect terminally ill patients from fraudulent or totally unsupported claims of efficacy in treatment or cure of their illnesses. In fact, quite the opposite was found in the plain language of the law and was affirmed prominently in the legislative history of laws passed in 1938 and 1962. In regard to the 1962 amendments that established the FDA's standards of therapeutic efficacy and requirements for clinical testing, the Supreme Court even quoted the most famous sponsor of the 1962 bill, Senator Estes Kefauver, as expressing on the floor of Congress the understanding that the amendments were intended to cover drugs used to treat cancer "in its last stages."[4] Justice Marshall also found that the FDA had followed the practice of regulating such drugs without interruption since 1962, and the practice had gone unchallenged by the drug industry. Furthermore, Congress had taken no action to alter this well-known administrative action.

Justice Marshall did not end his consideration of the regulatory policy at this point. He went on to examine the meaning of the term "safety" under the law in relation to drugs for persons alleged to be terminally ill. He held that safety in this context was not limited to the compound's inherent toxicity or lack of it. He asserted that an otherwise harmless drug (and Laetrile was not conceded to be inherently harmless) could nevertheless be dangerous to any patient if it did not produce its purported therapeutic effect. He said that if a patient with a potentially fatal illness rejects conventional therapy in favor of a drug with "no demonstrable curative properties, the consequences can be irreversible." Use of the ineffective remedy prevents or delays application of accepted modes of therapy. The Court pointed to the expert testimony received in the lower courts that showed that many patients eagerly seeking Laetrile or other mystery cures might not have the disease at that time, or might not be in an advanced stage of the disease, but would be discontinuing conventional treatment that might have achieved a complete cure or substantially prolonged survival. It was also noted that undisputed expert testimony had indicated that with diseases such as cancer, it is often impossible to identify a patient as terminally ill except in retrospect.

Justice Marshall recognized this case for what it was, an attack on the entire jurisdiction of the FDA over all drugs intended for use by seriously ill persons, not merely as a simple, one-time exception for this substance desired by desperate people in their last days. He reversed the case, but remanded it once more to the court of appeals for any further consideration of the issues of the FDA law and other constitutional points not reached in the court of appeals' opinion.

This litigation has not yet been brought to a close. However, it can be hoped that the forthright and outspoken directness of the Marshall opinion will lay to rest the embarrassment of the judicial support for this movement. It is understandable that judges have had trouble dealing objectively with the legal pleas of plaintiffs who are dying a painful death and whose only wish is to indulge in a harmless, although ineffective, gesture of hope. The courts have tried to dispense mercy, if not justice. Their error has been in abandoning the protection of law for these patients. These patients are entitled to the law's protection even in the depth of their illnesses. They are still human beings with all the rights of the living. This is the meaning of justice in our days.

REFERENCES

1. Suenram v. Society of Valley Hospital, 155 N.J. Super. 593 (1977).
2. 438 F.Supp. 1287 (1977).
3. U.S. v. Rutherford, 99 Sup. Ct. 2470, 61 L. Ed. 2d 68 (1979).
4. 108 Congressional Record 17399, 1962.

COMMENTS

I was particularly outspoken in this column. I could see no sense in the earlier decisions of the courts that allowed the sale of the worthless cancer drug Laetrile and forced doctors and hospitals to prescribe and administer it. The particular dispute reviewed in the column, the *Rutherford* case, had a prolonged history of negotiating its way up and down the federal court system and in the process had unleashed a disgraceful display of disregard for reasoned judgment and the protection of the population from charlatans and faith healers. Justice Marshall wrote one of his best opinions in stopping this nonsense in its tracks.

For law review articles tracing the history of the case and the constitutional arguments raised in the litigation, see H.J. Volzer, "Laetrile and the Right of Privacy in Decisional Responsibility" (*Medical Trial Technique Quarterly* 1980; 26:395-429); G. Lerner and J. Weeks, "The Laetrile Power Play in Drug Marketing" (*Hamline Law Review* 1980; 3:1-50); and J.F. Cannizzaro and M.M. Rosenfeld, "Laetrile and the F.D.A.: A Case of Reverse Regulation" (*Journal of Health Politics, Policy, and Law* 1978; 3:181-95).

The Patient's Bill of Rights Becomes Law

It is declared to be the public policy of this state that the interests of patients be protected by a patient's bill of rights.
Minnesota Laws of 1973, Chapter 688

During the past few years, hospitals and neighborhood health centers in the United States have been adopting documents called a "patient's bill of rights." Among the best known are the statements or booklets published by the Beth Israel Hospital in Boston and the Martin Luther King Health Center in New York City. In November 1972, the Board of Trustees of the American Hospital Association (AHA) adopted such a statement containing a list of 12 principles ranging from a right to considerate and respectful care, a right to informed consent before treatment, and on to a right to know the hospital's rules and regulations.

The AHA's statement on patients' rights was generally greeted with approval in the professional and popular press, but with the comment that the list seemed to contain little that was not already the legal and ethical responsibility of hospitals and medical professionals. The most controversial provision (Principle 4) asserted that the patient has a right to refuse treatment, but this was qualified by the phrase "to the extent permitted by law." Some thought that this would require the hospital to allow a dying patient to refuse further efforts to keep him alive, or to allow a suicidal patient to refuse security, or treatment, or to allow such a patient to leave the hospital. Another provision (Principle 9) required hospitals to advise all patients of proposals to engage them in any human experiment and to obtain their permission for such studies.

Not all commentators have greeted the AHA statement with approval, however. One physician characterized it as a document that

From the *New England Journal of Medicine*
1974; 290:32–33.

only returns to the patient some of the rights that hospitals have previously stolen from them. Dr. Gaylin asserted, "It is the thief lecturing his victim on self-protection – i.e., the hospital instructs the patient to make sure the hospital treats him according to the rules of decency and law to which he is entitled."[1]

None of these documents issued in the past have had any force of law behind them. In this day of fast-growing medical and hospital law, this condition could not remain for long. A state legislature, that of Minnesota, has passed, and the governor has signed into law, a "bill of rights" for patients and residents of "health care facilities." It is a part of a more general piece of legislation providing for the licensing and regulation of health care facilities by the state.

The Minnesota law is patterned after the AHA document, but seems to be considerably weaker. Neither of the controversial AHA provisions on refusal of treatment or experimental medicine is included. Even more seriously, it does not contain the AHA provision (Principle 3) on informed consent before treatment. Also missing are Principles 11 and 12 relating to a right to have an explanation of the hospital bill and to know all applicable hospital rules and regulations. What is included? It contains provisions on respectful care, privacy, continuity of care (undefined), a reasonable response to requests of the patient, and certain provisions on "information" to be given the patient. The patient is said to be entitled to know the name of the physician responsible for "coordination of his care." He is also entitled to obtain information about any relation of the facility to other health care and related institutions so far as his care is concerned. Also, the Minnesota law contains a somewhat modified version of the AHA's Principle 2 concerning the right of the patient to receive from his physician (not the hospital) complete and current information on diagnoses, treatment, and prognoses in terms that he can understand. However, the Minnesota law, like the AHA, qualifies this right when it is "not medically advisable." In such cases, it is said that "the information may" [the AHA said, "should"] be made available to an appropriate person on his behalf.

The Minnesota law requires that every patient and resident be given a copy of the patient's bill of rights, and it requires all licensed health care facilities to post a copy conspicuously in a public place in the institution.

Weak as they undoubtedly are, these statements of principles are steps in the right direction. Even when enacted as law, as in Minnesota, they are more related to the adoption of an attitude—a philosophy—than to a set of specific new powers in the human beings who enter occasionally and inevitably into that dependent status of "patient."

It is important, I submit, that it be declared publicly that patients have rights. The basic document is something to build on. It is the basis of a greater equality between patient and provider, as the Hippocratic Oath was the foundation of Greek medicine. But it must be admitted that these policy statements alone are of no great use to the many patients who will not understand them or who may, for many reasons, be unable to exercise them. An effective enforcement program may require a complaint system and a cadre of patients' representatives or advocates. Nevertheless, these representatives or advocates should not be viewed by the hospital staffs—or by themselves—as the sole protectors of patients' rights. It seems to me that these programs can only work if all medical personnel accept for themselves the professional ethical values inherent in the concept of patients' rights.

REFERENCE

1. Gaylin W. The patient's bill of rights. Saturday Rev Sci 1973; 1:22.

♦

COMMENTS

Many of the duties of physicians toward their patients in modern medical practice are set down not in textbooks on medical ethics, or even in medical licensure laws, but in legally adopted codes defining the rights of patients. This movement began in 1974, when Minnesota adopted the first legal code, or set of principles, relating to patients' rights. Most of this code, or bill of rights, was merely a restatement of already existing rights and duties in the field of medical and hospital practice. Nevertheless, the movement to codification was very important at the time and has continued ever since. Similar codes have been adopted in many other states. Some are general in coverage, whereas others relate to special categories of patients, such as the mentally retarded or developmentally disabled, mental patients, patients in nursing homes, and pediatric patients.

The subject of patients' "bills of rights" leads to the more general issue of the citizen's right to medical care services as a fundamental benefit in society. In several countries, the citizen's "right to health care" is listed among personal or human rights under the written constitution. Such formal statements are quite common in the constitutions of socialist countries in Eastern Europe, including the Soviet Union; however, the incorporation of such provisions into national constitutions is not limited to Eastern Europe. The Spanish constitution of 1980 contains a guarantee of "health protection and health care" to all Spanish citizens and to all foreign residents in Spanish national territory. The General Law on Health adopted on April 25, 1986, implements this constitutional provision under the authority of the National Public Health Administration. See General Law no. 14, 1986, the Official Bulletin of Spanish Law, 29 April 1986. See also the summary of provisions (*International Digest of Health Legislation* 1987; 38:1-4).

In the United States, no constitutional right to health care services is recognized, nor is there a universal health insurance system for all citizens. In this country, most of the current discussion about health care rights focuses on the issue of "equity" in the distribution of health care services, particularly to the parts of the population with little or no health insurance. See, for example, N. Daniels, "Equity of Access to Health Care: Some Conceptual and Ethical Issues" (*Milbank Memorial Fund Quarterly* 1982; 60:85-102); and L.A. Aday, R. Anderson, and D.V. Fleming, *Health Care in the United States: Equitable for Whom?* (Beverly Hills, Calif.: Sage Press, 1980). See also P.A. West, "Theoretical and Practical Equity in the National Health Service in England" (*Social Science and Medicine* 1981; 15:117-22). More recently, see W.K. Mariner, "Access to Health Care and Equal Protection of the Law: The Need for a New Heightened Scrutiny" (*American Journal of Law and Medicine* 1986; 12:345-80).

Official Torture and Human Rights: Medical Interests and Investigations

Physicians have a particular interest in the prevention of torture and in the effective punishment of barbarous acts of official torture by police and other government agencies. The profession of medicine is based fundamentally on the premise: do no harm. Physicians are often called on to examine the victims of torture. Competent medical evaluation is usually essential to proof of the use of torture on a person. Medical-ethics groups have condemned participation in official torture by the medical profession – or its tacit support – through supplying medical facilities or services to agencies conducting torture. The primary international pronouncement in this field is the World Medical Association's Declaration of Tokyo of 1975.[1]

Physicians have been particularly active in Amnesty International's efforts to seek out and expose official torture in various parts of the world.[2,3] Amnesty International–USA was one of a number of amici curiae in a recent landmark decision in the American federal courts, which is the subject of this "Law–Medicine Notes" column.

In *Filartiga* v. *Pena-Irala,*[4] the prestigious Second Circuit Court of Appeals in New York, after a long and exhausting series of court reviews, came down with a historic ruling that the deliberate, barbarous torture of a human being perpetrated by government agents under color of law in the home country of the victim at the time was a clear violation of universally accepted principles of the international law of human rights.

From the *New England Journal of Medicine*
1981; 304.1342-1343.

The plaintiffs were Dr. Joel Filartiga, a physician, and his daughter, Dolly Filartiga. The case concerned the alleged torture and death of Dr. Filartiga's 17-year-old son, Joelito. The Filartigas were described as longstanding opponents of the government of President Stroessner in Paraguay. Dr. Filartiga claimed that his son had been seized and tortured to death by the Inspector General of Police of Asunción, Paraguay, on or about March 29, 1976. The body had been displayed to Dolly Filartiga and later recovered by Dr. Filartiga. Autopsies had indicated the use of "professional methods of torture" leading to death. The plaintiffs had tried to bring legal action in Paraguay against the torturers. Their attorney had been taken into police custody by the same authorities, chained to a wall, and threatened with death if he continued the lawsuit. He had been disbarred as an attorney in Paraguay.

The Filartiga family left Paraguay and applied for political asylum in the United States. While in Washington, D.C., they learned that the police official in charge of the torture was in New York City on a visitor's visa. The visa had run out. The official was arrested and held for deportation at the Brooklyn Navy Yard, where the Filartigas were able to serve him with papers in their lawsuit. The complaint alleged that the defendant, Pena-Irala, had directed the torture of Joelito Filartiga and had caused his death. Compensatory and punitive damages totaling $10 million were claimed in the unprecedented action.

The lower court dismissed the claim on the grounds that the international law on which it was based excluded a nation's official police treatment of its own citizens within its own borders. The defendant was therefore ordered deported on his original overstayed visa. The plaintiffs tried to prevent the deportation by appeal to the court of appeals and then to the U.S. Supreme Court, but they failed in both attempts. The defendant was returned to Paraguay.

The merits of the claim of jurisdiction went on, nevertheless, to be heard in the Second Circuit Court of Appeals in New York. Circuit Judge Irving R. Kaufman, in a superbly crafted opinion, reversed the lower court's decision. The importance of the case is demonstrated by the fact that amicus curiae briefs were submitted to the court of appeals by five human-rights organizations and by the federal government's own Department of Justice and Department of State, all of which supported the Filartigas' claim.

The sources of international law are different from those of domestic law. For the former, courts can rely on international agreements and declarations, historical research concerning the practice of nations, and the writings of leading international legal authorities. The Court looked particularly at the Universal Declaration of Human Rights and the United Nations General Assembly Declaration against Torture. Both statements condemn all forms of torture as an instrument of national policy against criminals or political detainees. The Court also accepted affidavits from a number of recognized scholars of international law, all of whom agreed that official torture was a widely recognized breach of international human rights. Richard Falk of Princeton University concluded that in his judgment, "it was now beyond reasonable doubt that torture of a person held in detention that results in severe harm or death is a violation of the law of nations."

Judge Kaufman analyzed the American statutory and decisional law and applied the Federal Alien Tort Statute – a rarely used provision – to find jurisdiction in the federal system. He had no doubt about the substantive law: he found official torture by a national police agency of its own citizens to be a violation of international law, and thus a crime punishable in American courts. The police official, Pena-Irala, was found to be subject to this law and not immune from suit. Judge Kaufman concluded, "In the twentieth century the international community has come to realize the common danger posed by the flagrant disregard of basic human rights and particularly the right to be free of torture." In reference to the defendant, he ended his opinion with emphatic and eloquent clarity: ". . . the torturer has become – like the pirate and the slave holder before him – *hostis humani generis,* an enemy of all mankind. Our holding today, giving effect to a jurisdictional provision enacted by our First Congress, is a small but important step in the fulfillment of the ageless dream to free all people from brutal violence."

The horror of widespread torture of detainees as an instrument of official repression has been increasing in recent years, not declining. The civilized nations of the world must reach it, recognize it, and punish its perpetrators whenever and wherever they can be found. This historic decision will be a beacon for all courts of justice, and it should be applied with courage and vigor in the years ahead.

REFERENCES

1. World Medical Assembly. Guidelines for medical doctors. World Med J 1975; 22:87-90.
2. Danish Medical Group. Evidence of torture. London: Amnesty International, 1977.
3. Final report: Conference for the Abolition of Torture. London: Amnesty International, 1973.
4. Filartiga v. Pena-Irala. 630 F.2d. 876 (1980).

♦

COMMENTS

This was one of my most unusual columns. The question that it dealt with was not a medicolegal issue in the traditional sense, although it had medical overtones. In order to avoid the editor's eye, I stressed the interest of the medical profession in the prevention of official torture and the role of physicians in Amnesty International. In the main, however, I wanted to call the attention of physicians to the landmark decision that opened the American courts to lawsuits against individual defendants, not governments, for damages due to official torture. The plaintiff was a physician, a longtime opponent of the Stroessner dictatorship of the far right in Paraguay.

Mine was among the first articles to call attention to this decision and its implications in an American professional periodical. This was possible because the *Journal* is published weekly.

The importance of the decision in *Filartiga* v. *Pena-Irala* was readily apparent to contributors to the nation's law reviews. In the years that followed I found no fewer than 12 commentaries on the case in American legal periodicals. Some exemplary reviews were as follows: D.S. Dokos, "Enforcement of International Human Rights in American Courts after Filartiga versus Pena-Irala" (*Virginia Law Review* 1981; 67:1379-93); and L.A. Richard, "Filartiga versus Pena-Irala: A New Forum for Violations of International Human Rights" (*American Law Review* 1981; 30:807-33). A symposium on the decision was published in the *Georgia Journal of International and Comparative Law* (1981; 11:365-72). For a more recent discussion, see

P.L. Hoffman and L.W. Brachins, "The Elimination of Torture: International and Domestic Developments" (*International Law Review* 1985; 19:1351-64). For an article on related human-rights issues in South Africa, see J. Taitz, "Medical Mores, Judicial Review and the Last Days of Steve Biko" (*Modern Law Review* 1986; 49: 374-81).

6 • Legal and Moral Problems in Human Reproduction

Privacy, Birth Control, and "an Uncommonly Silly Law"

The Supreme Court of the United States has, after many years of on-again, off-again litigation, struck down as unconstitutional the Connecticut statute barring the *use* of contraceptive devices or drugs. The case before the court, *Griswold* v. *the State of Connecticut,*[1] involved a planned-parenthood clinic that was giving information and medical service to married couples on the best contraceptive materials for their personal use.

Connecticut is the only state in the union with a law barring the use of contraceptives. Furthermore, the Supreme Court treated the case throughout as involving the privacy of married couples, the very status of marriage itself, "an association," said Justice Douglas in concluding his majority opinion, "for as noble a purpose as any involved in our prior decisions." These two factors limit the significance of the case itself. It does not outlaw the controls on the sale or distribution of contraceptives that are imposed in many states. Also, it leaves somewhat in doubt the significance of the decision regarding the use of contraceptives by *unmarried persons.*

The majority of the Court based the invalidation of the statute on its invasion of "the right of privacy," which was found to be protected by the Constitution. The privacy involved here was the intimate relationship of husband and wife, the "association" of marriage itself. The right to maintain the privacy of this relationship was held to be a fundamental personal right, even though it is not mentioned specifically in the Bill of Rights. The justices asserted that the Constitution protects the individual's right "to marry, establish a home, and bring up children," and to educate them in schools of their choosing—"whether public, private, or parochial."

From the *New England Journal of Medicine*
1965; 273:322-323.

The two dissenters, Justices Black and Stewart, said that the Connecticut statute was "an uncommonly silly law" and "every bit as offensive" to them as to the majority. However, they did not concur in the wide-brush treatment given to "fundamental human rights" in the majority opinions. Said Justice Black:

> I get nowhere in this case by talk about a constitutional "right of privacy" as an emanation from one or more constitutional provisions. I like my privacy as well as the next one, but I am nevertheless compelled to admit that government has the right to invade it unless prohibited by some specific constitutional provision.[2]

As a matter of legal philosophy, Justice Black admitted that he was disagreeing with the trend in the Court's opinions to apply very broadly what he called the "mysterious and uncertain natural law concept." He argued against such formulas, which "require judges to determine what is or is not constitutional on the basis of their own appraisal of what laws are unwise or unnecessary."

The Supreme Court has raised the right of privacy, the right to be "let alone," as earlier legal scholars called it,[3] to a constitutionally protected status. It remains for future decisions to fill in the details of this area, and to draw the outline of intimacy beyond which the law cannot penetrate.

Physicians in general should be fairly comfortable with this action by the court, it seems to me. The code of silence regarding a patient's private life and his clinical involvement has been a part of medicine for over two thousand years. Later decisions of the courts will undoubtedly involve other medicolegal issues in this newly identified fundamental human right. What are some of these issues? Perhaps abortion, sterilization, autopsy, miscegenetic marriages, and confidentiality of medical information will be among the problems that will be raised in future cases. For a state to prohibit abortions or sterilization of married women may well be someday considered a similar breach of the privacy of the marriage relationship.

The difficulties in this area are compounded for the layman and legal scholar alike by the fact that constitutional guidelines are becoming more and more blurred, and the ruling that a law is unconstitutional seems to depend as much on the Supreme Court's interpretation of social mores of the times as on strict legal principles.

Nevertheless, in spite of the uncertainties that are spawned by this important decision, one thing is clear; the privacy within the marriage relationship is now given full recognition, and the right to privacy generally, a legal right that has been very slow in developing, has been given a significant boost toward its deserved prominence.

I might say a brief word about the effect of the Connecticut case on the statutes of other states; most of those statutes prohibit in some manner the giving of advice about contraception. This case casts considerable doubt on the constitutionality of such statutes. In this regard, Justice Black, even though dissenting, stated, "I can think of no reasons at this time why their [physicians' as well as nonphysicians'] expressions of views should not be protected by the First and Fourteenth amendments which guarantee freedom of speech."[4] However, the Court's opinion strikes only the Connecticut statute from the books, and it thus remains for the various state courts and legislatures to erase their statutes if they see fit to do so.

REFERENCES

1. 85 S. Ct. 1678 (1965).
2. 85 S. Ct. 1695 (1965).
3. Warren SD, Brandeis LD. Right of privacy. Harvard Law Rev 1890; 4:193.
4. 85 S. Ct. 1694 (1965).

♦

COMMENTS

This chapter, like several others in this collection, begins with one of my early columns. In this case the choice was not difficult. The *Griswold* decision in 1965 was one of the most important turning points in the history of our highest legal tribunal. It marked the first time that the Supreme Court had ever ruled invalid, on constitutional grounds, a state law prescribing personal morality in a manner consonant with traditional values, personal morality being an area of local law that the Court had hitherto not been in the habit of reviewing.

The *Griswold* decision also marked the first time the highest court recognized a constitutionally protected personal right of privacy, what was called "a right to be let alone." The decision was widely commented on in the legal literature, in most cases with emphasis on the implications of the recognition of a personal right of privacy. In those early years, very few commentators went as far as I did in this column – I honestly believe that I was among the first to predict that the decision would be applied to the criminal laws pertaining to abortion. Yet it was only two years later that the Supreme Court struck down the Virginia antimiscegenation law, which prohibited marriages between members of the white and black races, on the basis of the precedent set in the *Griswold* case. See *Loving* v. *Virginia,* 388 U.S. 1 (1967).

Columns examining the abortion decisions, all of which took *Griswold* as their major constitutional support, appear later in this chapter.

Birth Control, Judicial Surgery, and the Wonderful One-Hoss Shay

Have you heard of the wonderful one-hoss shay,
That was built in such a logical way
It ran a hundred years to a day,
And then, of a sudden, it – ah, but stay
I'll tell you what happened without delay,
. . . .
You see, of course, if not a dunce,
How it went to pieces all at once, –
All at once, and nothing first, –
Just as bubbles do when they burst.
End of the wonderful one-hoss shay
Logic is logic. That's all I say.

Oliver Wendell Holmes

Dr. Holmes' description of *The Deacon's Masterpiece* was composed in Massachusetts at close to the same time that the Good and General Court of the Bay State passed its famous anti-birth-control law of 1879.[1] Both the shay and the law were based firmly on irrefutable logic and were intended to last forever.

In 1966 a strong coalition of social forces succeeded in amending the anti-birth-control law.[2] They were not strong enough to win outright repeal. They used the strategy of creating large "exceptions" to the old law, leaving the 1879 statute on the books for all who believed in it to observe and admire, like the shay, seemingly intact, after so many years.

Under the exceptions of 1966, a registered physician is allowed to administer and prescribe to married persons drugs or articles for the prevention of conception. Registered pharmacists may furnish such

From the *New England Journal of Medicine*
1969; 281:546-547.

drugs or articles to married persons, and public health agencies, registered nurses, or maternity health clinics may furnish information to married people "as to where professional advice regarding such drugs or articles may be lawfully obtained."

After the passage of the law, there was an immediate response throughout the state in the establishment of a number of professionally operated birth-control programs. Many private physicians felt relieved in prescribing to their patients without the threat of illegality regarding their actions. But there was great discomfort over the remaining restrictions. It was not always easy to determine whether a patient was or was not married. Usually, the patient's word was taken, and her privacy was not invaded. In poorer neighborhoods, however, where privacy, like everything else, was hard to come by, the prohibition in the law seemed to be outright discrimination against hapless, desperate women who did not have the luxury of marriage.

Druggists were careful not to display contraceptives; this was well known to be a particularly offensive act to those who favored the old law. Educational programs favoring birth control through contraception continued to tread lightly and avoid open controversy.

The above might be described as the acquiescent reactions of the genteel—those who had wanted more change in the law, but who accepted what they got in the amendments of 1966. William R. Baird was not among them. He fought openly against the law as a curse and an abomination. On April 16, 1967, he addressed some 2000 students at Boston University. During his talk, he displayed various contraceptive devices "with diagrams" on two demonstration boards. After his address he gave away the devices to students who came up to him. On doing so, he was arrested and charged with violation of the 1879 statute and was found guilty in the lower court.

The Supreme Judicial Court has now upheld that conviction in a split (four-to-three) decision.[3] The majority found that, under the Supreme Court's *Griswold* decision[4] and other cases, the delivery of the Baird lecture itself advocating total abolition of the law and advising generally on contraception was fully protected as free speech under the First Amendment to the U.S. Constitution.[5] The display of the devices was also found constitutionally protected as a part of the speech and intended to clarify and illustrate it. However, the *distribution* of the devices indiscriminately to the youthful audience containing many unmarried persons was found a violation of the statute and not beyond the power of the legislature to prohibit.

The dissenting justices in two separate opinions (written dissents are unusual in Massachusetts) agreed with the finding about the address and the display, but thought the distribution was also constitutionally privileged as part of protest and speech. Justices Whittemore and Cutter asserted that the old statute, read with the 1966 amendments, was "so much eroded in the last half century as to be unconstitutionally vague" and that remaining "prohibitions" in the statute could not stand alone. They saw "no rational basis for using what little is left of a statute designed to prevent all assistance to all birth control merely to deter non-marital intercourse." Justice Speigel was of a similar opinion. He thought that what remained of the statute was a hodgepodge of uncertainties. He ended his opinion: "I am impelled to conclude that §21 [the old law] is incapable of being cut into segments which would be constitutionally valid without, in effect, performing judicial surgery."

The decision will undoubtedly be appealed to the Supreme Court of the United States, where, if the Court grants review, the next test of the 1879 law will be conducted. It will be seen whether the weakened vehicle, originally built of irrefutable logic, will survive as the majority of justices in Massachusetts have decreed, or will collapse all to nothing like the wonderful one-hoss shay.

REFERENCES

1. Laws of 1879, c. 159, Section 1; Mass. Gen. Laws, c. 272, 21.
2. Laws of 1966, c. 265.
3. Comm. v Baird, 247 N.E. 2d 574 (1969).
4. Griswold v. Conn., 381 U.S. 479 (1965).
5. Curran WJ. Privacy, birth control, and "an uncommonly silly law." N Engl J Med 1965; 273:322-23.

♦

COMMENTS

This is one of my favorite columns. It earned me a rare congratulatory letter from Franz Ingelfinger, who was then editor of the *Journal,* saying that it was the best column of mine that he had read up to that time. Most important, he let me keep the verses that led off the column, whereas hitherto, he had been uniformly adamant against beginning *Journal* articles with quotations. With this column I succeeded in breaking the rule, and this stood me in good stead on later occasions when I wanted to begin with a quotation. Of course, the fact that these lines were written by Dr. Oliver Wendell Holmes, venerable dean of the Harvard Medical School, may have helped my cause.

As I predicted in this column, the Supreme Court of the United States eventually—in 1972, as it turned out—reversed the Baird conviction. That opinion is reviewed in the next column in this collection.

In a later and even more dramatic decision in the same area, the Supreme Court struck down as invalid all state statutes prohibiting the advertising and display of contraceptives for sale and use. These laws were found to be in violation of the First Amendment right of free speech. The same decision, on less secure grounds, struck down state laws relating to the sale of contraceptives to minors.

These Supreme Court decisions concerning birth control and contraceptive methods paved the way for federal support of domestic and international family-planning services that included education and counseling on the use of contraceptives for purposes of birth control. These programs were well supported until the 1980s, when a conservative national government and Congress extensively reduced support for programs in this field. See also *City of Akron* v. *Akron Center for Reproductive Health,* 103 S. Ct. 2481 (1983).

Birth Control among the Unmarried in Massachusetts: The Supreme Court Speaks in Varied Tongues

> The commands of the Constitution cannot fluctuate with the shifting tides of scientific opinion.
>
> Justice White

> The teachings of Baird and those of Galileo might be of a different order; but the suppression of either is equally repugnant.
>
> Justice Douglas

> I am constrained to suggest that if the Constitution can be strained to invalidate the Massachusetts statute . . . we could quite as well employ it for the protection of a "curbstone quack" reminiscent of the "medicine man" of times past, who attracted a crowd of the curious with a soapbox lecture and then plied them with "free samples" of some unproven remedy.
>
> Chief Justice Burger

The Supreme Court of the United States has at last spoken on the Massachusetts anti-birth-control law as it was amended in 1966. The legally peripatetic William Baird has triumphed after his close-call loss (four to three) in the Supreme Judicial Court of Massachusetts. The U.S. Supreme Court found the statute unconstitutional in a seven-to-one vote, with Chief Justice Burger casting the lone dissent.[1] The Court's majority was widely divided in its reasons for finding the statute invalid. Justice Brennan wrote the "opinion of the court," but he had joining with him only Justices Stewart and

From the *New England Journal of Medicine*
1972; 286:1198-1199.

Marshall. Justice Douglas wrote his own concurring opinion, and Justices White and Blackmun joined another. The result is a confusion of voices of a quite unsatisfactory legal nature.

The case arose when Baird was arrested after a speech on birth control at Boston University in which he openly advocated breach of the law and the use of birth-control devices by both married and unmarried persons. Around him on the stage he displayed various birth-control devices. At the end of the lecture, he invited the audience to examine the display and to take anything they wanted. He handed a young woman a package of Emko vaginal foam and was promptly arrested by a policeman conveniently standing by for the purpose. Baird was charged with and convicted of violating the 1966 statute that allows only registered physicians to administer and prescribe birth-control drugs and devices to married persons. Registered pharmacists may fill such prescriptions, and public health agencies, registered nurses, and maternity health clinics may furnish information on birth control to married persons. Baird was admittedly in none of these classifications, and it was generally assumed that the student to whom he had given the foam was unmarried.

The Supreme Judicial Court of Massachusetts found that Baird's lecture itself was protected by the constitutional guarantee of free speech. The display of articles was also protected as intended to illustrate the speech. However, the majority found the distribution of the devices a violation of the statute, and it upheld the power of the legislature to outlaw distribution to unmarried persons as a legitimate legislative purpose.

In his majority opinion, Justice Brennan struck down the statute, after a laborious examination of its purposes, none of which he could find to be logically consistent. He accepted the reasoning of the dissenters in the Massachusetts court—namely, that the statute's discrimination against unmarried persons violated the equal protection clause of the Constitution.

In his concurring opinion, Justice Douglas saw no need for any such elaborate examination. He needed only the free-speech protection clause in the Bill of Rights to dispose of the case. He thought the distribution as well as the display were part of "the teaching techniques" of modern "educational lectures."

Justices White and Blackmun wrote the most complex opinion of all. They said that if Baird had been distributing "the Pill" they would have upheld the conviction. They reversed it because they could find no evidence in the record that Emko vaginal foam was dangerous or potentially dangerous if distributed by nonphysicians without prescription. The Massachusetts court had not even considered this issue. The two justices asserted that such a finding would be necessary to convict Baird because otherwise the statute would "impair the exercise of a constitutional right." It is not clear what this "constitutional right" was, but it was implied to be the right to use contraceptives. It is also not clear whether these two justices would apply this "right" only to married people, since they refused to answer what they called "the novel constitutional question whether a state may restrict or forbid the distribution of contraceptives to the unmarried." The justices rationalized their refusal to decide this issue by finding that the record did not contain any evidence of the marital status of the girl who took the foam from Baird.

This judicial reticence to face novel issues is most surprising in 1972. Mr. Baird was before the court because he wanted to test the constitutionality of the law. He even had with him the American Civil Liberties Union, the Planned Parenthood League of Massachusetts, and Human Rights for Women, all filing briefs as amici curiae. This was not a traditional criminal case in which questions of proof are commonly paramount. These two justices, after all this legal odyssey to reach the Supreme Court, used these technicalities to avoid facing the key issues in the case. In so doing, they accomplished nothing, since they left the decision in the hands of only three justices out of eight who were willing to be counted as finding constitutional invalidity in the limitation of the birth-control program in Massachusetts to married people.

I have reluctantly come to the conviction that the Supreme Court should be required to have at least a two thirds majority (six out of nine justices) to declare a statute unconstitutional and invalid when that law was passed by a legislature under proper procedures. The justices should be required to deliberate deeply enough – to discipline themselves firmly enough – to resolve such grave matters with the conviction of their members. The spectacle of five-to-four decisions striking down laws as unconstitutional has always struck me as the worst example of gamesmanship in our judicial system. In this Baird decision, we have something even worse. Not even a bare majority could agree on a single constitutional ground for invalidity of the law in restricting consultation and prescription to professionals and in restricting the program of birth control itself to married persons.

My critique of this case should not be misconstrued in the heady emotional atmosphere of medicomoral controversy. In my comment on the Massachusetts Supreme Judicial Court decision, I compared the Massachusetts law to "the wonderful one-hoss shay" made famous in Dr. Holmes' poem.[2] The original anti-birth-control statute was passed in the Bay State in 1879 by a very largely Protestant legislature, which believed in its irrefutable, moral–theological logic and intended it to last forever — just like the one-hoss shay. In 1966 the law was amended. But its logic was severely compromised, as the three-judge majority in the U.S. Supreme Court unmercifully pointed out. It does not hold together as a morality directive, either in preventing illicit sexual intercourse or in preventing the use of artificial methods of contraception. It is equally weak logically as a health measure, said Justice Brennan, since it makes no sense to protect the health of married persons while leaving the unmarried to shift for themselves. Dr. Holmes sang of the one-hoss shay, which just "went to pieces all at once." It seems to me that this was the fate of the 1879 law when its logical structure was destroyed by political compromises in 1966. In concluding his poem, Dr. Holmes said it well: "Logic is logic. That's all I say."

I must add a footnote to the case at hand, however. Almost unnoticed in Justice Brennan's opinion is a reference to the right-of-privacy concept set forth in the *Griswold* case that invalidated the Connecticut law prohibiting the use of contraceptives. The case involved a married couple, and the Court recognized a right of privacy in the marriage. The right has since been expanded to other aspects of marriage, including the right to marry interracially. Justice Brennan, in the *Baird* case, however, asserted, "If the right of privacy means anything, it is the right of the individual, married or single, to be free from unwarranted governmental intrusion into matters so fundamentally affecting a person as whether to bear or to beget a child." This sentence could be a sign of what the attitude of some members of the Court will be when the next and much more far reaching medicomoral issue is faced by the Court: the right of the woman, married or single, to have an abortion ("whether to bear or to beget a child") without governmental intrusion.

REFERENCES

1. Eisenstadt v. Baird. US Law Week 1972; 40:4303-14.
2. Curran WJ. Birth control, judicial surgery, and the wonderful one-hoss shay. N Engl J Med 1969; 281:546-7.

♦

COMMENTS

In reviewing the decision in the *Baird* case, I again called attention to the application of the *Griswold* decision and the law of privacy to this area. In view of Baird's aggressive platform tactics, it was only natural that the justices should concentrate on the right of free speech as his primary source of constitutional protection, but for the future of medicolegal cases like abortion, the right of privacy was to prove more crucial. Also in this decision, Justice William Brennan moved forward as the Court's foremost champion of freedoms in the area of human reproduction.

I was disturbed by the lack of discipline among the majority of the bench, as reflected in this decision, and this led me to make the suggestion that a two-thirds majority, not merely a plurality, of the Court should be required in order to declare a legislative enactment unconstitutional. I must report that over the years my recommendation has fallen on very deaf ears. This may be due not only to the difficulties that such a change would engender, but also to the fact that in many of the Court's more momentous decisions the members of the bench have been more disciplined and larger majorities, or unanimous opinions, have become somewhat more common, so that the problem has grown less acute. The fact that I am not a constitutional scholar did not deter me from making my suggestion, but it undoubtedly contributed to the relative lack of response from other legal quarters.

For important legal commentaries on the contraception decisions, see W. Friedman, "Interfering with Human Life: Some Jurisprudential Reflections" (*Columbia Law Review* 1970; 70:1058-77); and V.J. D'Ammora, "Infantile Privacy: A Minor's Right of Access to Contraceptives" (*Fordham Urban Law Journal* 1978; 6:371-87).

Abortion Law in the Supreme Court: A First Impression

> The subject of abortions—like cases involving obscenity—is one of the most inflammatory ones to reach the Court. People instantly take sides and the public, from which juries are drawn, makes up its mind one way or the other before the case is even argued.
>
> Justice Douglas

On April 21, 1971, the Supreme Court of the United States joined the abortion law debate. The "treacherous ground" has been entered, and the justices have begun to speak about morality, health, and the preservation of life. (The words are from Justice Jackson,[1] who in dissent, warned of "the treacherous ground we [the Court] tread when we undertake to translate ethical concepts into legal ones, case by case.")

In *United States* v. *Vuitch*[2] a very divided court has upheld the District of Columbia statute that outlaws all abortions except those performed by a competent, licensed physician for the purpose of preserving the mother's life or health. The majority held that these terms in the statute are not unconstitutionally vague. It was said that the term "health" had a meaning in general usage and understanding that includes psychological as well as physical well-being. The definition in *Webster's* was quoted approvingly: that health is a state of being sound in mind as well as in body. The Court left the determination of such matters up to attending physicians and concluded that the decision "whether a particular operation is necessary for a patient's physical or mental health is a judgment that physicians are obviously called upon to make routinely whenever surgery is considered."

From the *New England Journal of Medicine*
1971; 285:30-31.

The Court also examined the issue of the burden of proof and held that the burden is on the prosecution to prove beyond a reasonable doubt that an abortion performed by such a physician was not for the purpose of preserving the life or health of the mother.

The above-quoted majority opinion on the merits of the case was written by Justice Hugo Black, one of the Court's most outspoken liberals. It was concurred in by the chief justice and Justices Blackmun, Harlan, and White. Another member of the Court, Justice Stewart, upheld the statute, but would go farther in his interpretation than the majority. In a separate opinion, Justice Stewart asserted that he would bring the Court's reasoning to its logical conclusion and hold that any competent, licensed physician who has exercised his medical judgment in favor of performing an abortion is "wholly immune" from criminal prosecution under the statute. The justice came to this conclusion because, he said, "the practice of medicine consists of doing those things which, in the judgment of a physician, are necessary to preserve a patient's life or health."

The only expressed dissent from these views was offered by Justice Douglas. He would uphold the opinion of the District Court that the statute was "void for vagueness" under the Constitution. He gave a series of examples of situations that he thought unclear even with the Court's interpretation. He asked if an illegitimate pregnancy could be aborted for health reasons, or an unwanted pregnancy, or a pregnancy that in the judgment of the doctor would unduly tax the mother's physical well-being by reason of the additional work it would force on her. Justice Douglas also asserted that, given any latitude, juries might be apt to exercise their prejudices in abortion and to decide guilt or innocence on these grounds rather than on the law of the jurisdiction.

The unsatisfactory nature of the *Vuitch* case arises from many factors. First of all, the procedural questions in the case prevented (or were used to obscure) a clear confrontation on the merits for all the justices. The opinions of the minority, except Douglas, were never expressed, since they refused to agree that the Court should be hearing the case on the merits. They were of the opinion that the case should not have come directly to the Supreme Court on appeal from the District of Columbia Court. Secondly, the case on the merits only raised the "void for vagueness" objection to the statute and did not open up the issues of sexual and family-life privacy that were developed in *Griswold* v. *Connecticut*[3] and *Loving* v. *Virginia*.[4] Finally, the case, no matter what the decision, could be said to be specifically applicable only to the District of Columbia, not to the states.

All these complications are grist for expensive mills of constitutional lawyers. Many "counsel opinions" will be ground out of the big law firms, the civil-rights groups, religious organizations, and even pro-bono-publico storefront law practices in future months. They will not agree. Confusion will be confounded as the lawyers and the Supreme Court watchers guess at the next appeal, the realignment of the justices, and the next presidential appointments. On these medicomoral issues there are no clear-cut lines of liberal and conservative. The two elder liberals, Black and Douglas, split severely in this case and, in fact, wrote the two major opinions. Two other key justices, Marshall and Brennan, took no stand on the merits in the *Vuitch* case. Justice Marshall, the Court's only black member, is very difficult to predict. He wrote the *Powell* decision, considered quite conservative on medicolegal and medicomoral grounds. The black community is split over whether on-demand abortion laws are beneficial to minority groups. Justice Brennan, the Court's only Roman Catholic, is one of its strongest and most consistent liberals. Being considerably younger than Black or Douglas, he is more likely to remain on the Court when it hears later appeals on abortion law from the state courts. Brennan has been a liberal not only on economic issues but on so-called personal matters and moral questions. He wrote the Court's most liberal rulings on obscenity controls, for example. Actually, the only member of the Court who could clearly be said to be sympathetic to finding strict abortion laws unconstitutional on grounds of vagueness (which can be corrected by the legislatures, anyway) or on privacy grounds (which could open up very serious further issues) is Justice Douglas. Considering his age, Douglas is not the best ally the antiabortion law groups could have on the Court, unless the state-court appeals can reach the Court very quickly during the current term.

REFERENCES

1. Jordan v. De George 341 US 233.
2. 21 S. Ct. 1294 (1971).
3. 381 U.S. 479.
4. 388 U.S. 1.

COMMENTS

This case paved the way for the later landmark decisions of the Supreme Court on the subject of abortion, which are reviewed in the next column in this chapter. The *Vuitch* case concerned only the District of Columbia and therefore did not relate directly to the laws forbidding abortion in most of the 50 states. Furthermore, the decision was unusually complex, comprising not only the majority ruling, but also dissenting opinion and various concurring statements.

This first-impression decision furnished me with an occasion to predict the directions that individual justices would take in deciding future cases in the sensitive field of morality and reproductive freedoms. As prophesied in this column, Justice Brennan became a key spokesman in later decisions on this subject, and he was the most consistent in striking down attempts by the state legislatures to reestablish restrictions on personal choice in the field. I did not, however, foresee the importance that one of the newer appointees, Justice Blackmun, would assume in future developments in this area. It was he who would be chosen by the chief justice to write the majority opinions in both of the 1973 decisions. For an interesting, though much overdramatized, account of the roles of Justices Blackmun and Brennan (as well as that of the chief justice) in the abortion and birth-control decisions of that period, see the best seller by two reporters from the *Washington Post:* B. Woodward and S. Armstrong, *The Brethren: Inside the Supreme Court* (New York: Simon and Schuster, 1979).

The Abortion Decisions of 1973: The Supreme Court as Moralist, Scientist, Historian, and Legislator

There is a constant fascination in all of us concerning power and authority. One of the most successful of all human organizations in gathering to itself these vaunted objectives in modern times has been the Supreme Court of the United States. In two now very famous decisions, *Roe* v. *Wade*[1] and *Doe* v. *Bolton,*[2] these nine men have again displayed their prowess in this field.

By a strong majority (seven to two) the Court has struck down the abortion-control laws of most of the states as unconstitutional on the basis of their invasion of the privacy of the pregnant woman. The opinion of the Court, in each case, was written by one of the newer members appointed by President Nixon, Mr. Justice Harry A. Blackmun, of Minnesota. In his lengthy examination of the issues in the *Wade* case, Justice Blackmun discussed the historical development of antiabortion laws, the moral attitudes, the religious principles, and the current positions of the American Medical Association and the American Public Health Association.

The fundamental issue in the cases for those who favored the retention of legal controls over abortion was seen by the Court as the protection of human life from the point of conception. Justice Blackmun cut the ground from under this position by asserting, "We need not resolve the difficult question of when life begins."[3] As the basis for his refusal to rule, Justice Blackmun asserted that physicians, philosophers, and theologians were unable to arrive at a consensus on the question, so that the judiciary could not be expected to speculate

From the *New England Journal of Medicine*
1973; 288:950-951.

about it. On the other hand, the Court seized upon the concept of "viability" as a scientifically and philosophically accepted point of demarcation in fetal development. The Court defined viability as the time, at about seven months, when the fetus is "potentially able to live outside the mother's womb, albeit with artificial aid."

The Court reviewed earlier decisions concerning privacy in such matters as the selection of marital partners, the use of birth-control methods by married couples, and the use and dissemination of birth-control methods and information to unmarried persons and decided that the privacy concept does include the abortion decision. It was also decided that the unborn child is not a "person" for purposes of constitutional protection under the Fourteenth Amendment.

The majority now had all it needed to support its decision. It moved on to play the role of judicial legislator. It dealt first with the first trimester of fetal development. Justice Blackmun asserted that the danger of mortality from abortion during this period was less than that of mortality from childbirth. Therefore, the law could not step in and control the woman's decision. During this period, "the abortion decision and its effectuation must be left to the medical judgment of the pregnant woman's attending physician."[4] During the period from "approximately" the end of the first trimester to viability, the state is allowed to enact laws to protect the health of the mother. It may therefore regulate the abortion procedure in such matters as qualifications of the physicians and standards of the facilities where abortions are to be performed. In the stage after viability, the Court held that the interest of the state in protecting potential human life was now strong enough to override the mother's right of privacy. Therefore, the law could now, at this stage, limit the abortion decision to cases in which it is necessary to preserve the life or health of the mother.

The *Bolton* decision was also important, particularly for physicians and hospitals, in that it dealt with very specific matters of abortion procedure. The Georgia law in that case required abortions to be performed in hospitals approved by the Joint Commission on Accreditation of Hospitals, and also required that all abortions be approved by a hospital abortion committee. Both these requirements were struck down as unconstitutional invasions of the privacy of the woman and her physician in deciding whether or not, and how and where, to have an abortion. Obviously, these provisions were considered primarily a restriction on the judgment of the attending physician. On the same basis, a provision that the attending physician must seek consultation from two Georgia-licensed physicians and gain their concurrence in his judgment was struck down. Lastly, the Court went on to declare invalid the law's restriction of legal abortions performed in Georgia to pregnant women who were Georgia residents.

In a further effort to protect the opportunity of the attending physician to exercise his clinical judgment without legal interference, the Court upheld the Georgia statute's requirement that the physician's decision be based upon his best clinical judgment that the abortion is necessary. The appellants argued that the term "necessary" was restrictive. Justice Blackmun, however, cited *United States* v. *Vuitch,*[5] discussed in an early "Law–Medicine Notes" column,[6] the only other abortion decision of the Supreme Court, as controlling on this matter. He asserted that the *Vuitch* case had interpreted "health" in the broadest sense to include all factors — physical, emotional, psychological, familial, and the woman's age — relevant to the patient's well-being. It was observed that all these factors allow room to decide on an abortion for the benefit, not the disadvantage, of the pregnant woman.

The Court also upheld the Georgia law in the provisions that allow a hospital to refuse to admit patients for abortion procedures and also the separate provisions allowing physicians and any other hospital-staff members or employees to refuse to participate in abortion procedures (when the refusal is stated in writing and based on moral or religious grounds) and providing that such refusals shall not be the basis of any claim for damages or for any disciplinary or recriminatory action. A similar provision in the New York law was discussed in another "Law–Medicine Notes" column.[7] Justice Blackmun called attention to these provisions in his opinion and asserted that they were "obviously" intended to protect individuals and denominational hospitals.[8] However, the Georgia statute allows any hospital to refuse to admit patients for abortions, not merely religiously affiliated institutions.

The abortion decisions are already under a good deal of attack by constitutional lawyers, not so much for their result as for their reasoning. The Court seems to exercise more legislative initiative than judicial restraint in determining what types of public interests the state legislatures may choose to protect. Scientists may also quarrel with the Court's heavy reliance on a naturalistic concept of "viability" as tied to a particular time in a woman's pregnancy.

It remains to be seen what the reaction of medicine and public health will be to these decisions. It seems clear, however, that physicians are not required to help women obtain abortion "on demand," as it were. Chief Justice Burger makes this point specifically in his concurring opinion when he asserts: "I do not read the Court's holding today as having the sweeping consequences attributed to it by the dissenting Justices; the dissenting views discount the reality that the vast majority of physicians observe the standards of their profession, and act only on the basis of carefully deliberated medical judgments relating to life and health. Plainly, the Court today rejects any claim that the Constitution requires abortion on demand."[9]

REFERENCES

1. 93 S. Ct. 705 (1973).
2. 93 S. Ct. 739 (1973).
3. Roe v. Wade, p. 730.
4. *Idem,* p. 732.
5. 402 v. 62. 91 S. Ct. 1294 (1971).
6. Curran WJ. Abortion law in the Supreme Court. N Engl J Med 1971; 285:30-1.
7. *Idem.* Medical ethics – malpractice and the conscience of the practitioner. N Engl J Med 1971; 285:1306-7.
8. Doe v. Bolton, p. 750.
9. *Idem,* p. 756.

♦

COMMENTS

The 1973 abortion decisions have proved to be among the most controversial in Supreme Court history. As the next column in this chapter indicates, the state legislatures made extensive efforts to restrict the application of *Roe* v. *Wade* and to reinstate various forms of antiabortion legislation. In later decisions, the Supreme Court has consistently supported the principles laid down in the 1973 opinions. See, in particular, *Planned Parenthood of Kansas City* v. *Ashcraft,* 103 S. Ct. 2517 (1983); *City of Akron* v. *Akron Center for Reproductive*

Health, 103 S. Ct. 2481 (1983); *Simopoulos* v. *Virginia,* 103 S. Ct. 2532 (1983); *Colanti* v. *Franklin,* 493 U.S. 379 (1979); and *Bellotti* v. *Baird,* 443 U.S. 662 (1979). Of particular medicolegal interest is an important decision exploring the medical procedures for abortion: *Planned Parenthood of Central Missouri* v. *Danforth,* 98 S. Ct. 2831 (1976).

Since the *Roe* v. *Wade* decision, the Supreme Court's response to almost all appeals relating to abortion has favored the proponents of wider access to the procedure, the only major exception having been in the matter of the so-called Hyde Amendment, the legislation that barred federal funding for abortions under Medicaid except in limited circumstances (e.g., rape, incest, or a threat to the life of the mother). In a series of decisions, a majority of the Court has held that Congress was acting within its legitimate powers in refusing federal funding when none of these circumstances obtained. See the leading decision, *Harris* v. *McRae,* 100 S. Ct. 2671 (1980), which was closely divided, five to four. As might be expected, Justices Blackmun and Brennan, the leaders in the majority opinions in the cases decided in 1973, were in dissent in the *Harris* case. On the abortion funding issue, see S. Altman, "Abortion Funding and the Indigent" (*Journal of Social Philosophy* 1980; 11:5); W. Cates et al., "The Health Impact of Restricting Public Funds for Abortion: October 10, 1977–June 10, 1978" (*American Journal of Public Health* 1979; 69:945-7); and M.J. Perry, "Abortion Funding Cases: A Comment on the Supreme Court's Role in American Government" (*Georgetown Law Journal* 1978; 66:1191-245).

The Aftermath of the Abortion Decisions: Action in the Legislatures and the Courts

It has become a cliché to say that the abortion decisions of the U.S. Supreme Court in 1973 left more questions unanswered than they answered. The basic holdings in the two cases were outlined in an earlier column.[1]

The American people were just about evenly, but very fiercely, divided about abortion, particularly abortion on demand, at the time of the decisions. Since the cases came down, the state legislatures have been very active in considering and in passing legislation.

During the 1973 sessions, some 200 abortion bills were introduced in over 40 of the states. Twenty-eight states considered bills setting up regulation of the abortions in the second and third trimesters, but not in the first, in accordance with the Supreme Court decisions. Laws were actually passed of this type in at least 10 states. Some states, such as Massachusetts, adopted health department regulations to control abortion practice, rather than statutes.

Some the regulatory statutes were also attempts at clarifying unanswered issues. For example, Idaho, Indiana, Nevada, South Dakota, and Utah required the consent of the husband to a wife's abortion. In Indiana, Nevada, South Dakota, and Utah, the consent of the parents was required for an abortion on a minor. Under California law, a court decision had ruled parental consent unnecessary for minors before the Supreme Court decision.[2]

So-called conscience laws, which allow physicians and other medical personnel and hospitals to refuse to participate in abortions, were

From the *New England Journal of Medicine*
1973; 289:955.

considered in over 30 states and passed in at least 12, including Massachusetts.

Some states, such as Rhode Island, have attempted to reinstate strict abortion laws. A statute was enacted declaring that human life begins at the moment of conception and allowed "therapeutic abortion" only to save the life of the mother. The U.S. District Court in Rhode Island has issued an injunction against enforcement of the statute as clearly unconstitutional. North Dakota seems to have taken a course similar to that in Rhode Island by enacting a therapeutic-abortion law allowing abortion only when the mother's life is seriously threatened.

There have also been important court decisions. The Federal Court of Appeals for the Seventh Circuit refused to rule that private hospitals must perform abortions as a "constitutional right" of women.[3] The petitioners had argued that the hospital was bound under the Civil Rights Act of 1871 and the Hospital Survey and Construction (Hill–Burton) Act. On the other hand, the First Circuit Court of Appeals in Boston, in a very far-reaching decision, ruled that the Worcester City Hospital, a municipal institution, could not refuse to allow sterilization operations.[4] The court interpreted the Supreme Court's abortion rulings as applying to sterilization procedures as well. The decision was also based on the Equal Protection Clause. The court noted that the hospital placed no such total ban on other surgical procedures.

I am sure that we have not seen the last of the legal activities in the abortion and related fields. The dust has not settled around this area, the most explosive medicolegal issue in modern times.

REFERENCES

1. Curran WJ. The abortion decisions: the Supreme Court as moralist, scientist, historian and legislator. N Engl J Med 1973; 288:950-1.
2. Ballard v. Anderson, 12 Cal. App. 3d 846, 90 Cal. Rptr. 468 (1970).
3. Doe v. Bellin Memorial Hospital, No 73-C-230, June 1, 1973.
4. Hathaway v. Worcester City Hospital, 475 F.2d 701 (1 Cir. 1973).

♦

COMMENTS

In later years the legislatures and the courts have continued the battle over abortion legislation. The courts, both federal and state, have generally followed the principles laid down in the two Supreme Court decisions of 1973, although there have been signs of some weakening in the mid-1980s. On the other hand, since 1973 it has proved possible to save more babies of very low birth weight delivered early in pregnancy, and this aspect of medical progress has affected the concept of "viability," as defined in *Roe* v. *Wade,* in obvious ways. Moreover, the Supreme Court has recently upheld state statutes requiring that second-trimester abortions be performed in licensed clinics and hospitals. See *Simopoulos* v. *Virginia,* 103 S. Ct. 2532 (1983). For more recent comment, see N. Ford, "The Evolution of a Constitutional Right to an Abortion" (*Journal of Legal Medicine* 1983; 4:271-322); and C.W. Tyler, Jr., "Public Health Implications of Abortion" (*Annual Review of Public Health* 1983; 4:223-58).

For a survey of attitudes taken by women toward abortion in the 1980s, see K. Luther, "The War between Women" (*Family Planning Perspectives* 1984; 16:105-10). For a survey of the attitudes and practices of obstetricians, see M.S. Goldstein, "Abortion as a Medical Care Choice: Entrepreneurs, Community Physicians, and Others" (*Journal of Health and Social Behavior* 1984; 25:211-29).

For an international perspective, see S.L. Isaacs, "Reproduction Rights in 1983: An International Survey" (*Columbia Human Rights Law Review* 1983; 14:311-53); and R.J. Cook and B.M. Dickens, "A Decade of International Change in Abortion Law" (*American Journal of Public Health* 1978; 68:637-44).

On issues pertaining to the "personhood" of the fetus, one of the most controversial aspects of the Supreme Court's ruling in *Roe* v. *Wade,* see W.J. Curran, "A Historical Perspective on the Law of Personality and Status with Special Regard for the Rights of the Human Fetus and the Rights of Women" (*Milbank Memorial Fund Quarterly* 1983; 61:58-69).

Sterilization of the Poor: Judge Gesell's Roadblock

> There is uncontroverted evidence in the record that minors and other incompetents have been sterilized with federal funds and that an indefinite number of poor people have been improperly coerced into accepting a sterilization operation under the threat that various federally supported welfare benefits would be withdrawn unless they submitted to irreversible sterilization.
>
> Judge Gerhard A. Gesell

Federal Judge Gerhard Gesell, who sits in the U.S. District Court in Washington, D.C., is known to the bar as an activist liberal judge. He has amplified his reputation once again in a very forceful decision that strikes down the validity of Department of Health, Education, and Welfare (HEW) regulations for sterilization under federally supported welfare medical-care programs.[1] The quotation from the opinion that heads this column is the actual key to the decision. Judge Gesell was apparently shocked and affronted by the revelations by witnesses and by sworn affidavits of the extensive application of sterilization procedures to the poor of America under federal programs. He found that in the last few years some 100,000 to 150,000 poor persons were sterilized annually with federal welfare support.

The aggressive use of sterilization against poor black people, some of whom were alleged to be mentally retarded, was dramatically revealed some six months earlier on national television. The result was Congressional hearings before Senator Kennedy's health subcommittee and new regulations by HEW. These regulations were intended to place controls on sterilization, but did allow what were termed "voluntary" sterilizations of competent adults and of minors and incompetent persons. It was undoubtedly the belief of HEW that they provided very stringent safeguards to protect the two latter groups.

From the *New England Journal of Medicine*
1974; 291:25-26.

The written informed consent of the minors and incompetents was specifically required in the regulations. Also, a special review committee was required of independent persons from the community to determine whether the sterilization was in the best interest of the person, taking into consideration the expected mental and physical effect of pregnancy and motherhood on the person, if female, or the expected mental impact of fatherhood, if male, and the expected immediate and long-term mental and physical results of sterilization on the person. The review committee was also required to examine medical, social, and psychological information about the person, alternative family-planning methods, and the adequacy of consent by the person, and to interview the person, the person's parents, and such other persons as deemed necessary. In addition, the sterilization had to be approved by a state court of competent jurisdiction acting in the best interests of the child.

As for competent adults, the regulations required their informed consent to the procedure and that the written and signed consent document indicate that the patient was made aware of the costs and benefits of sterilization and the fact that he or she could decline the operation without losing federal benefits.

On a class-action challenge to the regulations by certain poor people threatened with involuntary sterilization and the National Welfare Rights Organization, these sections were found invalid, and an injunction was issued against their enforcement. Judge Gesell found that the regulations for competent adults were not adequate in ensuring that no coercion was used by doctors or project officers. He required that the regulations be amended to provide that persons be informed at the outset that no federal benefits can be withdrawn because of a failure to accept sterilization. This guarantee must appear prominently on the top of the consent form.

Regarding minors and incompetents, however, the judge was much more restrictive. He held that because the statute covered only voluntary sterilization under federal funds, no sterilizations at all could be carried out on minors and incompetents, even with their consent, and with the other safeguards provided in the regulations.

Judge Gesell asserted that he had made his finding solely on the basis of the lack of statutory authorization and without invoking any constitutional rights of the people concerned. Nevertheless, he also asserted that involuntary sterilization procedures would be a violation of the constitutionally protected right of privacy. He concluded that no minor and no incompetent could meet the dictionary standard of voluntariness, which requires free will and precludes coercion or force. He asserted that minors and incompetents "appear to lack the knowledge, maturity and judgment to satisfy these standards with regard to this important issue ['irreversible sterilization'] whatever may be their competence to rely on devices or medication that temporarily frustrates procreation. This is the reasoning that provides the basis for the nearly universal common law and statutory rule that 'minors cannot consent to medical operations.'"[2]

Judge Gesell ends his examination of the law with this statement. His interpretation of the law is unusual, however. When a parent consents to beneficial medical procedures on a minor child, the treatment is not generally viewed as "involuntary," particularly if the child also consents, as is required in these regulations. A court order is not required for an involuntary procedure every time a parent or guardian takes a minor or an incompetent to a physician or to a hospital for medical treatment of clear benefit to the child. Judge Gesell seems, in fact, to be using two different standards. He says that a minor and an incompetent cannot consent to a sterilization, but may be able to consent to the use of devices or medication to frustrate procreation temporarily. Yet his last sentence says such persons cannot consent at all to medical treatment. Judge Gesell is really disturbed about sterilization, not all medical treatment. He lays down a flat rule that minors and incompetents can never fully understand the detrimental effects of such a procedure. Therefore, it is always involuntary.

The decision has been greeted with widespread approval. It seems quite clear that too many medical programs of sterilization have been used in a coercive manner to achieve highly questionable goals of population control among poor people on welfare.[3] Sterilization has been a handy tool in the hands of the privileged against the underprivileged through most of this century. Groups that in earlier decades sponsored programs of involuntary sterilization have now changed their slogans to "voluntary sterilization," but there has apparently been little change in their basic motivations. Judge Gesell has put a serious roadblock in the path of these groups.

REFERENCES

1. Relf v. Weinberger. Civil Action no. 73-1557. National Welfare Rights Organization v. Weinberger. Civil Action no. 74-243, 1974.
2. *Idem.* p. 9.
3. Slater J. Sterilization: newest threat to the poor. Ebony 1973; 28:150-3.

COMMENTS

As a result of the Gesell opinion, a moratorium was imposed on Medicaid funding for sterilization procedures on persons under 21. This moratorium was not lifted until new regulations were adopted, requiring a 30-day "waiting period" and stricter standards for informed consent in the case of minors. For a commentary on the ethical implications of the regulations, see R.P. Petchesky, "Reproduction, Ethics, and Public Policy: The Federal Sterilization Regulations" (*Hastings Center Report* 1979; 10(6):29-41).

In other important decisions pertaining to the involuntary sterilization of incompetent persons, in some instances after parental or guardian consent had been obtained, the courts, in a series of cases, have required "clear and convincing" proof that sterilization is necessary and in the best interests of the person. This proof must include evidence that the person lacks either understanding in regard to sexual intercourse and birth control or the ability and understanding needed to care for and raise children, or that sterilization is advisable for other reasons, such as the consideration that it would otherwise not be feasible to allow the person greater freedom than he or she could enjoy in a closed institution. See, in particular, *In re Grady,* 426 A.2d 467 (1981), and *In re Penny N.,* 414 A.2d 541, N.H. (1980). For recent legal commentary, see R.M.J. Gould, "Procreation: A Choice for the Mentally Retarded" (*Washburn Law Journal* 1984; 23:359-78); and D.J. Bays-Beinart, "Exclusive Juvenile Jurisdiction to Authorize Sterilization of Incompetent Minors" (*Indiana Law Review* 1983; 16:835-60).

In a decision that was upheld in the Supreme Court, a trial-court judge has been found civilly liable for improperly ordering the sterilization of a minor on petition of the parents. The trial judge had no statutory authority for his action, and it was held that the court did not have inherent common-law powers to issue such an order. In addition, the judge had issued the order in an informal hearing without the knowledge of the minor or the appointment of a guardian to represent the interest of the minor. See *Stump* v. *Sparkman,* 435 U.S. 349 (1978).

Experimentation Becomes a Crime: Fetal Research in Massachusetts

In the aftermath of the Supreme Court's abortion decisions in early 1973 there has been a rash of legislative action in the states and a rush to the courts by proponents on both sides of the issues to seek clarification of the many unanswered questions that remain in the wake of these historic pronouncements of the law.[1]

Among the most serious questions raised by the decisions is the fate of the human fetus involved. The Supreme Court held that the fetus, before a vaguely defined stage of viability, is not a "person" subject to the protection of the Fourteenth Amendment to the Constitution.[2] Most importantly for this discussion, the Court did not consider and did not seem even to be aware of the importance of the fetus, alive and dead, to scientific study and experimentation.

It has been argued by some commentators that if the Supreme Court's thesis were followed, fetal research would be entirely uncontrolled and outside the scope of legal protection. It must be realized that "human experimentation" has acquired a highly suspect connotation in some circles in American society and in mass literature. The image could be conjured up very quickly of hideous experiments on human fetuses in Frankensteinesque laboratories and hospitals, none of it useful to mankind or contributing to the understanding of human life, growth, or development.

There has been a rapid reaction in the U.S. Congress regarding this field of research. A law has been enacted imposing a four-month moratorium on all federal support of fetal research and on all fetal research in federal establishments pending an investigation and report by the National Commission for the Protection of Human Sub-

From the *New England Journal of Medicine*
1975; 292:300-301.

jects of Biomedical and Behavioral Research, which is also set up by the same legislation.[3]

Late in the 1974 legislative session, the Massachusetts Legislature passed a law entitled, "An Act Prohibiting Experimentation on Human Fetuses."[4] It was signed by Governor Sargent on June 26, 1974. Violation of this law is a crime, a felony, carrying a penalty of up to five years in a state prison.

It should not be assumed that all the people, including legislators, who supported this law also opposed the liberalization of the abortion laws. It is possible to separate the issues. However, as enacted, these issues clearly and inherently overlap, as an analysis of the law demonstrates.

As first drafted, the fetal-research bill was more restrictive than it now appears in the enacted form. Its advocates were found to be open to some objections by the medical-research community. Much of the credit for getting the parties together must go to Representative Lois M. Pines, of Newton, and the speaker of the House of Representatives, David M. Bartley, of Holyoke.

The law as enacted is intended to prohibit, not merely to regulate, experimentation on live human fetuses, within the womb or outside, with certain exceptions.

A "live fetus" is defined as one showing "evidence of life" as determined by the same medical criteria as are used in determining life in a spontaneously aborted fetus of the same gestational development. No specific tests or findings are required, but are left to the "best medical judgment of a physician." A fetus includes an embryo or neonate.

There are three exceptions to the broad application of the law:

(1) The law does not apply to the use of diagnostic tests to determine the state of health of the fetus, or to determine whether it is alive. This exception was specifically intended to cover such procedures as amniocentesis seeking information on birth defects, including genetic disorders.

(2) The law does not apply to the use of "remedial procedures" intended to preserve the life or health of the fetus or of the mother.

(3) The law allows "procedures incident to the study of a human fetus" within the womb to be conducted if such procedures do not "substantially jeopardize" the life or health of the fetus, and if the fetus is not the subject of a "planned abortion."

This exception allows research to be conducted on the live fetus, despite the title of the act. The limitation ("does not substantially jeopardize the life or health of the fetus") is less demanding than it might have been. In the literature of experimentation on children much more restrictive standards could have been found.[5] In the first place, all research could have been prohibited that was not directly "beneficial" to the fetus. Alternatively, all research involving any possibility of harm to the fetus, or to the mother, could have been outlawed.

The second restriction on the allowable area of fetal research indicates the law's inherent relation to the abortion issue. Such research is not allowed if it is part of an abortion planned in advance of the procedure. The law is thus designed to prevent researchers from seeking out women who are planning abortions and then obtaining their consent to experimentation on the live fetus. It is alleged that this is the type of study that resulted in the criminal indictments at Boston City Hospital. Of course, the indictments related to the alleged deaths of the fetuses at abortion, not to the study itself.

Another concession was made to the medical researchers regarding this last restriction. A sentence was added that makes a signed statement by the mother at the time of the experimental study that she is not planning an abortion a "conclusive presumption" of such lack of planning in any later criminal proceeding. The practical effect here is that no evidence could be admissible in court to rebut this presumption, even the testimony of the mother, and even if she decided to have an abortion later and actually had it.

The most serious problem of interpretation regarding these three exceptions is whether experimental procedures are allowed under (1) and (2) above. It has been indicated to me by one of those who drafted the law that the intention was not to exclude experimental procedures from these two exceptions. However, the experimental procedure would have to be intended to provide the mother with specific information diagnostically about the health or life status of the particular fetus, or be intended to be "remedial" (presumably therapeutic) to this particular fetus or mother. Under this interpretation, a researcher could not try to perfect his diagnostic technique without regard to the information that it produced concerning the particular fetus.

The law also regulates, but does not prohibit, research on dead fetuses. "Experimentation," undefined, can be performed on dead fetuses with the consent of the mother, who must be 18 years of age or older. This provision appears to include research on fetal tissues capable of metabolism, provided the fetus is dead and the consent requirement has been satisfied.

There is another important restriction, which again is related to abortions. Researchers must not offer to perform or actually perform any abortions wherein part of the "consideration" for the abortion service is that the researcher will be allowed to keep the fetus for research. The intent here is similar to that noted earlier. The law is designed to prohibit researchers from seeking out women, particularly poor women, who are planning an abortion and offering them free service in return for experimentation on the dead fetus, often including some study and testing while the fetus is in the womb. Actually, the legal term "consideration" includes anything of value, not merely money, or anything the researcher was not legally obliged to do at the time. This language could be a trap for the unwary obstetrical service that has any contact with the mother before the abortion, whether planned or not.

The law also prohibits "any person," seemingly including the mother and any obstetrical service, from selling, transferring, distributing, or giving away any fetus for "a use which is in violation" of this law. This proviso may sound restrictive, and perhaps it was intended to be, but a full perusal of the law reveals no restrictions on "use" of a dead fetus for "experimentation" other than obtaining the consent of a mother over 18 years of age. It also seems advisable that the restriction mentioned above concerning "consideration" be observed.

As a further indication of the overlap between abortion law and the fetal-research prohibition law as enacted in Massachusetts, it should be noted that the same session of the General Court also enacted a new abortion law placing various restrictions on abortions performed in the state.[6] The abortion law requires hospitals to have life-supporting equipment present in the room where abortions are performed. It also requires physicians performing abortions to take reasonable steps during and after the abortion to preserve the life and health of a fetus that is 24 weeks old or older. It should be apparent that there is a consistency in these two

Massachusetts laws in opting to support life in the human fetus wherever it is possible to do so.

It seems clear that sponsors of the fetal-research–prohibition law were open to some compromise in all areas but one: the basic thrust of the law preventing fetal research from being used to encourage "planned abortions."

I am concerned about the fact that this law leaves a number of important terms such as "dead fetus" and "consideration" undefined and leaves a great deal of uncertainty about the scope of the first two exceptions noted above. Most importantly, however, the terms "experimentation" and "procedures incident to study of a human fetus" are left totally undefined. This ambiguity may have seemed advantageous to researchers consulted at the time in that any attempt at definition might well have added restrictions on investigation or on research procedures. Yet these are the key terms in the bill, the very actions that are declared criminal under the law. The American Constitution requires that criminal laws be sufficiently clear that those who are being restricted may know what they cannot do. Researchers who wish to do investigative studies in fetal development in Massachusetts will be in very uncertain territory where a wrong step may result in egregious criminal prosecution and a ruined career. Unlike the abortion law of the past, on the statute books for decades and rarely enforced against violators, these new laws will apparently receive vigorous enforcement in the presence of the ever watchful media. I am also disturbed that the advocates of this law thought it necessary to make its violation a felony of such serious criminal consequences. Would not a noncriminal penalty have accomplished the objectives of the law? I must say that I come away from laws of this type with a very uneasy feeling.

REFERENCES

1. Curran WJ. Aftermath of the abortion decisions: action in the legislatures and in the courts. N Engl J Med 1973; 289:955.
2. *Idem.* The abortion decisions: the Supreme Court as moralist, scientist, historian and legislator. N Engl J Med 1973; 288:950-1.
3. Public Law 93-348, Section 213.
4. Massachusetts Acts of 1974, Chapter 421.
5. Curran WJ, Beecher HK. Experimentation in children: a reexamination of legal ethical principles. JAMA 1969; 210:77-83.
6. Massachusetts Acts of 1974, Chapter 706.

COMMENTS

The Massachusetts statute on fetal research was amended in order to mitigate some of the problems that I mentioned in this column. The offense was reduced from a felony to a misdemeanor, but the penalty remained harsh: imprisonment in a county jail for not less than one year nor more than two and one-half years, plus a fine of up to $10,000 – an unusually high amount to be charged in the case of a misdemeanor.

For similar statutes prohibiting or controlling medical research on fetuses in other states, see California Health and Safety Code, Sections 25956–25957; Pennsylvania Consolidated Statutes Annotated, Title 18, Section 3216. California law treats "experimentation on a live fetus except to protect or preserve the life and health of the fetus" as a misdemeanor, whereas in Pennsylvania it is a felony to conduct "any type of nontherapeutic experimentation on an unborn child." Experimentation on "children who have died during the course of an abortion" may be conducted only with the written permission of the mother.

Quite obviously, the statutory protections enacted to control or prevent experiments on fetuses reflect philosophical positions regarding the "personhood" of the developing human life. See the series of excellent papers on personhood collected in a symposium on the subject in the *Milbank Memorial Fund Quarterly* (1983; 61:1-147).

The Thalidomide Trial in Germany: The End of Innocence in the Use of Drugs in Pregnant Women

On December 18, 1969, the longest trial in the history of West Germany ended. It was the legal action brought against Chemie Grünenthal, the German pharmaceutical company, and some of its officials concerning the manufacture and sale of the drug, thalidomide, which was alleged to be responsible for the tragic birth deformities of from 5000 to 6000 babies, some 4000 of them in West Germany itself. None of the courtroom cases of war criminals after World War II took longer or required more of the judicial system.

The thalidomide trial began in Alsdorf, West Germany, on May 27, 1968. It ended with a financial settlement of nearly $30 million.

Over $27 million, plus interest, was paid by the company to the parents of 2000 surviving children, or approximately $19,000 per child, and $1.1 million was paid to some 800 adults who suffered nervous disorders as a result of taking the drug. The company also met court costs of $1.6 million.

The case was not a personal-injury trial. It was a criminal action based on violation of West German drug laws and upon charges of homicide and criminal negligence. Originally, there were nine officials of the company under charges, but two were dismissed from the case for reasons of health. In the 283 days of trial, 120 witnesses were heard, 60 of them experts drawn from all over the world. The case was heard by a five-judge bench. After the financial settlement was agreed on, the court dismissed the criminal charges, holding that a criminal intent had not been proved. It was found that the company and its

From the *New England Journal of Medicine*
1971; 284:481-482.

officials were not aware of the extremely grave consequences of their product until most of the damage was done. Thalidomide was an over-the-counter, prescription-free drug in Germany from late 1957 until 1961. It was an extremely popular tranquilizer without noticeable side effects and was used extensively by women in the early months of pregnancy. It was not until May 1960 that Dr. Ralf Voss, a Düsseldorf neurologist, first called attention publicly to the disturbing relation of the drug to the rise in birth defects. Further reports followed over the next year until the drug was removed from the market.

Thalidomide was never commercially released in the United States, thanks largely to the alertness of Dr. Frances O. Kelsey, of the federal Food and Drug Administration (FDA). She had read some of the warnings about its possible dangers in European medical journals and had held up the American drug company's "new drug application" long enough for further investigation to prove the truth of the reports. Nevertheless, there have been 17 cases of phocomelia in the United States that have been claimed to be related to thalidomide. In most of them the drug was obtained by the mothers from foreign countries. However, some cases may be related to the clinical investigational use of the drug in this country. Testing in the United States was far more extensive than the FDA had thought it was before the American company withdrew its new drug application. At first, the FDA believed that only about 40 or 50 doctors had been involved in clinical trials of thalidomide. By August 1962, however, the FDA had discovered that over 2,500,000 tablets had been distributed by 1267 physicians to 19,822 patients, including 3760 women of childbearing age.[1] The public outcry concerning thalidomide was responsible in large part for the passage by Congress of the so-called Drug Amendments Act of 1962, with its much stricter laws concerning the conduct of drug testing in the United States and the control of the marketing of new drugs.[2]

The story of thalidomide is a tragic chapter in the generally progressive development of drug therapy in medicine. Its lessons are many on an international scale. In its way, it was a turning point, an end of innocence. It marked the beginning of a new, greater sense of responsibility in clinical pharmacology, clinical investigation, and medicolegal relations.

REFERENCES

1. Press release of the Department of Health, Education, and Welfare, Food and Drug Administration. August 23, 1962.
2. Curran WJ. Governmental regulation of the use of human subjects in medical research: the approach of two federal agencies. Daedalus 1969; 98:542-95.

♦

COMMENTS

Over the years I have written very few columns commenting on trials held in foreign jurisdictions in which medicolegal issues were dealt with. The American courts and legislatures have provided me with more than enough material for my contributions to the *Journal*'s crowded pages. This decision in West Germany was most unusual and most compelling. Although it received little, if any, recognition in American law reviews, it was heavily covered in the mass media and in professional periodicals all over Europe.

As indicated in the column, the thalidomide tragedies in Europe helped greatly to encourage Congress to pass the therapeutic-drug reform legislation of 1962. That legislation completely revolutionized the regulation of therapeutic drugs, requiring proof of efficacy as well as safety before new products could be marketed. In later years, programs regulating the clinical trial of drugs have been particularly protective of pregnant women and women of childbearing age. Moreover, the FDA requires extensive preclinical laboratory testing and testing in animals to guard against the marketing of drugs with the potential to damage the growing human fetus. For a historical review, see M. Sherman and S. Straus, "Thalidomide: A Twenty-Five Year Perspective" (*Food, Drug, and Cosmetics Law Review* 1986; 41: 458-66).

7 • Life and Death

LIFE AND DEATH IN THE LAW

Until very recent years, it seemed quite settled in American law that no legal rights attached to a person until he was born – that is, he could not bring an action for injury when *en ventre sa mère.* This rule was based on a Massachusetts decision in 1884 by Justice Oliver Wendell Holmes that refused to recognize a fetus as having a legal existence.[1] After World War II, however, this rule was abrogated in many states, and the person, after birth, was given a right to bring an action for damages against a wrongdoer who caused injury to him during the fetal period. The Court of Appeals of Maryland, in a recent case (*Maryland* v. *Sherman*[2]), has gone a step farther: in a split decision, with a vigorous dissent, the court allowed an action for prenatal injury in which the "plaintiff" was stillborn. Thus, a legal action has been recognized for a person who was *never born.*

When Justice Holmes rendered his opinion against these actions, perhaps he was thinking of some of the puzzling situations that can arise when rights are recognized in the unborn. Perhaps he was speculating about the fact that if a right of action for injury is recognized, the child may eventually sue the mother! Such an action has not been brought, but something close to it and just as disturbing legally has appeared in the courts. In Illinois, an illegitimate child sued his natural father for damages. His mother was married to another man at the time of the conception and birth of the plaintiff. The plaintiff claimed that his father induced his mother to have intercourse on the basis of a fraudulent promise to marry her. The damage claim was based on the deprivation of the plaintiff's alleged right to legitimacy, to a normal home life, and to inheritance rights from his father and paternal ancestors, and for the mental anguish of being stigmatized as a bastard.

The trial court dismissed the suit, and the plaintiff did not indicate that he would appeal. However, the court asked a law professor

From the *New England Journal of Medicine*
1964; 271:1006.

to write an amicus curiae brief on the law to bring the case to the higher court so that an opinion would be rendered. It was admitted that the case was "novel," and no such claim had ever been brought in Illinois, in any common-law jurisdiction, or in any civil-law country either.

Professor Rheinstein did his best, but the upper court, in an agonizing reexamination of the cases concerning prenatal rights, denied the plaintiff's claim to what might be called his "wrongful life."[3] The court reviewed the cases that had recognized a right of action in the unborn child for injuries sustained only after viability, calculated as the time from which the child might be said to be capable of life separate from the mother. The court then noted cases that allowed actions for injuries before this viability stage. In the case at hand the Illinois judges said that they were now being asked to push back the right of action to the moment of conception. The court then said it was willing to entertain such a view in a proper case, but would deny recovery in the action before it. The court noted that the plaintiff was protesting not only the act that had caused him to be born but birth itself. The court was unwilling to recognize this new tort (civil action for damages) for a wrongful life. Quite openly, the judges shrank from the possibilities of litigation to which this claim, if allowed, could give rise. They lifted the lid of this legal Pandora's box, peeked in, and saw that: "One might seek damages for being born of a certain color, another because of race; one for being born with a hereditary disease, another for inheriting unfortunate family characteristics; one for being born into a large and destitute family, another because a parent has an unsavory reputation."

This is the sort of thing the courts are faced with when they begin to redefine human existence.

During the same period the courts of this country have had some highly significant cases raising questions on the other end of the life cycle: the "right" of death. Can a human being decide to die rather than receive blood transfusions?

REFERENCES

1. Dietrick v. Northampton, 138 Mass. 14 (1884).
2. Court of Appeals of Maryland, 234 Md. 179, 198 A.2d 71 (1964).
3. Zepeda v. Zepeda, 41 Ill. App.2d 240 (Appellate Court of Illinois, First District, 1963).

COMMENTS

This chapter is made up of a number of columns on medicolegal issues of life and death, beginning with my 1964 essay on the *Zepeda* case, the first for which I used the words "life and death" in the title. The range of subjects that I touch on under this heading is very broad, and the individual essays relate to a variety of fields, ranging from forensic pathology to obstetrics, neurology, organ transplantation, and internal medicine. Theoretically, all of the columns dealing with the care of dying patients could have been included here, but I chose to place those of the discussions that center on the legal and ethical responsibilities of physicians in Chapter 5 and to restrict this last chapter to essays that focus on the role of the courts as arbiters of the rights of the dying.

The opening column clearly brings out the momentousness and complexity of the issues that are raised in litigation of this kind. Since this essay was written, several other jurisdictions have followed the precedent set in the *Zepeda* case and have denied recovery for a "wrongful life" in instances in which the plaintiff was born illegitimate but healthy. See *Williams* v. *State,* 18 N.Y. 2d 481 (1966), and *Stills* v. *Gratton,* 127 Cal. Rptr. 652 (1976).

State courts across the country are still grappling, however, with the sensitive issues of public policy raised in claims for damages in cases of "wrongful life" in which the child was born physically or mentally defective or with multiple handicaps and, often, a greatly shortened life expectancy. The sympathy of the court is always with the child and the parents. The financial burdens, let alone the personal anguish that the family suffers, create strong pressure to find legal liability when a third party, a physician, is alleged to have breached a professional duty to advise against pregnancy or to discuss the possibility of an abortion. However, in *Becker* v. *Schwartz,* 46 N.Y. 2d 401 (1978), a precedent was set for refusing to recognize a cause of action in the birth of a child with Tay–Sachs disease.

A few later decisions seemed to indicate a trend toward allowing recovery in some cases of this kind, but there now appears to be a nationwide trend to reject the "wrongful life" argument firmly on the grounds that judgments assessing the benefits of nonlife as compared to existence are beyond judicial competence and financial evaluation. See *Smith* v. *Cote,* 513 A.2d 341, N.H. (1986); and

Azzolino v. *Dingfelder,* 315 N.C. 103 (1985), *cert. denied,* 107 S. Ct. 131 (1986).

As predicted in this column in the 1960s, there is continued interest in the concept of taking legal action against mothers who do not care for themselves adequately during pregnancy. Such actions could consist of efforts either to force the pregnant woman to change her ways or to remove the child from the mother's custody after birth. For a general review of the legal issues involved, see C.J. Dougherty, "The Right to Begin Life with a Sound Body and Mind: Fetal Patients and Conflicts with Their Mothers" (*University of Detroit Law Review* 1985; 63:89-117). For a useful comprehensive review of issues in this field, see Student Note, "Legal Rights and Issues Surrounding Conception, Pregnancy, and Birth" (*Vanderbilt Law Review* 1986; 39: 597-650).

THE BIRTH OF A HEALTHY CHILD BECAUSE OF NEGLIGENT FAILURE OF "THE PILL": BENEFIT OR HARM TO THE PARENTS?

The inevitable has occurred. A physician prescribed an oral contraceptive. The pharmacist made a mistake. He filled the prescription with a tranquilizer. The patient, mother of seven children, took the "pill" faithfully, continued to have intercourse with her husband, became pregnant, and was delivered of a fine, healthy, unwanted eighth child.

The husband and wife brought an action against the pharmacist, not against the physician, for money damages alleging four separate bases of recovery: the economic cost of rearing an eighth child; the pain and anxiety of the pregnancy and childbirth; medical and hospital expenses; and the wife's loss of wages owing to the pregnancy, childbirth, and child rearing.

The trial court judge dismissed the case summarily, asserting that the birth of a healthy child was a benefit that offset all losses sustained and that the public policy of the state could not be otherwise.

The parents appealed the case to a higher court. On the basis of precedent, the plaintiffs could not have expected much in the way of a recovery, at least for the actual bringing up of the child. Other courts have refused recoveries for so-called "wrongful life," at least where the person was healthy. However, the suits have usually involved action by the child himself rather than the parents and

From the *New England Journal of Medicine*
1971; 285:1063-1064.

have alleged more unusual bases of damages, such as the anguish involved in being illegitimate.[1,2]

In the instant case, *Troppi* v. *Scarf,*[3] the Michigan Court of Appeals reversed the lower court and held all four bases of recovery in the case to be valid and actionable under Michigan law. The case must now go before a jury, which will be ordered to assess damages on these allegations, if they are found true.

The higher court found that it was not against Michigan law to encourage family planning. In fact, two recent legislative actions were cited in the state to indicate that the Michigan legislature favored such programs. Clear negligence was shown on the pharmacist's part. Under the law, pharmacists owe a very high degree of duty in filling a prescription, and this duty was violated here. The pharmacist is liable for the harm done. The court had no trouble with the last three items of damage. Most of the discussion revolved around the first item: the economic cost of rearing the child.

The defendant alleged that the benefit test should at least apply here – that the joys of bringing up a child outweigh the expenses. The court rejected the argument. It held that in modern times, the value of the "services" of a child are largely illusory. In an earlier agricultural society, the child might have contributed direct services to the family, but in today's culture, he is almost entirely supplied with all needs, and many luxuries if they can be afforded, until almost into adult life. The court had little regard for any value in a child's "companionship" either. In any event, the court said it was up to the jury to weigh the evidence of the cost of raising the child against these rather evasive "benefits" and to come up with a verdict.

Perhaps the most problematic question raised in the case was the defendant's contention that, if the negligence of the pharmacist was actionable at law, the plaintiff-parents had a legal obligation to mitigate the damages in the case either by having an abortion or by letting the child out for adoption. The court examined both grounds seriously and at length, but rejected both. The court asserted, "The [pharmacist] does not have the right to insist that the victim of his negligence have the emotional and mental makeup of a woman who is willing to abort or place a child for adoption." The court ruled as a matter of law that no mother, wed or unwed, can reasonably be required to abort (even if legal) or place her child for adoption.

This case is difficult to offer comment on in any meaningful sense without an examination of the very basis of money damages for so-called civil wrongs or torts. Originally, the money damages were intended as compensation for actual, out-of-pocket losses for property stolen or damaged, or for medical expenses and wage loss in personal injury. In recent years, the more liberal courts have applied what is called "social engineering" to torts and have allowed very large verdicts for much more indirect and less measurable "losses" such as pain and suffering, mental anguish, and loss of reputation. They have also found many more "losses" actionable. Physicians are well aware of this in the field of medical malpractice. Reforms such as the Massachusetts "no-fault" law on automobile torts are moving against both these trends in the courts.

In this case, the pharmacist is left with a damage-award principle under which he is basically required to furnish the funds to bring up another person's child. The family has the child, does not have to abort it or place it for adoption, but, nevertheless, does not want it and considers it—legally and publicly—a burden it wants someone else to pay for to bring up. Just what kind of family relation does this establish between child and parents? In a facetious way, we might almost ask if the pharmacist has visitation rights with the child. Only the existence of liability insurance, which may well pay the verdict, makes this an impersonal situation. Would the court have arrived at its conclusions if large-coverage liability-insurance policies did not exist? Are insurance money and "shifted losses and benefits" of high finance really what were needed here?

Note: In 1971, another state appellate court, the Delaware Superior Court, has come to the same general conclusion as the above Michigan court, citing the *Troppi* case. The Delaware case involved a negligently performed sterilization procedure on the wife, who was pregnant with an unwanted fifth child at the time of the suit. The court also found that the damages could include the cost of another sterilization operation.[4] The two cases are the first such decisions in American courts.

REFERENCES

1. Life and death in the law—Part I. N Engl J Med 1964; 271:1006.
2. Life and death in the law—Part II. N Engl J Med 1964; 271:1206-7.
3. Troppi v. Scarf. 187 N.W. 2d 511 (Mich. 1971).
4. Coleman v. Garrison. 281 A.2d 616 (Del. 1971).

COMMENTS

This was another of my strongly worded essays critical of court decisions that I found unreasonable. The worst of the policies endorsed in this case was, of course, rewarding the parents of a healthy child for publicly and permanently branding the infant "unwanted." The triumph of greed for money, on the grounds that "it is only the insurance company's loss," was only too apparent.

The determination in the *Troppi* case remains the leading decision made in the United States awarding damages for a "wrongful life" due to failure of contraceptive services or a sterilization procedure. See also *Hackworth* v. *Hart,* 474 S.W.2d 377 (1971); and *Jones* v. *Malinowski,* 299 Md. 257 (1984).

The Gift of Life: The Uniform Anatomical Gift Act Is Adopted

One of the most important medicolegal developments of 1968 was the adoption of the Uniform Anatomical Gift Act by the National Conference of Commissioners on Uniform State Laws on July 30, 1968, and its approval by the American Bar Association on August 7, 1968. This draft legislation will be presented to each of the state legislatures for consideration this year.

The Commissioners on Uniform State Laws is an official national body composed of three representatives from each state and appointed by the governor for three-year terms. The Uniform Anatomical Gift Act is the product of over three years of work. The preparation of the draft legislation is one of the finest examples of interprofessional cooperation between medical and legal groups that I have ever witnessed in this country.

The proposed act authorizes donation by any person 18 years of age or older before death and donation by next of kin after the death. The gift can be of all or any part of the human body to a variety of donees, including a hospital, a particular physician or dentist, an educational or research institution, or a storage bank. Any physician or other person acting in good faith to carry out the anatomical gift made under the act is specifically protected from any suit against him either civilly or criminally.

The third and final draft of the uniform act is particularly significant in the clarification it provides concerning the rights of the next of kin. The next of kin may make a gift by a simple written document, without witnesses, by a telegram, or by a "recorded telephonic or other recorded message." The next of kin may not, however, interfere

From the *New England Journal of Medicine*
1969; 280:36-37.

with a donation made by the donor during his lifetime. These provisions are very important. Though 39 of the states have at least some law authorizing anatomical gifts by a living donor, only 16 states have statutes clearly authorizing next-of-kin donations.

The act also contains an important provision concerning the death of the donor. It provides that the time of death shall be determined by the physician who attends the donor at his death, or if no physician is in attendance, by the physician who officially certifies the death. However, this physician "shall not participate in the procedures for removing or transplanting a part."

Only three of the New England states (Massachusetts, Connecticut, and Rhode Island) have general anatomical donation laws. Maine authorizes donation only of eyes. New Hampshire and Vermont have no laws of this type at all. None of these statutes, even that of Massachusetts, is as comprehensive and desirable from a medical and surgical point of view as the Uniform Anatomical Gift Act.

As a person deeply interested and involved in the medicolegal aspects of transplantation for over 10 years, I would strongly support the enactment of this Uniform Anatomical Gift Act in each of the New England states and throughout the nation. I urge that this step be taken not only because this is the best piece of legislation ever produced on this subject in this country or in any other country, but also because uniformity is essential in this field if transplantation programs are to be developed effectively in the future. Nearly all clinical programs in this field must serve patients and use donors from various states, not merely their own states. Serious legal and logistical problems can be avoided if the state laws concerning anatomical donation are the same in every state. Federal law cannot be enacted to cover these issues; they are exclusively within the domain of the states. Also, national educational campaigns cannot be launched to encourage donations when the laws of the states are different and confusing, or completely ineffective in this field. A uniform law across the country can be used as the touchstone of a national program of anatomical donation, not only for transplant purposes but also for medical, dental, and other scientific education and research. Physicians and medical organizations in this country should play an important part in encouraging their state legislatures in 1969 to consider very seriously this important proposed legislation.

COMMENTS

The adoption of the Uniform Anatomical Gift Act by the National Conference of Commissioners on Uniform State Laws was a significant event in medicolegal history in this country, marking the first instance in which legislation relating to medicine was ever prepared and supported by this prestigious interstate body.

The new law was not, however, entirely without precedent. The first anatomical-gift legislation, enacted in Massachusetts a few years earlier, was based on a bill that I had drafted and submitted, with considerable support from Boston hospitals involved in kidney transplantation programs. See Massachusetts Acts of 1967, Chapter 353.

The Uniform Anatomical Gift Act won enthusiastic support in all parts of the country. At present, all 50 states have adopted the act's provisions, in some cases with minor variations. In recent years, more than half the states have also adopted laws authorizing motor-vehicle drivers to indicate their willingness to make postmortem anatomical donations through a notation on their driver's licenses. See, for example, Massachusetts Acts of 1975, Chapter 879, and Virginia Acts of 1976, Chapter 57.

The main effect of these laws has been to increase public support for transplantation programs. In practice, hospitals have been reluctant to allow anatomical donations solely on the basis of the donor's intentions as evidenced by a donation card or a suitably endorsed driver's license. Almost without exception, hospitals and transplantation programs also require the written permission of the next of kin, when available. In order to encourage hospitals actively to seek donations of needed organs from appropriate donors, states have recently been amending their anatomical-gift legislation so as to require hospitals and treating physicians to request donations from next of kin. There also have been nationally publicized cases in which parents of sick children have made public pleas for organ donations to save the lives of their children. "Organ bank" programs organized across the country have attempted to bring order and fairness to the process of procuring organs and tissues for transplant purposes and to their utilization.

For a general review of the legal aspects of the subject, see R.D. Cotton and A.L. Sadler, "The Regulation of Organ Procurement and Transplantation in the United States" (*Journal of Legal Medicine*

1985; 7:55-84); and J.M. Prottas, "The Rules for Asking and Answering: The Role of Organ Donation" (*University of Detroit Law Review* 1985; 63:183-93). For a policy-oriented review of methods of organ procurement, see H.S. Swartz, "Bioethical and Legal Considerations in Increasing the Supply of Transplantation Organs: From UAGA to 'Baby Fae'" (*American Journal of Law and Medicine* 1985; 10:397-437). See also an excellent series of papers on a broad range of issues related to organ transplantation in *Law, Medicine and Health Care* (1985; 3:4-40).

In October 1986, Congress adopted legislation that will require hospitals in all states to seek donations of organs from appropriate patients. The law also authorizes the establishment of a national organ-sharing network with federal funding support. See R. Pear, "New Law May Spur Organ Donations" (*New York Times,* September 6, 1987:1). The federal law grew out of the work of the 25-member Task Force on Organ Transplantation established by the National Organ Transplant Act of 1984. Organized in 1985, the task force was asked to conduct a comprehensive examination of the medical, legal, ethical, economic, and social issues involved in the procurement and transplantation of human organs. Its recommendations are reported in *Organ Transplantation: Issues and Recommendations, Report of the Task Force on Transplantation* (Rockville, Md.: Department of Health and Human Services, 1986).

An Enigma Wrapped in Swaddling Clothes: Congress and Crib Death

Congress has just published the report on the first congressional investigation in American history devoted to what is called "sudden infant death syndrome," commonly known among physicians as "crib death."[1] The objective of the investigation was to determine what the federal government's medical research program was doing about this problem.

The findings were not encouraging, to say the least. The federal medical research establishment in 1971 was supporting only one research project directly related to the field. In the past seven years only five such research efforts were supported, all small by any relative criteria. It was generally agreed that there are approximately 10,000 such deaths every year in the United States. They occur between the second month of life and the end of the first year, and constitute the highest single cause of death in that period of life.

A number of witnesses came to the hearing representing the National Foundation for Sudden Infant Death. Some were physicians, but many were parents who had lost children in this way. They were among the most knowledgeable witnesses about the entire subject and obviously impressed the Senate investigators. The story was told of how death came, so quietly, so unexpectedly. A beloved baby, now just becoming old enough to be past the first few fragile weeks of life, gives such new joy to its parents each day. Then, the mother goes in during the night to check on the child, or to make an early morning visit to the cribside, and finds the child still and cold. Life is gone, joy is dead, tragedy has begun.

From the *New England Journal of Medicine*
1972; 287:235-237.

In some families the tragedy was expressed in words of blame and panic that cannot now be forgotten: husbands who are no longer willing to trust their wives with children; mothers who are made neurotic, pathetic shadows of their former selves, by the cancerous voices of guilt and self-doubt; young siblings who found the child and now cannot get the memory out of their minds, even with the purges of the most able and understanding counselors and therapists.

But this is a medicolegal column. What is the medicolegal issue here? It is plain enough in the stories of these parents. They told of being questioned suspiciously by police and of being unable to get autopsies performed by medical examiners, or, when autopsies were performed, of not getting the results for months and months.

A father from Chicago told of severe questioning by police and about Chicago-style medicolegal investigation. He testified as follows:

> The cruelest part of this whole nightmare was the inquest. . . . The supposition is that a panel of experts, forming a jury, is to listen to all the facts associated with the death of the child and then decide whether the evidence warrants prosecution. In actual fact, the coroner's jury consists of aging political appointees who are neither expert in law nor medicine and who rubber-stamp the conclusions made by the state attorney's office. . . . My feeling is that it is a crime to subject loving parents grieving for their child who has been stricken with crib death, to such treatment.

But conditions were reportedly no better in a large metropolitan area with a medical-examiner system. A mother testified that her baby was left in the house in a closed room with a policeman guarding the door until late in the day when an "investigator" from the Medical Examiner's Office appeared and viewed the infant and questioned the parents. Such questions were asked as "How many times did you hit the baby?" "Did your other child choke or in any way abuse the infant?" "Did you let your dog bite the baby?" Eleven months later, having received no report on the death or any results of any autopsy, the parents called the Medical Examiner's Office. The answer given was apparently that no record existed of such an investigation and no record existed of the birth or death of the child.

The government witnesses at the hearing were not able to provide current information on autopsies on such deaths or on the work of competent forensic pathologists in the field. They promised to provide further information at a later time. The committee report contains that further information. It is a collection of gross inaccuracies on medicolegal autopsies in this country and on the number of statewide medical-examiner systems.

It reported that the latest annual figures of the National Center for Health Statistics on autopsies on all deaths is for the year 1958. It goes on to say that 19.1 percent of all deaths were autopsied in that year. It is then observed, "However, all states required that sudden deaths, including sudden infant deaths, be autopsied, so it may be assumed that the percentage of those deaths which are autopsied approaches 100%." This statement and the assumption made are astonishingly incorrect. No state, not one, requires by law that all sudden deaths be autopsied. Certain classes of sudden, unexplained death are reportable in all states to some legal authority—whether police, coroner, or medical examiner. It is the decision of these officials whether the case will be investigated at all, a view taken of the body, or an autopsy ordered and performed. In actual fact, medicolegal cases constitute 20 to 30 percent of deaths in any community, depending upon the breadth of the definition used in that jurisdiction. Some 25 to 30 percent of these deaths are actually investigated, and no more than 10 percent or so are autopsied on a national average. Some jurisdictions have a high ratio of autopsied cases to reported cases, but these are few and far between among the bulk of jurisdictions that do not choose to spend the money on such procedures, or do not have the personnel to perform them. Crib deaths are not high on the priority list of medicolegal autopsies in most states. Emphasis is placed on cases involving the potential for criminal trials, especially when the bill is being paid by county judicial authorities. In autopsies performed in crib deaths, particularly those performed by inadequately trained personnel, useful findings are rarely produced, except to rule out foul play. After paying for a few of these, the authorities are reluctant to go to the expense of having more done. The coroners and medical examiners are quietly told to avoid such procedures in future. The parents are thus left with the inconclusive results and their own feelings of guilt forever unresolved.

In many communities, crib deaths are written off in unthinking cruelty as suffocation, pneumonia, and undifferentiated accidental death. It is a serious medicolegal problem that the "sudden infant death syndrome" is not a reportable cause of death in this country and has no code in the *International Classification of Diseases.* It was reported at the hearing that the federal government is working toward establishing the classification based on the definition set forth in the Second International Conference on Sudden Infant Death Syndrome.

The reason for the vast ignoring of this syndrome, which claims so many infant lives, by the medical scientific research community was a mystery to the U.S. Senate. It is not to anyone who knows the environment of medical research, its methodology, and its system of rewards and promotions. Research is established in hospitals and laboratories. It is disease-oriented and patient care–oriented in health care settings. Crib deaths do not occur in hospitals; they occur in homes. They are not now associated with any known entity treated in hospitals. Little, if any, instruction is given in the problem in medical schools, and none at all in the hospital-based residencies from which the profession grows. Crib deaths are associated with accidents, with legal investigation, with forensic medicine — none of which are very palatable to the American medical research community.

Self-help groups are often the key to keeping national attention on serious health problems. The National Foundation for Sudden Infant Death, a relatively new self-help group, was given its first real test in this congressional investigation. It passed the test and got the result it wanted. A joint congressional resolution has been introduced by Senator Mondale and 15 other senators calling on the National Institute of Child Health and Human Development to make investigations into crib deaths "one of the top priorities" of its intramural and extramural research and research training efforts.[2] This quiet infant killer will now receive some of the attention that it clearly deserves. That attention cannot be given and will not be given until methods of medicolegal death investigation in this country are also improved.

REFERENCES

1. Examination of the Sudden Infant Death Syndrome. Hearing before the Subcommittee on Children and Youth. United States Senate, 92nd Congress. Washington, D.C.: Government Printing Office, 1972.
2. Senate Joint Resolution no. 206 (1972).

COMMENTS

This column received considerable attention from parents' organizations interested in promoting programs to prevent crib death. I also heard from federal officials seeking support for the report reviewed in the column. The interest expressed in this subject in the early 1970s gave me another occasion to "beat the drum" for improved medicolegal death-investigation systems across the country. Other columns that I wrote on this subject in the early 1970s have been collected in Chapter 5.

As a result of this persuasive report to Congress, comprehensive legislation was enacted in 1974, providing financial assistance for state programs to inform the public about crib death, counseling services for the bereaved families, and federal and state research into the causes of the syndrome and possible means of preventing it. For a comprehensive review of the problem, see A.P. Cleveland, "Sudden Infant Death Syndrome (SIDS): A Burgeoning Medicolegal Problem" (*American Journal of Law and Medicine* 1975; 1:55-68).

In the conservative political climate of the 1980s, federal support for state programs relating to crib death was repealed. The only provision retained was the authority given to the Department of Health and Human Services to continue to support research in the field from other funds available to it for purposes of biomedical research (see Public Law 97-35, 1981).

Some state legislatures have continued support for public-information programs and for family counseling in cases of crib death. For a general historical review of service and research programs in the field, see D.H. Kelly and D.C. Shannon, "Sudden Infant Death Syndrome and Near Sudden Infant Death Syndrome: A Review of the Literature 1964–1982" (*Pediatric Clinics of North America* 1982; 29: 1241-61). See also J.D. Brady, "Sudden Infant Death Syndrome: The Physician's Dilemma" (*Advances in Pediatrics* 1983; 30:635-72).

Legal and Medical Death: Kansas Takes the First Step

Come away, come away, death
  And in sad cypress let me be laid;
Fly away, fly away, breath;
  I am slain by a fair cruel maid.
My shroud of white, stuck all with yew,
  O prepare it!
My part of death, no one so true
  Did share it.

Twelfth Night

Shakespeare said it well: no one else shares in a person's death. Yet we all prepare for it and the living "pronounce" the death of the individual. The Bard spoke of death as the flight of breath. In a medical sense it has been defined in the past as the cessation of all vital signs. The law, in individual cases, has accepted this definition and has left it to the attending physician to determine death as a matter of fact, of his own clinical determination.[1] My colleague, Henry Beecher, has spoken in the pages of the *Journal* of "death of the heart, so dear to some lawyers and the editors of Black's Law Dictionary."[2] In practice, the law has never taken the cessation of one vital system as the definition of death. It has required the irreversible stoppage of all systems that could be detected by the clinician in his examination at the scene.

But the law is built upon evidence and assumptions concerning the real world. When conditions change in the real world, the law, if it is to remain relevant, must also change. The first step in changing the conditions concerning the concept of death took place at Harvard in 1968 with the report of the Ad Hoc Committee to Examine the Definition of Brain Death.[3] The committee, under the chairmanship of

From the *New England Journal of Medicine*
1971; 284:260-261.

the same Dr. Beecher, involved a number of specialties of medicine and other disciplines, including law. The committee proposed a new definition of death based on irreversible coma. Since the publication of the report, the clinical recommendations have been accepted and followed on a worldwide basis in a most gratifying fashion.

Now, the first legal step has been taken. The state of Kansas has enacted a statutory definition of death, the first legislative definition of death in the history of our nation and of the common-law world.[4] The statute is skillfully drafted. It adopts two separate and alternative criteria for determining death. It leaves the determination of either in the hands of the attending physician at the scene of death. In the first, the older or classic definition of death is set out requiring "an absence of spontaneous respiration and cardiac function" and a hopelessness of attempts at resuscitation. Death is said to occur at the time "these functions" cease.

In the second alternative definition a person is considered dead, medically and legally, if there is "an absence of spontaneous brain function; and if, based upon ordinary standards of medical practice, during reasonable attempts to either maintain or restore spontaneous circulatory or respiratory function in the absence of aforesaid brain function, it appears that further attempts at resuscitation or supportive maintenance will not succeed, death will have occurred at the time when these conditions first coincide." This would have been a useful first effort even if it had stopped here. But it did not. It went on in clear, specific fashion: "Death is to be pronounced *before* artificial means of supporting respiratory and circulatory function are terminated and before any vital organ is removed for purposes of transplantation [emphasis supplied]."

This last sentence adopts the primary legal recommendation of the Ad Hoc Committee. At the time, it was considered a radical proposal. It was admittedly without precedent in the law, in the United States, or anywhere else in the world. It was adopted by the committee as a means of protecting the attending physician and his associates from being accused of being the last instrument of death if they turned off the heart–lung machine on a person who was still "legally alive." Such actions did take place in the heart-transplant cases in South Africa and in other places in those first frantic months in late 1967 and early 1968. The machines were turned off, and the attending physician and transplant teams waited while the last sign slowly ebbed away in the next 10 minutes and more. Not only were these grisly reports, but further irreparable damage was being done in these minutes to transplantable organs. The donor was not helped by this grotesque death watch, and salvageable organs that could save lives were being endangered or sacrificed. The new Kansas law eliminates this macabre limbo of law and medicine.

The statute is commendable also in what it does *not* require. It does not require that two physicians pronounce the death, as recommended by the World Health Assembly. Also, the statute does not spell out detailed clinical procedures for determining the various aspects of the definition. This is left to clinical standards developed by the medical profession.

This field is still developing and should not be locked into strict legal requirements that could hamper the development of this work and result in damage to the very objectives being sought by transplant medicine: the prolongation of salvageable lives.

REFERENCES

1. Thomas v. Anderson, 96 Cal. App. 2d 371, 211 P.2d 478 (1950); Smith v. Smith, 229 Ark. 579, 317 S.W.2d 275 (1958).
2. Beecher HK. After the "definition of irreversible coma." N Engl J Med 1969; 281:1070-1.
3. A definition of irreversible coma: report of the Ad Hoc Committee of the Harvard Medical School to examine the definition of brain death. JAMA 1968; 205:337-40.
4. Kansas Session Laws of 1970, Ch. 378.

♦

COMMENTS

As I mentioned earlier, it was a source of great satisfaction to me when the *Journal* editor allowed me to open my discussion of the *Baird* case with a quotation from Oliver Wendell Holmes' "one-hoss shay," and I got by with leading off my reflections on legal and medical death with a snatch of verse as well. Once again the authorship of the lines proved rather helpful to my cause, but it was mainly Shakespeare's reference to death as the flight of breath that made the quotation relevant to the subject under discussion, since over the centuries stoppage of respiration and heartbeat were the classic signs of death. Physicians of earlier times were guided by this criterion and were usually not aware how little was contained in formal law, especially in statutes, on the subject of what constituted death in a human being.

This 1971 essay provoked the only full-length article ever written in reaction to one of my columns. See I.M. Kennedy, "Kansas Statute on Death—An Appraisal" (*New England Journal of Medicine* 1971; 285:946-50). The author did not oppose the legal movement for the recognition of brain death, but took the position that such changes in definition should come about only through case law, not legislation. An editorial submitted by a well-known medicolegal specialist and published in the same issue of the *Journal* expressed agreement with my standpoint that legislation was appropriate and necessary at that time in order to encourage transplantation programs and to protect surgeons performing transplantations from vexatious lawsuits claiming that the surgeons had caused the death of the donor by removing the organ. See D.H. Mills, "Kansas Death Statute: Bold and Innovative" (*New England Journal of Medicine* 1971; 285:968-9).

Strong support for statutory definitions of brain death has developed in response to subsequent events. In 1978 the National Conference of Commissioners on Uniform State Laws selected this subject for its next major effort in the medicolegal field: a Uniform Brain Death Act, which was adopted in many states but did not receive the immediate endorsement of legislative bodies as readily as the earlier uniform bill on anatomical donations. Opposition to the brain-death legislation came mainly from right-to-life organizations, in whose view such bills were manifestations of a movement to withhold medical care and life support from handicapped persons.

In 1980, the National Commissioners abandoned the draft bill of two years before and worked together with the American Medical Association and the American Bar Association to develop a new version. Efforts to have this second proposal enacted have met with more success in the America of the 1980s than had been accorded the earlier version in its time. In its new form the model bill has been adopted, with some modifications, in at least 15 states. For a review of opposition views on brain-death legislation, see P.A. Byrne, S. O'Reilly, P.M. Quay, and P.W. Salsich, "Brain Death: The Patient, the Physician, and Society" (*Gonzaga Law Review* 1983; 18:429-516). See also Student Note, "The Bell Tolls for Thee: But When?

Legal Acceptance of 'Brain Death' as a Criterion for Death" (*American Journal of Trial Advocacy* 1985; 9:331-45). The concept of brain death was the subject of a superb report by the President's Commission on the Study of Ethical Problems in Medicine and Biomedical and Behavioral Research. See *Defining Death: A Report on Medical, Legal, and Ethical Issues in the Determination of Death* (Washington, D.C.: Government Printing Office, July 1981).

Brain-Death Statutes and Court Review

Whenever the brain-death concept as a compulsory or alternative method of determining human death has come before the courts in the United States, the United Kingdom, or Canada, it has inevitably been all or part of the defendant's appeal of a homicide conviction in which the attempt has been to throw the responsibility for causing the death on the physicians who have declared the person, the alleged homicide victim, to be dead owing to brain death and have then removed support systems. Most cases, but not all, have also involved removal of some organs for transplantation purposes.

In every case of this type, the basic medical criteria for determining brain death, usually in strict accordance with the recommendations of the Harvard Ad Hoc Committee on Brain Death, have been followed, and the defendant's attorneys have not claimed otherwise. In every single case the defendants have lost their appeals, and the courts have uniformly upheld the physicians' actions as medically proper, ethically justified, and legally sound. Nevertheless, criminal-defense attorneys continue to be undaunted; they have challenged the application of the brain-death concept at every opportunity in a desperate attempt to use any available defense for their clients in these most serious of criminal cases. It may be suggested, however, that after a time, the legal ethics of the defense counsel can be challenged in these increasingly futile appeals. The reputations, the time, and the finances of the physicians and hospitals are constantly placed in jeopardy in these cases. They are charged by these attorneys with improperly and illegally "causing" the death of these persons, all of them victims of brutal assaults or gunshot killings in whom brain functions were lost. Often, the families of the victims are led to believe the physicians were at fault. Newspaper and television cover-

From the *New England Journal of Medicine*
1978; 299:31-32.

age, to present a dramatic confrontation, also tries to make the challenge a serious issue in which physicians could be found "guilty" and could be called body snatchers, or organ snatchers, or worse.

There are now two important appellate-court cases that could help to put the legal issues in these appeals to rest nationally and put an end to this questionable litigation. The first was the *Golston* case in Massachusetts reported on in this column in May.[1] In that opinion Massachusetts, which does not have a statutory definition of brain death, accepted the Harvard Ad Hoc Committee definition as applied to a homicide victim and dismissed the argument that the physicians caused his death. This case was highly influential because it applied common-law doctrines. The Ad Hoc Committee was based in Massachusetts and used data from experience in Massachusetts hospitals. Now, only a few weeks after the *Golston* case was passed down, the Kansas Supreme Court has, for the first time, judicially reviewed the Kansas Brain Death Statute.[2] It is a very important decision because Kansas was the first state in the United States, and the first legal jurisdiction in the world, to enact a statutory definition of death. The law was enacted in 1970. The provision, reviewed in a previous "Law–Medicine Notes" column,[3] is an admirable piece of legislative drafting. It allows the application of the brain-death concept as an alternative means of declaring human death. It does not contain technical requirements that quickly could become outdated. It essentially leaves the application and further development of the content of the standard for brain death to medical practice and science.

In *State* v. *Shaffer*[4] the court refused to find the action of the physicians to be the legal, intervening cause of the death in which the defendant had admittedly shot the victim in the head in the course of a robbery in a gasoline station. The defendant first challenged the application of the statute to a criminal-homicide case. The court pointed out that the statute, by its very language, applied "for all purposes in this state, including trials of civil and criminal cases." The appeal on this ground was boldly frivolous. The second and more serious attack was based on the constitutional claim that the statute was "void for vagueness" in allowing physicians to apply an alternative method of finding human death, one being the traditional method of cessation of the cardiac-respiratory system, and the other being the brain-death concept. This challenge was also dismissed on the grounds that the alternative method was clearly supported by modern medical science and practice, and there was no constitutional requirement that a single standard be applied for determining death. Next, the defendants asserted that the statute was unconstitutionally vague because it allowed for medical determinations on the basis of "ordinary standards of medical practice." The court upheld this language as an adequate legislative policy in areas in which medical scientific standards are subject to change and progress. It was not necessary that the technical requirements be spelled out in detail in the law.

Also of great importance for organ-transplant practice was another finding of the court, which was made almost in passing and not in response to a defense challenge. The court expressly recognized the need to make a pronouncement of death on a brain-death standard, but to keep the heart-lung apparatus functioning and otherwise to prepare the body for useful harvest and transplant of organs. To quote directly from the opinion of Justice McGarland:

> The increasing number of organ transplant operations complicates the situation further as organs such as kidneys may become too damaged for transplant within five minutes after respiration ceases. So for kidney transplants, respiration must continue almost uninterrupted until the kidney is removed.

The Kansas opinion is as admirable as the Kansas statute. It even has the rare quality that Justice Holmes called judicious brevity. The Massachusetts opinion, though excellent, is not as important or as far-reaching in its scope as this Midwest opinion — strange as that may sound on this myopic Atlantic shore. The *Golston* opinion did not mention the issue of organ transplantations. It did not discuss or lay at rest constitutional challenges. It did not reach the issue of alternative definitions of death; it even tried to limit its scope to criminal-homicide appeals, leaving broader attacks to later cases or legislative remedy. The Kansas court dealt with all these issues and did not seek limitations of scope. The ethical and scientific support for the brain-death concept and properly administered organ transplants from such patients has now received strong judicial support in the best traditions of American jurisprudence.

REFERENCES

1. Curran WJ. The brain-death concept: judicial acceptance in Massachusetts. N Engl J Med 1978; 298:1008-9.

2. Kansas Session Laws of 1970, Chapter 378.
3. State of Kansas v. Shaffer 574, P.2d. 205 (Kansas, 1977).
4. Curran WJ. Legal and medical death – Kansas takes the first step. N Engl J Med 1971; 284:260-1.

♦

COMMENTS

The *Shaffer* decision in Kansas made the use of advanced surgical techniques in organ transplantations more acceptable across the country. The same case came before the Kansas Supreme Court for a second time in 1981. The views of the court on the constitutionality of the law did not change.

The major change in the amended version of the legal criteria in the model act of the National Commissioners on Uniform State Laws was that it required medical evidence (based on accepted medical standards) of permanent cessation of brain-stem function, not merely cortical function. See P.L. Ryan, "The Uniform Determination of Death Act: An Effective Solution to the Problem of Defining Death" (*Washington and Lee Law Review* 1982; 39:1511-21).

The *Saikewicz* Decision in Massachusetts: A Questionable Role for the Courts

After a delay of some 16 months, the Massachusetts Supreme Judicial Court has issued a full opinion concerning life-death decisions on patients.[1]

The decision has caused great consternation among Massachusetts physicians and hospitals. Physicians involved in intensive care of infants and adults alike, physicians in burn centers, and physicians and hospitals caring for terminally ill patients are frankly reacting in disbelief at the news reports about the case; lawyers representing medical clients waited to read the decision and, after reading it, could only respond that the news reports were correct. The court really did mean that all decisions on either removal of life-support systems or continuation of life-extending therapy in otherwise dying patients who are incompetent because of mental retardation or incapacity or who are under the age of maturity in the state (age 18) must go before a probate court for approval. In these petitions, no rapid decision can be expected, not only because of usual court delays, but because the *Saikewicz* decision strongly suggested that in all cases of incompetency, the judge appoint "a guardian *ad litem*" to represent "the interests" of the person and to be specifically charged to present to the judge all reasonable arguments against the petition being sought. Thus, each case is required to be an adversary proceeding.

After reading the 41-page opinion, I am convinced that the Massachusetts court did not intend its decision to have the devastating effect that it has had on the medical community. The opinion is

From the *New England Journal of Medicine*
1978; 298:499-500.

thoughtfully written by one of the newer members, Justice Paul Liacos. There were no dissents. Most of the opinion, until the very end where these medicolegal procedures in the probate court are introduced, is in keeping with most of the enlightened jurisprudence of the field in recent years.

To go back to the actual case, the patient was a 67-year-old man with profound mental retardation. He could not talk; communication with him was through gestures and physical contact only. He was physically strong and ambulatory and had been in a state school most of his life. He was terminally ill with acute myeloblastic monocytic leukemia, but was not in pain. The school was concerned about whether to place him on a course of chemotherapy, which might prolong his life for a few months to over a year.

The side effects of the chemotherapy could be severe. Also, a number of blood transfusions would be required. The patient would not understand what was happening to him except that he would go through months of pain and discomfort and would be very sick. It was highly doubtful if he could cooperate in the treatment; he might, in fact, require restraint.

The school was unsure of what to do. The only relatives who could be located, two sisters, were told of the situation and did not want to become involved or to attend the subsequent court hearing.

The school superintendent and a staff attorney at the facilities brought a petition in the probate court for the appointment of a guardian to be given authority to make a decision. The judge appointed a guardian *ad litem,* who investigated the matter and recommended that it was not in the best interests of the ward to undergo treatment. The probate court entered an order agreeing with the recommendation. The Supreme Judicial Court affirmed the order in early July 1976, indicating that a full opinion would be forthcoming. It came on November 28, 1977.

Of particular importance in the body of the opinion is its ruling that a competent adult who was in this terminal condition could refuse further treatment. In so deciding, the court was making new law in the commonwealth, since there was no precedent or statutory law on the subject.

The above ruling was a foundation point for the actual decision on Mr. Saikewicz, since a guardian for an incompetent person could not do for the person what the person, if competent, could not do for himself. The court also indicated its concurrence in the medical ethical position that "extraordinary means" should not be used to prolong life, or its semblance, when after careful consideration, consultation, and the application of well-conceived therapy, it becomes apparent that there is no hope of recovery. The court also seemed to look with favor on the use of informed consent and even a living will as a means of avoiding civil liability on the part of a hospital or a physician withholding treatment, though this possibility was merely noted in passing in one of the references in the opinion. Legislation would be necessary in Massachusetts to make living wills legally binding.

It was the concluding part of the opinion that presented the difficulty for implementation of the decision. Justice Liacos compared the case of Mr. Saikewicz with the famous Karen Ann Quinlan case in New Jersey. He indicated that the appointment of a guardian, the father in that case, was similar to the petition in Massachusetts and that the basic law applied was consistent with his opinion. However, Justice Liacos indicated the Massachusetts court's disagreement with the part of the New Jersey opinion that, Justice Liacos said, entrusted the decision whether to continue artificial life support to the patient's family, attending doctors, and a hospital ethics committee. The Massachusetts court ruled that this "awesome question" of either continuing life support or withholding potentially life-prolonging treatment was one for the courts of law and could not be granted to any other group.

Thus, the court covered both forms of decision making: those in favor of life and those pertaining to turning off the machine. Both will require court approval if the patient is incompetent and perhaps also when the patient is unconscious or unable to communicate.

The court also offered a ruling on issues of the quality of life to be expected if a patient is continued on treatment. The court asserted that "To the extent that this formulation equates the value of life with any measure of the quality of life, we reject it." This statement seemed to apply to Mr. Saikewicz's condition of mental retardation. The court seemed to want to make it clear that a mentally retarded person's life was fully worth saving. This ruling could mean that brain damage to an infant or very serious burns and disfigurement and limited bodily functioning could not be taken into consideration in offering or withholding resuscitation or intensive care to a patient.

This interpretation could present very serious implications for medical care decision making.

One does get the impression that the court thought that the decisions covered by its opinion are rare and can await a studied and deliberate decision-making process in the courts of law. Nothing seems further from the truth, if the decision is to be applied literally to all situations that its language covers.

It seems a shame that the Massachusetts court was so disturbed with the comments of the New Jersey court about leaving these decisions with families, attending physicians, and ethics committees. First of all, it displays a lack of understanding and a distrust of the current medical care system to handle life–death matters with any degree of equity and sensitivity. Secondly, it assumes that the decisions of such ethical groups are not appealable to the courts when there is disagreement by any parties or interested groups or any indication of abuse of their discretion. As an earlier "Law–Medicine Notes" column pointed out, I never interpreted the New Jersey decision to bar court relief in appropriate cases.[2] Also, the hospital committees are not really deciding ethical or legal matters; they are, as I pointed out in that column, mainly aiding in the medical determination of the patient's condition. I am glad to say that New Jersey hospitals call these groups "prognosis committees," not ethics committees. The point here is that the families and physicians, aided by a prognosis (or ethical) committee composed partly of persons outside the treating group and usually outside the hospital, should be able to act in most cases quickly and equitably when there is no doubt about the need to take action. Delays do not always mean a stable condition, as this court seemed to assume; delays mean that the decision is made to continue treatment, often to produce a nonfunctioning or minimally functioning person. The court procedure suggested in the *Saikewicz* case is clearly too slow and cumbersome to fit most of the decisions made in intensive care units. The result will tend to be the prolongation of treatment, with little if any chance for good results — a definite move to prolonging tragedy and suffering for families and patients and increased strain and cost for the medical and nursing-home systems.

The *Journal* earlier published two thoughtful papers on procedures, including the use of committees, set up in two teaching hospitals in Boston to deal with cases involving decisions not to resuscitate.[3,4] These articles were accompanied by a highly laudatory editorial by a law professor who did not anticipate this action of the Massachusetts court.[5] These professional plans will now need to be reevaluated in full for teaching hospitals and for all health care facilities in Massachusetts.

REFERENCES

1. Superintendent of Belchertown State School v. Saikewicz 370 N.E.2d 417 (Mass. 1977).
2. Curran WJ. The proper and improper concerns of medical law and ethics. N Engl J Med 1976; 295:1057-8.
3. Rabkin MT, Gillerman G, Rice NR. Orders not to resuscitate. N Engl J Med 1976; 295:364-6.
4. Clinical Care Committee of the Massachusetts General Hospital. Optimum care for hopelessly ill patients. N Engl J Med 1976; 295:362-4.
5. Fried C. Terminating life support: out of the closet! N Engl J Med 1976; 295: 390-1.

♦

COMMENTS

I am glad to be able to report that the prior court review required by the Massachusetts court in *Saikewicz* has not been adopted in any other jurisdiction in the United States since the decision was passed down in 1977 and that the *Saikewicz* approach was also rejected by the Law Reform Commission in Canada when that body drew up its report on cessation of life-support systems. See the discussion of this report in Chapter 5 ("Quality-of-Life and Treatment Decisions: The Canadian Law Reform Report").

The harshness of the *Saikewicz* decision was somewhat mitigated in a later opinion, written by another justice, in *Matter of Earl N. Spring,* 405 N.E.2d 115 (Mass. 1980). As pointed out in this column, the *Saikewicz* opinion was not all bad; in fact, the court was quite reasonable in its approach until it reached the matter of prior review by lower courts in future cases. Particularly encouraging was the court's recognition of a standard of "substituted judgment" under which, if the person concerned had earlier expressed the preference not to be continued on life-support systems under particular circumstances, the court could be guided by his or her wishes. The reason that this section of the decision was of no practical relevance in *Saikewicz* was that the patient involved had been severely retarded from birth. No "substituted judgment," based on prior stated wishes while competent and communicative, could possibly apply to Mr. Saikewicz. The only alternative standard that could be applied was the "best interests" of the person as determined by the court or a guardian, as applied in the case of small children.

In a very important later case, *Brophy* v. *New England Sinai Hospital,* 398 Mass. 417 (1986), the high court applied the "substituted judgment" test in authorizing the removal of a feeding tube from a patient in a persistent vegetative state, citing *Saikewicz* as precedent. See the review of this case and the related *Conroy* decision in Chapter 5 ("Care for the Dying Patient: Legal Standards for Denying Nutrients and Hydration").

A series of papers, now all somewhat dated, attempting to clarify the implications of the decision was published in one important medicolegal journal. For a favorable reaction to the prior court-review approach, see C.H. Baron, "Assuring 'Detached but Passionate Investigation and Decision': The Role of Guardians Ad Litem in Saikewicz-type Cases" (*American Journal of Law and Medicine* 1978; 4:111-30). See also G.J. Annas, "Reconciling Quinlan and Saikewicz: Decision-making for the Terminally Ill Incompetent" (*American Journal of Law and Medicine* 1979; 4:367-96). Another paper expressed disagreement with both earlier viewpoints. See A. Buchanan, "Medical Paternalism or Legal Imperialism: Not the Only Alternative to Handling Saikewicz-type Cases" (*American Journal of Law and Medicine* 1979; 5:97-117).

Several states have adopted so-called "living wills" as a means of ensuring that formal written statements by competent adults expressing the wish not to be continued on life-support systems will be honored at a later time. As of 1987, such legislation has been adopted in 39 states. Also, some states have adopted legislation authorizing the appointment by competent adults of other persons as proxies, representatives, or attorneys in fact under a document of power of attorney, to act for them in such matters should they become incapacitated or incompetent to act for themselves. These various legal instruments are becoming more important in the face of the epidemic of the acquired immunodeficiency syndrome (AIDS), which is causing large numbers of young patients slowly to become very seriously ill and – in later stages of the illness, which are often marked by mental deterioration due to dementia – eventually to lose the capacity to act for themselves. See R. Steinbroak and B. Lo, "Decision Making for Incompetent Patients by Designated Proxy: California's New Law" (*New England Journal of Medicine* 1984; 310:1598-601). See also J.K. Fackler, "Living Wills, Organ Donation, and Durable Powers of Attorney" (*Tennessee Bar Journal* 1987; 23:15-23); and L.A. Marsh, "Living Will Legislation in Colorado: An Analysis of the Colorado Medical Treatment Decision Act in Relation to Similar Developments in Other Jurisdictions" (*Denver University Law Review* 1987; 64:5-31).

Court Involvement in Right-to-Die Cases: Judicial Inquiry in New York

> Jarndyce and Jarndyce drones on. This scarecrow of a suit has, in course of time, become so complicated that no man alive knows what it means.
>
> Charles Dickens

The American courts continue to involve themselves – perhaps to become irrevocably entangled – in issues of clinical decision making for certain incompetent patients who might die without vigorous treatment. In the popular press, these complex legal cases are all grouped under the colorful and emotional description of the "right to die."

One of the most publicized of the cases has been that of Brother Joseph Fox, an 83-year-old member of a religious order, who was on a respirator after a cardiac arrest in which substantial brain damage was sustained. The case has gone through three judicial opinions in the New York court system and has already resulted in considerable commentary in medical, ethical, and legal journals in response to the lower courts' opinions. Most of this rather ponderous commentary has now been rendered largely obsolete as a result of the final decision of New York's highest court.

The court of appeals joined its opinion and decision in the Brother Fox case, which was actually called *In the Matter of Father Eichner,* with another case, *In the Matter of John Storar,* which dealt with similar issues.[1]

Surprising as it may seem, the joining of the two cases has provided a clearer result than we could have expected if the court of appeals had reviewed only the *Eichner* matter.

From the *New England Journal of Medicine*
1981; 305:75-76.

In its progress through the lower courts, the *Eichner* case was heavily influenced by the other two major decisions in the field, the *Quinlan* case in New Jersey and the *Saikewicz* decision in Massachusetts.[2] In fact, the intermediate court passed down what was undoubtedly the most intricate and complex opinion of any court that has reviewed these issues. The opinion seemed to take the good and the bad from both earlier cases and to mix them in a witches' brew of procedural ingredients that would, if ever followed step by step, exhaust all the resources and patience committed to individual litigation since the Jarndyce and Jarndyce case of Dickens' *Bleak House.* Mercifully, perhaps, most of the terminally ill patients would have died before these quixotic efforts to protect the patients' dignity and lives were completed.

The lower courts' suggestions were not even discussed in detail by the court of appeals. Justice Wachtler noted only that they were "an elaborate set of procedures to be followed by doctors, hospitals, family members, parties, and the courts before future applications of this nature may be entertained or granted."

The court of appeals refused to apply elaborate procedures for the handling of right-to-die cases in the future. In both cases the court applied consistent and fairly simple rules of personal determination to accept or refuse medical treatment.

In *Eichner,* the court found that the controlling circumstance was the undisputed fact that Brother Fox had made known his personal desire not to be treated in an extraordinary manner (as on a respirator) just before his hospitalization for the operation during which he had his cardiac arrest. The discussions were not casual; they were a part of serious discussions within the religious group about moral obligations and medical treatment, occurring around the time of the *Quinlan* case in nearby New Jersey. Brother Fox's announced preference not to be treated further in such circumstances was in accordance with the teachings of his church. As far as New York's highest court was concerned, this fact settled the matter. The hospital could not continue to provide treatment or use the respirator against the will of the patient. The proof of the patient's refusal, in the view of the court, was based on "clear and convincing evidence." This degree of proof was deemed adequate in such cases. The court refused, quite sensibly, to impose a higher burden of proof ("beyond reasonable doubt") on petitioners seeking termination of treatment, as requested by the district attorney involved in the case. The court concluded,

> In this case the proof was compelling. There was no suggestion that the witnesses who testified for the petitioner had any other motive but to see that Brother Fox's stated wishes were respected. The finding that he carefully reflected on the subject, expressed his views, and concluded not to have his life prolonged by medical means if there were no hope of recovery is supported by his religious beliefs and is not inconsistent with his life of unselfish religious devotion.

The court based its decision on the common-law right of a competent person to refuse treatment, enforceable even during that person's incapacity (due to the illness) to express such wishes further. It was not necessary to embroider the finding with fanciful constitutional doctrines, such as the right to privacy. The court also placed no great stress on the exercise of vicarious authority on behalf of the patient by a third party, such as a guardian or petitioner.

If all we knew about the law on these issues in New York were the *Eichner* opinion, our enlightenment would be quite circumspect. The court was reluctant to lay down general rules. I believe that this reluctance was a legally proper and refreshing approach in these days of increased judicial overstepping and overstating of the necessary premises for court decisions. A little reticence in the development of broad principles in the common law that are not applicable and not required by the case at hand has always been advisable, as most good judges learn in their years on the bench.

More substantial guidance about New York common law was immediately provided by the unexpected but welcome addition of the opinion in the *Storar* matter. John Storar was a profoundly retarded man of 52 who was being treated for bladder cancer; the tumor had been clearly determined to be terminal in nature. He had been a lifelong resident of a facility for the retarded. His only close relative was his 77-year-old mother, who was a frequent visitor to the facility. After his hospitalization, when permission to institute radiation therapy was believed to be necessary, the mother was judicially appointed as his guardian to give consent. She did so, and the radiation resulted in some remission. The patient subsequently needed frequent blood transfusions to prevent shock and to control his condition. His mother at first consented to each transfusion. She later became discouraged, convinced that her son was dying and that the transfusions were only prolonging his suffering. She refused further consent. Because they believed that the patient would die "within weeks" if the regimen of transfusions was interrupted, hospital officials brought suit to obtain authorization to continue treatment.

The New York Court of Appeals in this case granted this petition and in effect refused to allow the legally appointed guardian to prevent further treatment.

The court distinguished the *Storar* case from *Eichner* by pointing out that the patient's prior wishes and prior consent to treatment (or refusal) could not be assumed clearly, as it had been with Brother Fox. Storar had never been competent to give consent or to withhold it. Therefore, the court decided that the common-law rule that a parent or guardian can only act for the benefit of the ward had to be applied. The court would not allow the guardian's refusal to result in the patient's bleeding to death.

Actually, the above is all we learn from the *Storar* matter. Any other comment is speculation. In both *Eichner* and *Storar,* the court could have discussed "substituted judgment" or "the best interests of the patient." Neither doctrine was described as the basis of decision. In *Eichner,* a substituted judgment – that is, applying the known wishes or judgment of the person as he or she would have done if able to – could have been used, because the wishes of Brother Fox were discoverable and had been clearly ascertained. The court apparently did not consider this step necessary. It applied the wishes of Brother Fox directly without the need to substitute for them through a surrogate or guardian, although it allowed the petitioner, Father Eichner, to plead the wishes of the patient successfully.

In *Storar,* on the other hand, no such application of a substituted judgment could have taken place. The court rejected any effort to explore what a person with lifelong profound retardation would have wanted if he could have made a rational decision. Again, I find this conclusion refreshingly clear and wholly convincing. It is directly contrary to the contrived argumentation of the *Saikewicz* case, in which the Massachusetts court seemed to assert, as its rule of decision, that it was embarking on a search for the wishes of a man with exactly the same kind of lifelong profound retardation. The logical vulnerability of this spurious pursuit of substituted judgment—and, even worse, the discovery of such a judgment—have been ably exposed by the ethicist Paul Ramsey.[3]

The unusual nature of this matter is also found in the fact that of all the right-to-die cases that have been brought to court around the country up to this writing, *Storar* is the only major decision of a highest court that has refused to allow the patient's death to occur as a result of judicial inquiry. Despite their often impassioned rhetoric about protecting life and requiring courts to intervene, the *Quinlan, Saikewicz, Perlmutter, Spring, Severns,* and *Eichner* cases—the series of decisions that provoked the broadside of medical, ethical, and legal commentary—have all approved actions to remove treatment that was presumed to result in death. The *Storar* matter may well be a turning point in judicial intervention in this field.

REFERENCES

1. N.Y. Law Journal. April 2, 1981:2-9.
2. Curran WJ. The Saikewicz decision. N Engl J Med 1978; 298:499-500.
3. Ramsey P. The *Saikewicz* precedent: what's good for an incompetent patient? Hastings Cent Rep 1978; 8(6):36-42.

♦

COMMENTS

I sought the help of Charles Dickens and his comments on the interminable case of Jarndyce and Jarndyce (in his novel *Bleak House*) to admonish the American courts a century later to stay out of the sticky quagmire of deciding issues of life and death.

The New York cases examined in this column were the most influential, after *Quinlan* in New Jersey and *Saikewicz* in Massachusetts, in spelling out a role for the courts in this sensitive area. Since 1981, several further decisions have dealt with criteria for the removal of nutritional and hydration support. Columns dealing with these cases are collected in Chapter 5 (see particularly "Care for the Dying Patient: Legal Standards for Denying Nutrients and Hydration").

Before the decisions reported on in this column, hospitals in New York had been so greatly intimidated by the threat of criminal actions for homicide voiced by several local district attorneys that transplantation programs had broken down and reasonable guidelines were not developed for dealing with brain-dead patients. See J.J. Paris, "Brother Fox, the Courts, and Death with Dignity" (*America* 1980; 143: 282-5). For another view of the cases, see G.J. Annas, "Help for the Dead: The Cases of Brother Fox and John Storar" (*Hastings Center Report* 1981; 11:19-20). See also a view of the role of criminal prosecutors in New Jersey: D.G. Collester, "Death, Dying and the Law: A Prosecutorial View of the Quinlan Case" (*Rutgers Law Review* 1977; 30:304-28).

The district attorneys were not bluffing when they threatened to take action for homicide in connection with the intentional withdrawal of life support. See *Barber* v. *Superior Court,* 195 Cal. Rptr. 483 (1983), in which the Los Angeles district attorney brought murder charges against two physicians who, at the request of the family, removed a respirator and later a feeding tube from a comatose patient who had suffered cardiac arrest and brain damage in an operative procedure two days earlier. On appeal, the criminal charges were dismissed on the grounds that the physicians had no criminal intent and, in view of the patient's condition, had no medical duty either to set up or to maintain a life-support system.

Appendix

Original Publication Dates of "Law–Medicine Notes" in the *New England Journal of Medicine*

Note: The titles of the articles in this book differ in some cases from the titles used when the articles were originally published in the *New England Journal of Medicine.* The following appendix lists the original titles, along with the bibliographic citations for the articles and the page numbers on which they begin in this book.

Chapter 1 ♦ Medical Malpractice

PAGE

CHAPTER 2 ♦ HOSPITALS: THE NEW LEGAL DOCTRINES

Chapter 3 ♦ Forensic Medicine and the Law

Chapter 4 ♦ Insanity, Psychiatry, and the Armor of the Law

Chapter 5 ♦ Ethics in Medical Practice

CHAPTER 6 ♦ LEGAL AND MORAL PROBLEMS IN HUMAN REPRODUCTION

CHAPTER 7 ♦ LIFE AND DEATH

Index

A

B

C

D

E

F

I

M

N

O

Q

R

T

U